ANATOMY AND MRI OF THE JOINTS

A Multiplanar Atlas

ANATOMY AND MRI OF THE JOINTS
A MULTIPLANAR ATLAS

Editors

William D. Middleton, M.D.   Thomas L. Lawson, M.D.

Department of Radiology
Medical College of Wisconsin
Milwaukee, Wisconsin

RAVEN PRESS • NEW YORK

Raven Press, 1185 Avenue of the Americas, New York, New York 10036

© 1989 by Raven Press, Ltd. All rights reserved. This book is protected by copyright. No part of it may be reproduced, stored in a retrieval system, or transmitted, in any form or by any means, electronic, mechanical, photocopying, or recording, or otherwise, without the prior written permission of the publisher.

Printed and bound in Hong Kong

Library of Congress Cataloging-in-Publication Data

Anatomy and MRI of the joints.

   Includes bibliographies and index.
   1. Joints—Anatomy—Atlases. 2. Joints—Imaging—
Atlases. 3. Magnetic resonance imaging—Atlases.
I. Middleton, William D. II. Lawson, Thomas L.
[DNLM: 1. Joints—anatomy—atlases. 2. Magnetic
Resonance Imaging—atlases. WE 17 A535]
QM331.A53   1989   611'.72   87-42729
ISBN 0-88167-455-9

The material contained in this volume was submitted as previously unpublished material, except in the instances in which credit has been given to the source from which some of the illustrative material was derived.

Great care has been taken to maintain the accuracy of the information contained in the volume. However, neither Raven Press nor the editors can be held responsible for errors or for any consequences arising from the use of the information contained herein.

9 8 7 6 5 4 3 2 1

*This book is dedicated to my parents,
William and Joyce*

W.D.M.

Preface

As techniques that are used to image the human body improve, our knowledge of anatomy must expand and adapt to enable us to accurately interpret the images. In the 1970s, the development of computed tomography (CT) forced us to become intimately familiar with axial cross-sectional anatomy. The current development and continuing refinement of magnetic resonance imaging (MRI) makes it necessary to understand cross-sectional anatomy in multiple planes. In general, this understanding requires only a reorientation of thinking since we are already well acquainted from our experience with CT with the anatomic structures and their axial relationships.

However, the imaging of the joints is more involved. The lack of respiratory motion and the use of small surface coils allows for images of extremely high contrast and resolution, resulting in a clarity of visualization of many anatomic structures not previously achieved. Therefore, not only are we imaging the joints in orientations that are unfamiliar, but we are seeing structures that we have not been able to see in the past. The resulting displays of anatomy can be as intimidating as they are impressive.

The ability to image the complex multiplanar anatomy of the joints with MRI and the resulting need to understand this anatomy served as the motivation for the development of this atlas. Our intent was to produce an atlas to be used as a ready reference for the identification of articular and periarticular structures seen on MR images. To accomplish this we have imaged live volunteers on a 1.5 Tesla system. All images were obtained using commercially available surface coils and standard spin-echo pulse sequences. For all the joints except the vertebral column, T-1–weighted images were obtained since they showed the overall anatomy best. Two excitations were used for all the images. The slice thickness was 3 mm for the smaller joint and 5 mm for the larger joints (the vertebral column and hip). The imaging field of view varied depending on the size of the joint.

To confirm the identity of the structures seen on the MR images, we carefully compared the images with actual anatomic sections obtained from frozen cadavers. The joints of these cadavers were cut into tissue blocks and mounted on the stage of a cryomicrotome unit. The frozen tissue specimens were then sequentially cut and photographs of the surface taken at less than 1-mm intervals. Representative color photographs of these serial sections have been included in the atlas, not only to allow for MR-anatomic correlation but, more importantly, to guard against obsolescence. The MR images are state-of-the-art. Although MR imaging will undoubtedly continue to improve, the cryomicrotomes, however, cannot be improved upon, and will remain a valuable reference regardless of advances in MRI or other imaging techniques.

William D. Middleton
Thomas L. Lawson

Acknowledgments

Many people contributed to the preparation of this atlas and their efforts have been greatly appreciated.

Dr. Victor Haughton was instrumental in obtaining cadavers for anatomic sections as well as providing the cryomicrotome unit used to cut the sections. Without his help, this book would not have been possible.

The cryomicrotomes were produced and photographed by Bruce Nowicki. Their beauty is the result of his skilled work.

The MR images were obtained with the excellent assistance of the technologists in the MRI facility at the Medical College of Wisconsin. They include Beth Beck, Marie Bye, Steve Censky, Lisa Klotz, and Julie Strandt.

The artwork was provided by Robert Fenn at the Medical College of Wisconsin and Leslie MacConnell-Clubbs at the Mallinckrodt Institute of Radiology.

Preparation of the manuscript was the result of the tireless efforts of Marilyn Bell and Lynn Losse.

Finally, the support, assistance, and advice that was received from Dr. Mary Middleton throughout the preparation of this atlas provided constant encouragement for its ultimate completion.

Contents

1. The Temporomandibular Joint 1
   J. Bruce Kneeland, M.D.

2. The Shoulder 13
   William D. Middleton, M.D.

3. The Elbow 49
   Stephan J. Macrander, M.D.

4. The Wrist 83
   William D. Middleton, M.D.

5. The Finger 121
   Scott Erickson, M.D.

6. The Vertebral Column 139
   Lowell Sether, Ph.D.

7. The Hip 153
   Thomas L. Lawson, M.D. and William D. Middleton, M.D.

8. The Knee 205
   Gary W. Hinson, M.D. and William D. Middleton, M.D.

9. The Ankle 251
   William D. Middleton, M.D.

   Recommended Reading 293

   Subject Index 297

Contributors

Scott Erickson, M.D., *Medical College of Wisconsin, Milwaukee County Medical Complex, 8700 West Wisconsin Avenue, Milwaukee, Wisconsin 53226*

Gary W. Hinson, M.D., *Menorah Medical Center, Kansas City, Missouri 64110*

J. Bruce Kneeland, M.D., *Medical College of Wisconsin, Milwaukee County Medical Complex, 8700 West Wisconsin Avenue, Milwaukee, Wisconsin 53226*

Thomas L. Lawson, M.D., *Medical College of Wisconsin, Milwaukee County Medical Complex, 8700 West Wisconsin Avenue, Milwaukee, Wisconsin 53226*

Steven Macrander, M.D., *Medical College of Wisconsin, Milwaukee County Medical Complex, 8700 West Wisconsin Avenue, Milwaukee, Wisconsin 53226*

William D. Middleton, M.D., *Mallinckrodt Institute of Radiology, 510 South Kingshighway, St. Louis, Missouri 63110*

Lowell Sether, Ph.D., *Medical College of Wisconsin, Milwaukee County Medical Complex, 8700 West Wisconsin Avenue, Milwaukee, Wisconsin 53226*

ANATOMY AND MRI OF THE JOINTS

A Multiplanar Atlas

CHAPTER 1

THE TEMPOROMANDIBULAR JOINT

J. Bruce Kneeland, M.D.

The temporomandibular joint (TMJ) is relatively simple compared to other joints in this atlas. Figure 1–1 illustrates the important articular structures. The osseous portion consists of the articular eminence and mandibular fossa of the temporal bone above and the mandibular condyle below. The articular surfaces are covered with fibrocartilage. Within the joint is an ovoid plate consisting of fibrous tissue called the disc. The disc has a biconcave structure with thick anterior and posterior bands connected by a thin intermediate zone. The joint is separated into two synovial spaces (superior and inferior) by the disc.

Attached to the posterior band is the bilaminar zone which consists of a superior lamella of fibroelastic tissue and a lower lamella of fibrous tissue. These two lamellae are attached to the posterior margin of the mandibular fossa and the posterior margin of the condyle, respectively. Anteriorly the disc is attached to the lateral pterygoid muscle.

In "normal" individuals the posterior margin of the posterior band of the disc is located at the highest point of the condyle (approximately 12 o'clock) with the jaw closed, although it may be anteriorly displaced a few degrees. With jaw opening, the condyle moves anteriorly under the disc.

Although not a part of the TMJ, the external auditory canal is a useful landmark that permits an evaluation of the degree of opening of the jaw. With closed jaw the posterior surface of the condyle abuts the canal. As the jaw opens the condyle moves anteriorly away from the canal.

As previously noted, the disc is attached anteriorly to the lateral pterygoid muscle.

The lateral pterygoid has two parts: a superior head which arises from the sphenoid and temporal bones and inserts on the disc, and an inferior head which arises from the lateral pterygoid plate and inserts on the neck of the mandible. Although not directly attached to the joint, the medial pterygoid muscle is located anterior to the lateral pterygoid. It attaches to the ramus and angle of the mandible.

The TMJ is supplied by the superficial temporal artery, which is one of two terminal branches of the external carotid artery and originates in the parotid gland posterior to the neck of the mandible. Also seen in this region is the maxillary artery, which is the second terminal branch of the external carotid and likewise originates in the parotid gland.

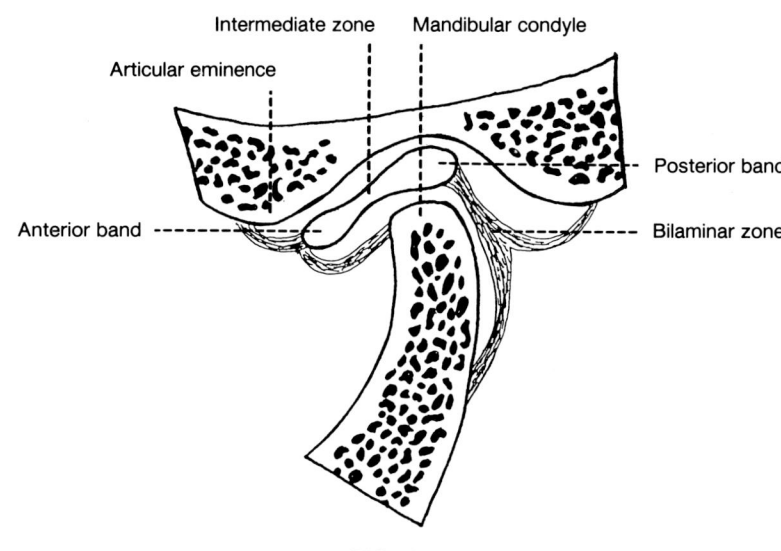

FIG. 1–1

THE TEMPOROMANDIBULAR JOINT

AXIAL
    Cryomicrotome.........................FIG. 1–2
    MR Image..............................FIG. 1–3

SAGITTAL
    Cryomicrotomes........................FIGS. 1–4 to 1–5
    MR Images.............................FIGS. 1–6 to 1–7

CORONAL
    Cryomicrotome.........................FIG. 1–8
    MR Image..............................FIG. 1–9

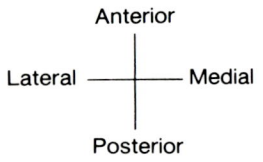

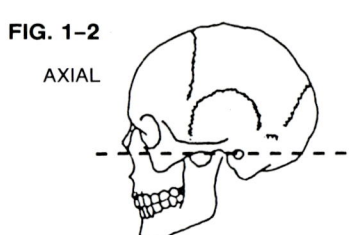

FIG. 1-2
AXIAL

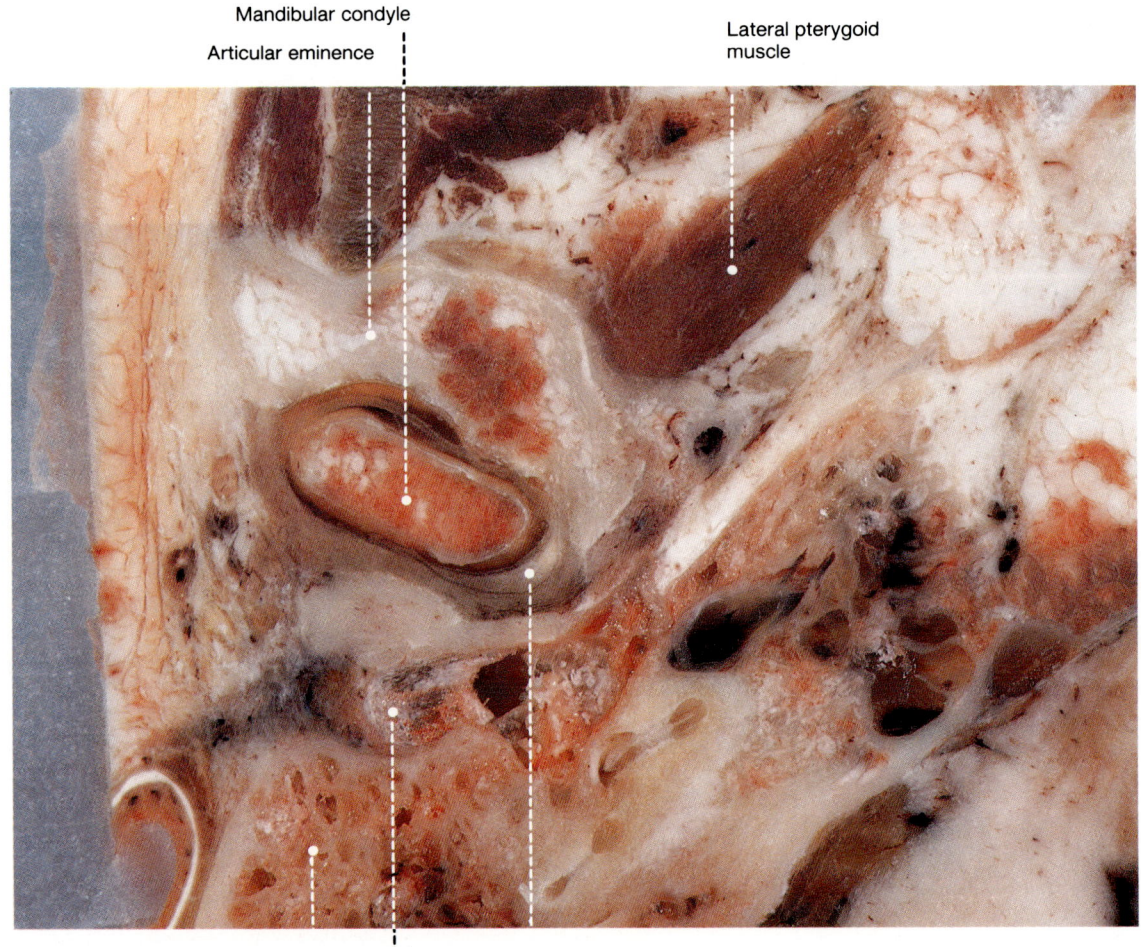

THE TEMPOROMANDIBULAR JOINT

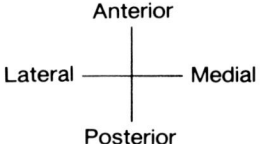

FIG. 1-3

AXIAL

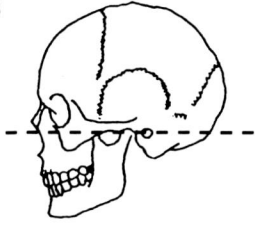

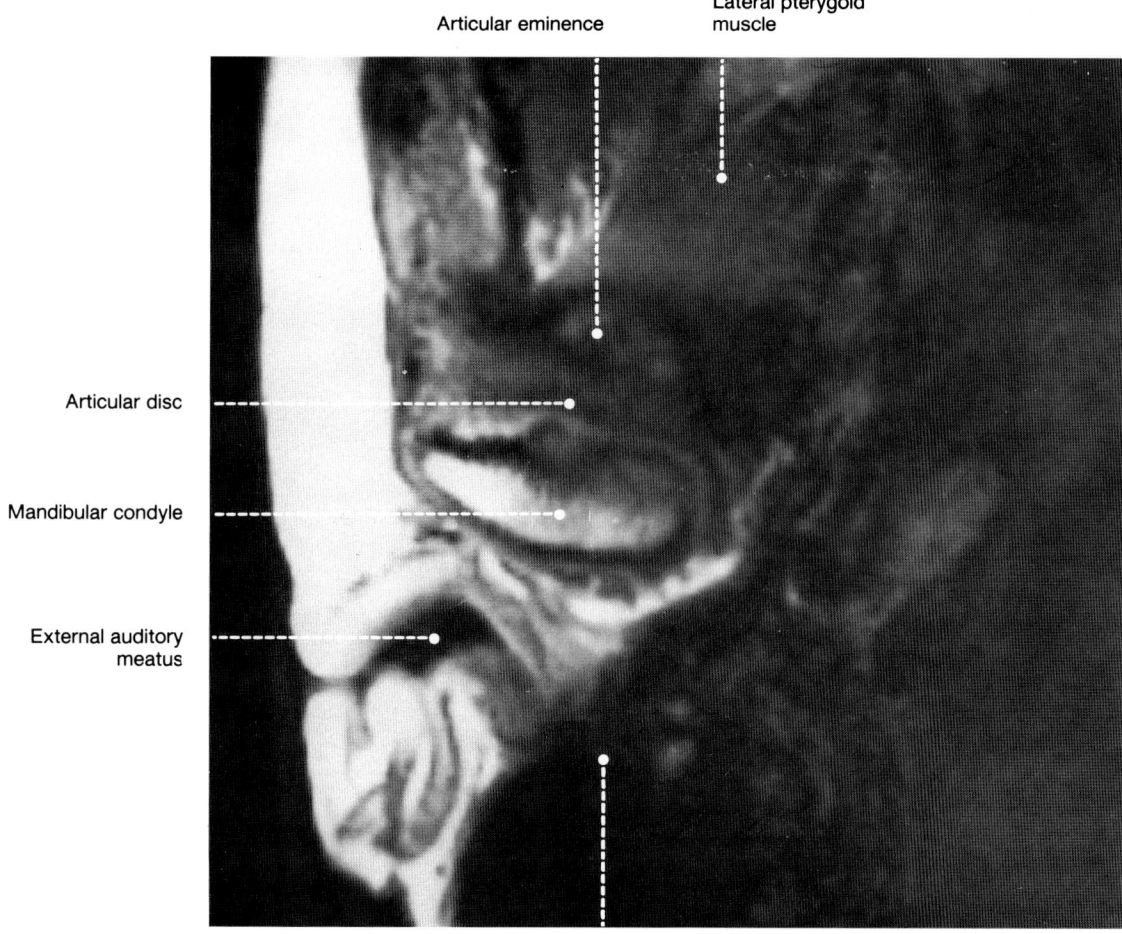

- Articular eminence
- Lateral pterygoid muscle
- Articular disc
- Mandibular condyle
- External auditory meatus
- Mastoid process

Anatomy and MRI of the Joints

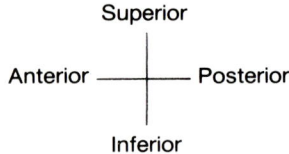

FIG. 1-4
SAGITTAL

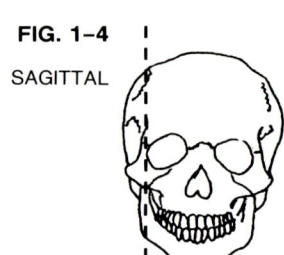

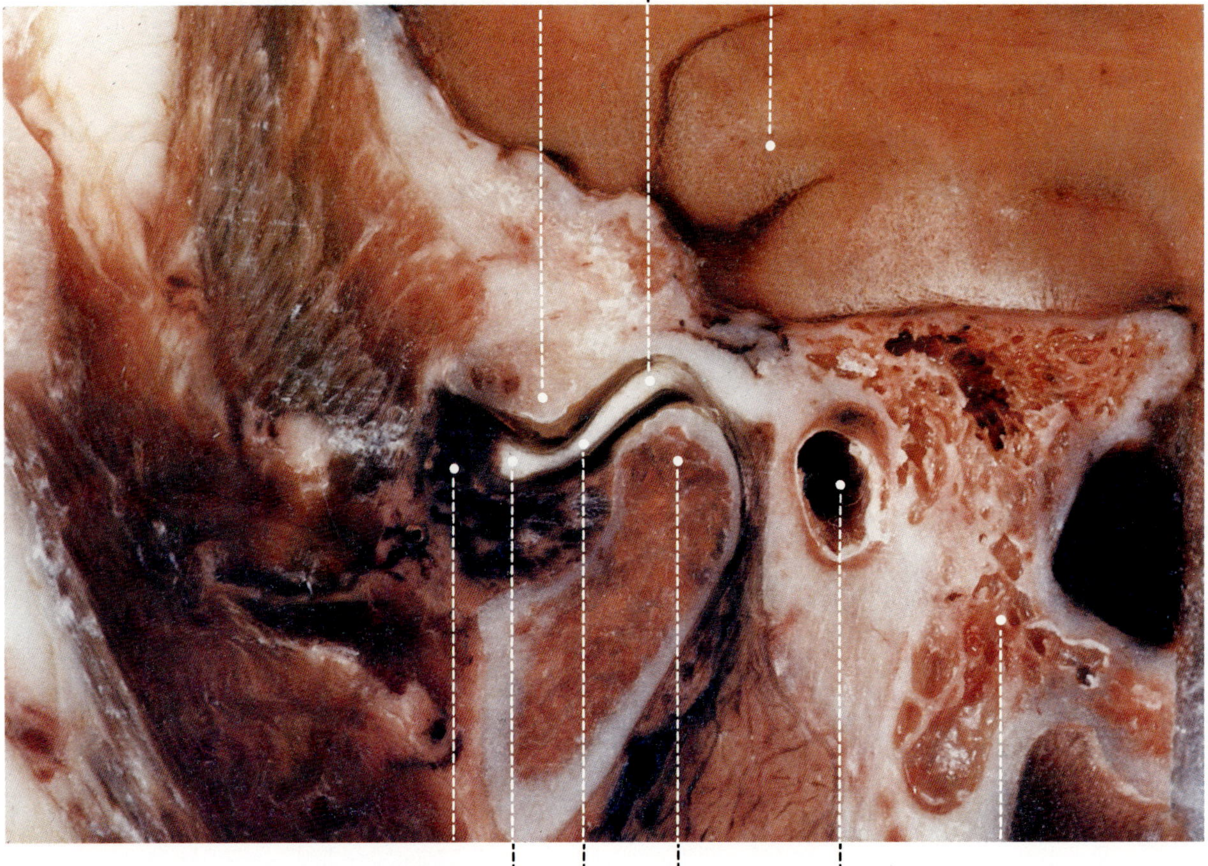

Labels: Articular eminence, Posterior band, Temporal lobe, Lateral pterygoid muscle, Anterior band, Intermediate zone, Mandibular condyle, External auditory meatus, Mastoid

Superior
Anterior
Posterior
Inferior

FIG. 1–5

SAGITTAL

Temporalis muscle
Articular eminence
Temporal lobe
External auditory meatus
Anterior band
Intermediate zone
Mandibular condyle
Posterior band
Mastoid process

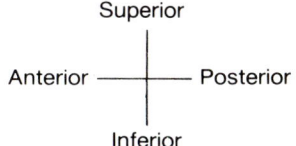

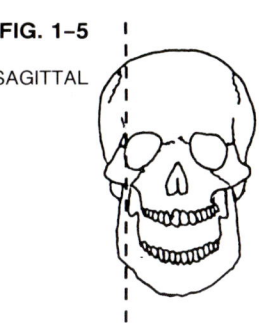

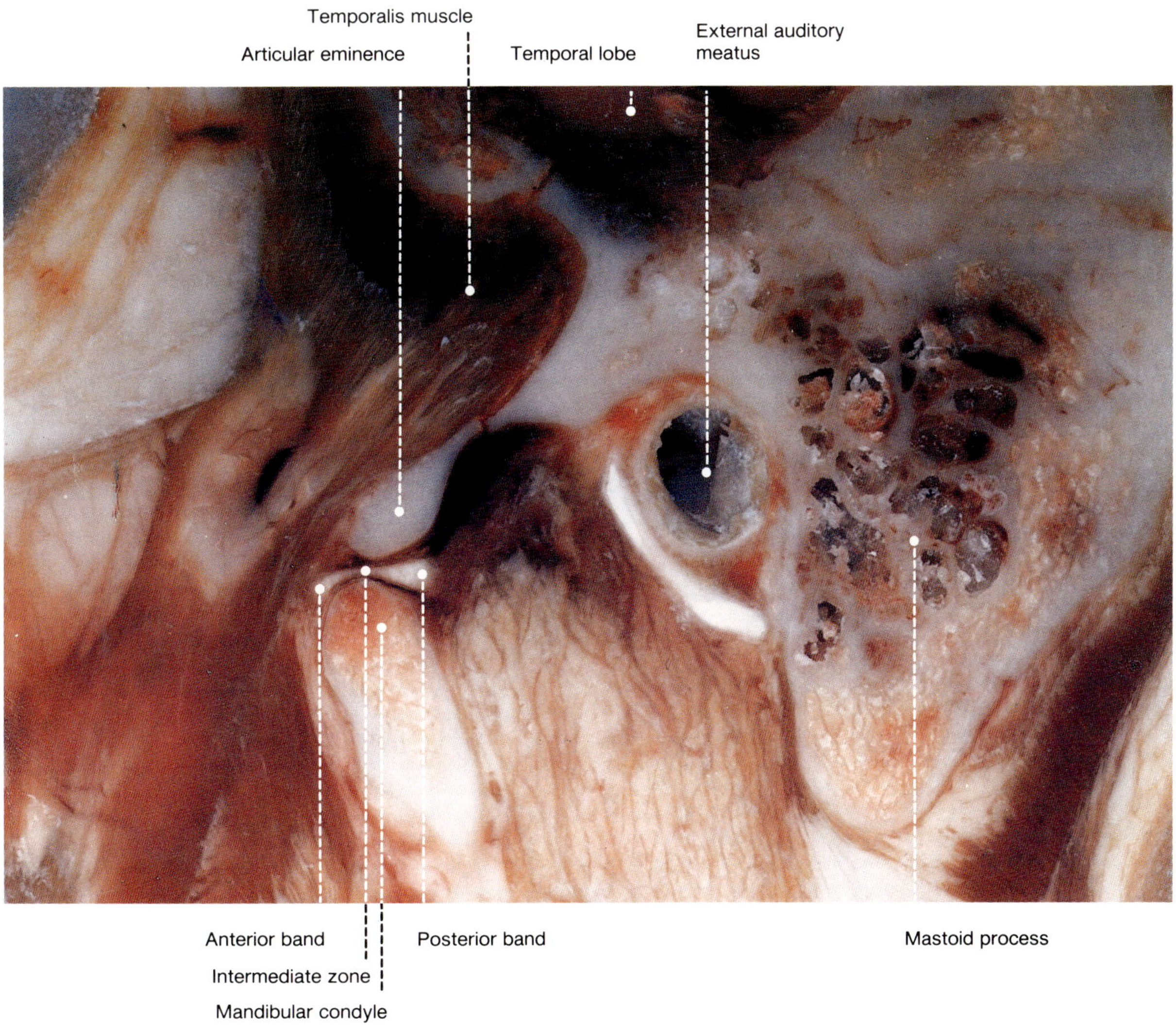

Anatomy and MRI of the Joints

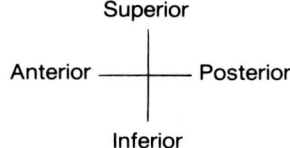

FIG. 1-6
SAGITTAL

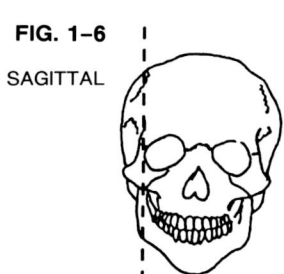

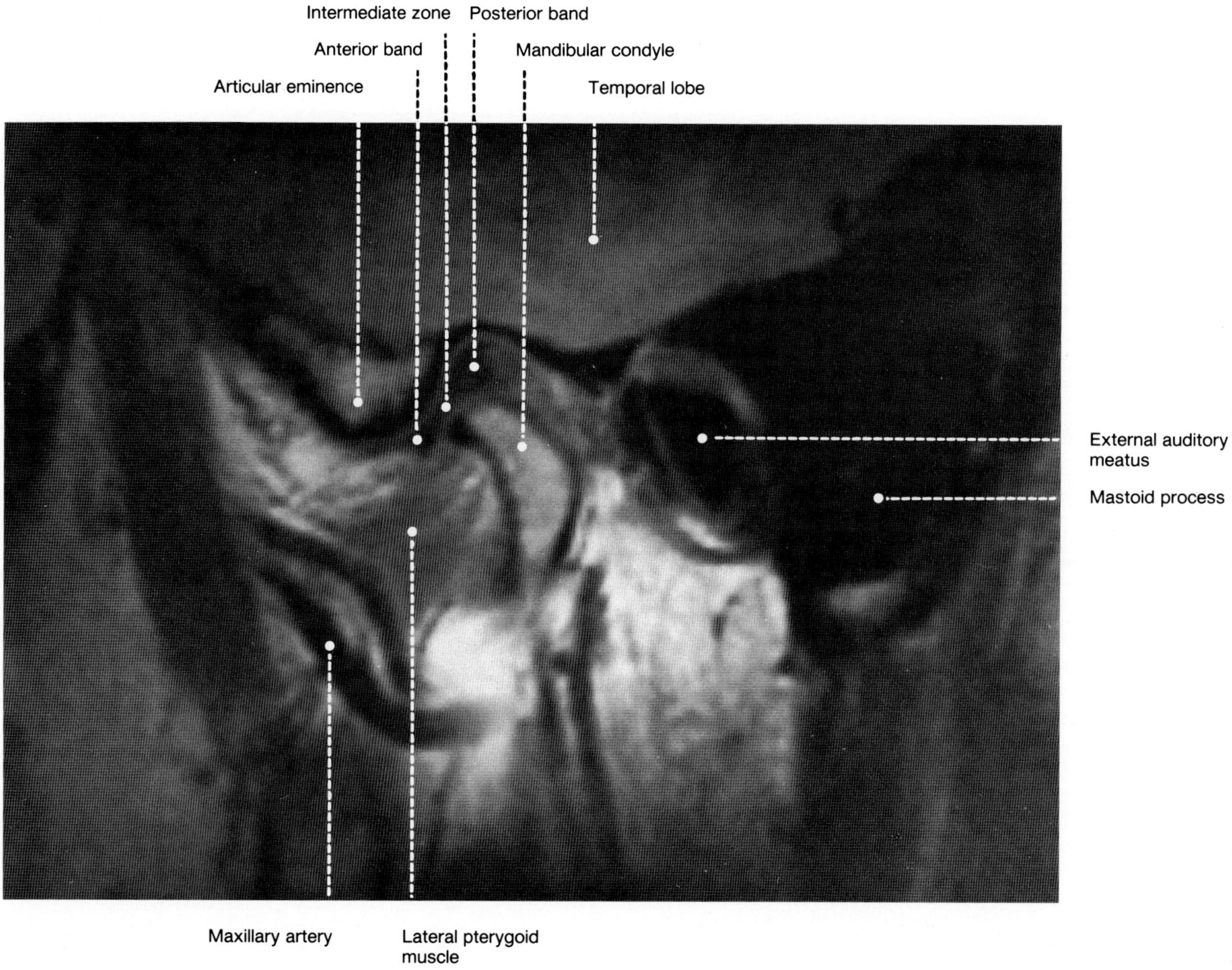

Articular eminence · Anterior band · Intermediate zone · Posterior band · Mandibular condyle · Temporal lobe

External auditory meatus

Mastoid process

Maxillary artery · Lateral pterygoid muscle

THE TEMPOROMANDIBULAR JOINT

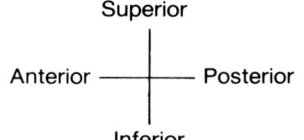

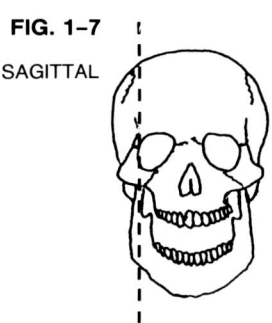

FIG. 1-7
SAGITTAL

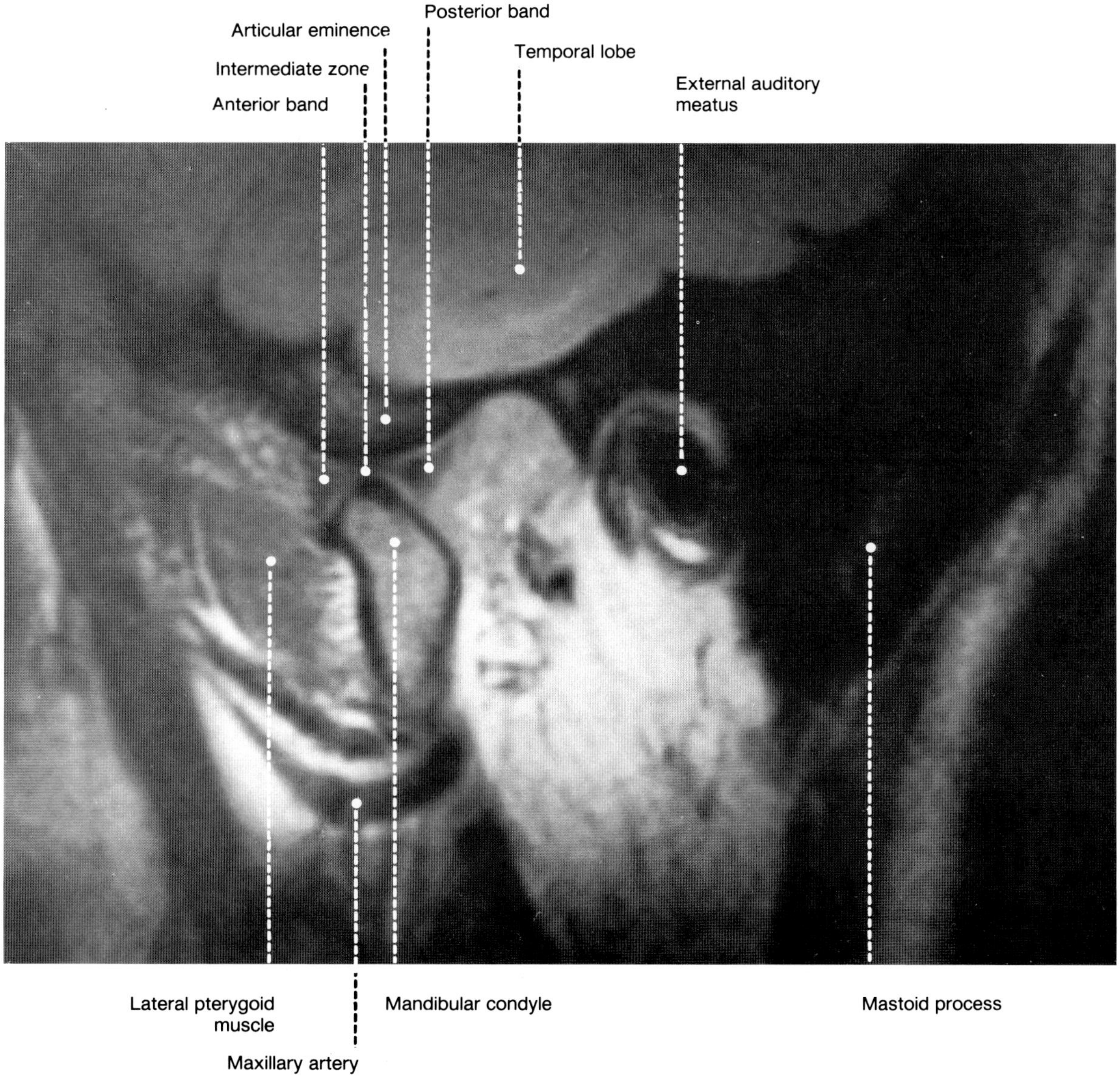

Labels: Articular eminence, Intermediate zone, Anterior band, Posterior band, Temporal lobe, External auditory meatus, Lateral pterygoid muscle, Maxillary artery, Mandibular condyle, Mastoid process

Anatomy and MRI of the Joints 10

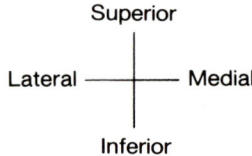

FIG. 1-8
CORONAL

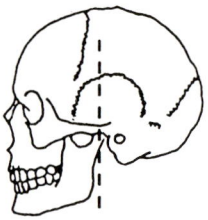

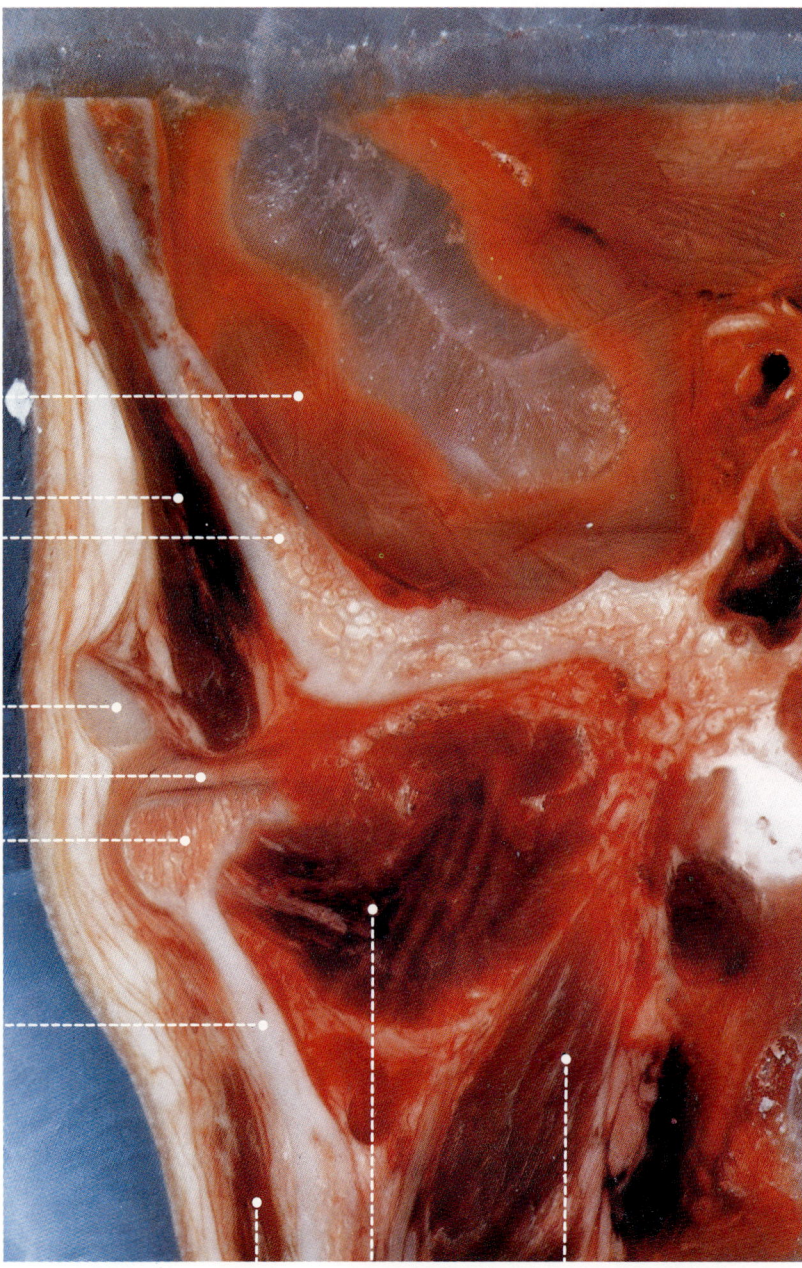

- Temporal lobe
- Temporalis muscle
- Temporal bone
- Zygomatic arch
- Articular disc
- Mandibular condyle
- Mandibular ramus

Masseter muscle   Lateral pterygoid muscle   Medial pterygoid muscle

THE TEMPOROMANDIBULAR JOINT

FIG. 1-9
CORONAL

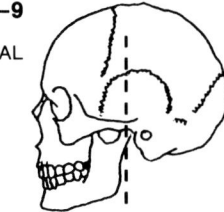

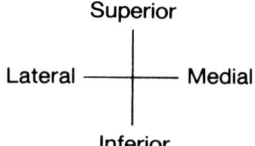

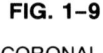

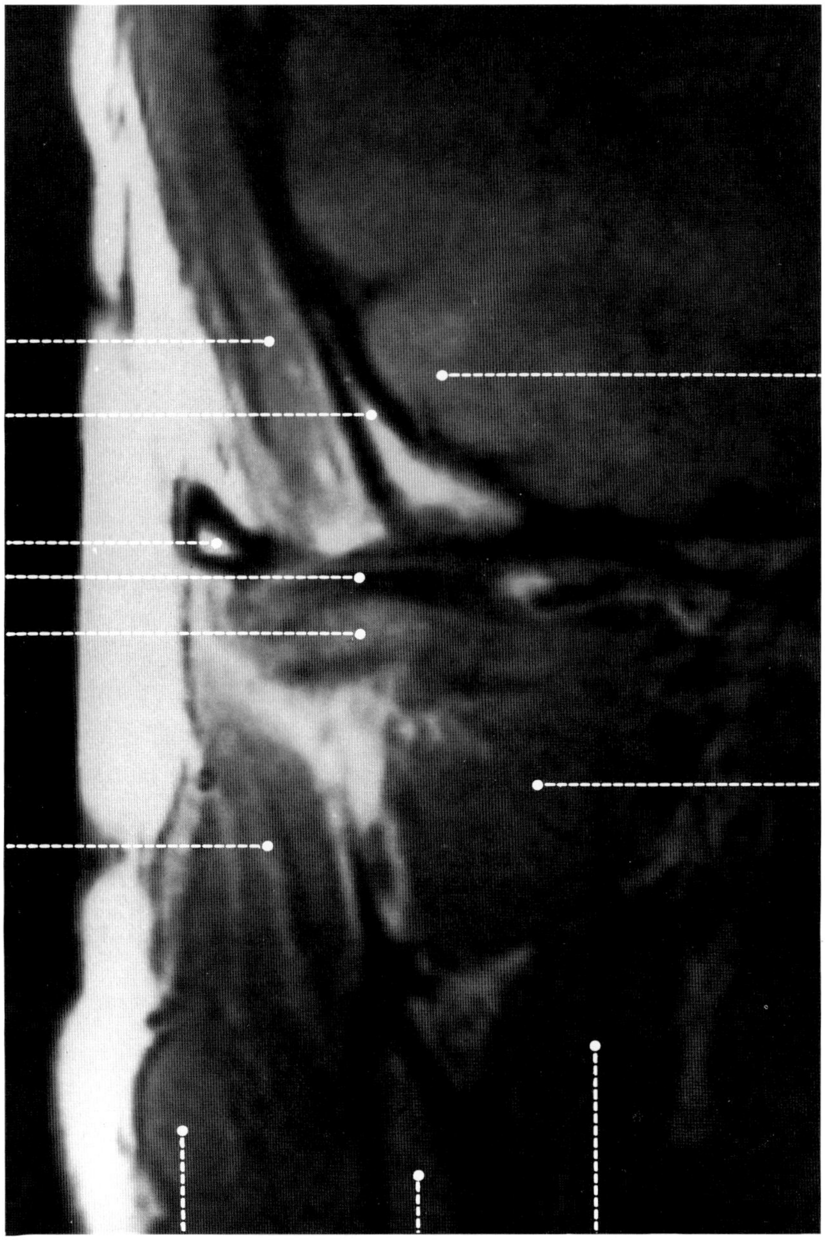

- Temporalis muscle
- Temporal bone
- Zygomatic arch
- Articular disc
- Mandibular condyle
- Masseter muscle
- Temporal lobe
- Lateral pterygoid muscle
- Parotid gland
- Mandibular ramus
- Medial pterygoid muscle

CHAPTER 2

THE SHOULDER
William D. Middleton, M.D.

The shoulder is defined as the area of junction of the arm and the trunk. This includes all the bony and soft tissue structures in this region. This chapter describes the important articular and periarticular anatomy.

The glenohumeral joint is a ball and socket joint, with the glenoid functioning as an extremely shallow socket for the humeral head. The glenoid surface is roughly elliptical with a shallow concavity that functions as the socket for the humeral head. The long axis of the glenoid is oriented vertically with its surface angled approximately 45 degrees anteriorly from the sagittal plane.

The shallow glenoid cavity is deepened slightly by the glenoid labrum, which is a fibrocartilaginous ring surrounding the edge of the glenoid. The labrum is triangular in cross-section and can be seen on axial sections buttressing the anterior and posterior portions of the glenoid.

The other articulation of the shoulder is the acromial clavicular joint. This is a gliding joint formed by the medial margin of the acromion process and the lateral aspect of the clavicle. An articular disc, which is often absent, separates the two bones superiorly. Rarely the disc extends completely across the joint and separates it into two synovial cavities. The acromial clavicular joint is oriented vertically with its long axis in the sagittal plane.

A number of ligaments assist in support of the bony structures of the shoulder. The superior, middle, and inferior glenohumeral ligaments cross the anterior aspect of the glenohumeral joint, originating from the anterior glenoid and inserting on the lesser tuberosity and inferior anatomic neck of the humerus. These ligaments actually represent thickenings in the joint capsule that can be palpated but are difficult to visualize on anatomic sections or magnetic resonance images. The subscapularis recess (bursa) commonly communicates with the joint cavity via a capsular defect between the superior and middle glenohumeral ligament.

Another ligament that crosses the glenohumeral joint is the coracohumeral ligament (Fig. 2-1). This ligament arises from the base of the coracoid process laterally and inserts on the anterior aspect of the greater tuberosity. Laterally it blends with the supraspinatus tendon superiorly and the joint capsule inferiorly; because of this it is difficult to see laterally.

The coracoacromial ligament arises with a broad base from the lateral border of the coracoid process. It narrows as it extends laterally and attaches to the anterior aspect of the acromion (Fig. 2-1). Generally, the central portion of the tendon is thinner than the anterior and posterior margins, and it may be completely absent.

The third ligament arising from the coracoid is the coracoclavicular ligament (Fig. 2-1). This is actually composed of two portions: the posteromedially located conoid and the anterolaterally located trapezoid ligaments. The conoid fasciculus is triangular, with its base attached to the inferior aspect of the clavicle and its apex to the coracoid process. The trapezoid fasciculus is thinner and has a quadrilateral shape. The posterior edge of the trapezoid ligament is attached to the anterior edge of the conoid ligament.

Because of the minimal bony stability of the shoulder, the muscles that act on the glenohumeral joint are extremely important in providing dynamic stability to the joint. The four rotator cuff muscles are the most important stabilizers of the shoulder. The most anterior of the rotator cuff muscles is the subcapularis (Fig. 2-1). It is a triangular, multipenate (multiple tendons) muscle that has a broad origin from the deep surface of the scapula. As it extends laterally across the glenohumeral joint, the multiple tendons fuse into one thick tendon that inserts on the lesser tuberosity. The subscapularis is separated from the rest of the rotator cuff by the tendon of the long head of the biceps and the coracohumeral ligament.

The supraspinatus is the most superior muscle of the rotator cuff (Fig. 2-2). It arises from the supraspinous fossa of the scapula and crosses the superior aspect of the glenohumeral joint to insert on the anterior-most portion

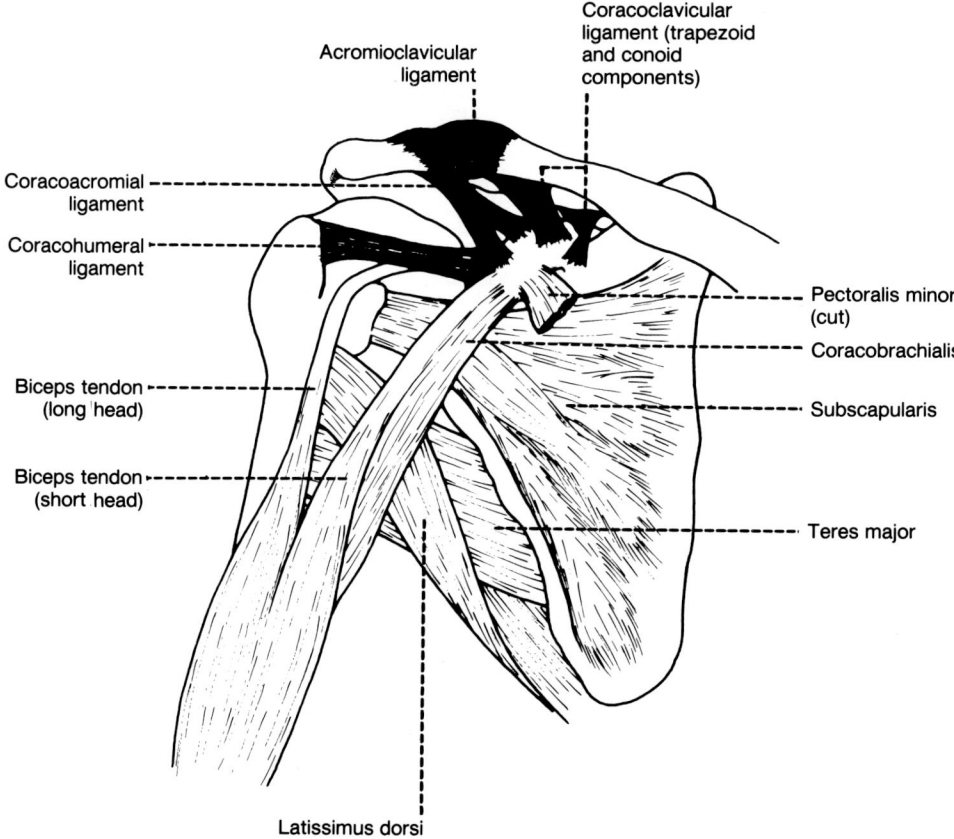

FIG. 2-1

of the greater tuberosity. The supraspinatus has a single, central tendon that originates in the deep substance of the muscle belly. As the muscle extends laterally, the central tendon migrates to the anterior surface of the muscle.

Posterior and inferior to the supraspinatus is the intraspinatus (Fig. 2-2). It arises on the superficial surface of the scapula in the infraspinous fossa. Like the subscapularis, it is a triangular-shaped, multipenate muscle. As the central tendons converge laterally, they form a single flattened tendon which is the most prominent tendinous structure covering the humeral head. This tendon inserts on the lateral aspect of the greater tuberosity just posterior to the supraspinatus.

The final rotator cuff muscle is the teres minor (Fig. 2-2). This is the smallest of the rotator cuff muscles and some anatomists consider it as part of the infraspinatus. It arises from the superficial surface of the scapula just inferior to the intraspinatus. The teres minor crosses the posterior surface of the glenohumeral joint to insert on the posterior-most aspect of the greater tuberosity.

The rotator cuff is covered by the deltoid muscle. The deltoid is a bulky muscle that has a broad origin from the lateral aspect of the clavicle, the acromion process, and the spine of the scapula. It extends inferiorly to insert on the deltoid prominence of the humerus. The multiple tendons of the deltoid are prominent structures which are well seen on all planes. The deltoid is actually separated from the rotator cuff by the subdeltoid/subacromial bursa. This bursa allows for a smooth, gliding motion of the rotator cuff under the deltoid muscle and the coracoacromial arch.

A prominent intraarticular structure within the glenohumeral joint is the tendon of the long head of the biceps (Fig. 2-1). This tendon arises from a tubercle at the superior aspect of the glenoid and runs within the joint capsule, but outside the synovial cavity, between the supraspinatus and subscapularis. It exits the joint at the biceps tendon groove.

The short head of the biceps arises from the tip of the coracoid process along with the more medially positioned coracobrachialis muscle (Fig. 2-1). Both muscles extend inferiorly; the short head of the biceps joins with the long head to form the distal biceps muscle and the coracobrachialis inserts on the medial aspect of the mid-humerus.

The other muscle attaching to the coracoid is the pectoralis minor which originates from the chest wall (ribs 3, 4, and 5) and inserts on the medial aspect of the coracoid (Fig. 2-1). The pectoralis major runs superficial to the pectoralis minor. It originates from the sternum and the medial half of the clavicle. The clavicular head extends inferiorly and laterally in close apposition to the clavicular head of the deltoid.

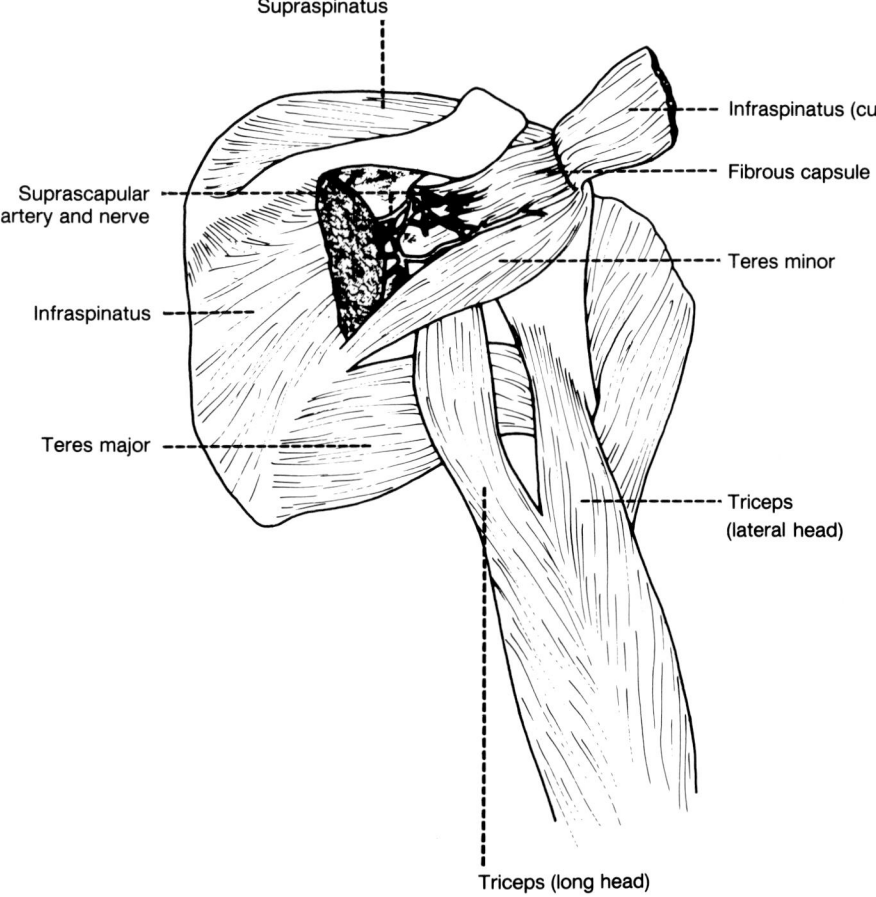

FIG. 2-2

The only major neurovascular structure in the shoulder is the axillary artery and vein and the brachial plexus. The axillary vessels are arranged with the artery superior and posterior to the vein. In the axilla the brachial plexus is composed of multiple cords and divisions which are seen adjacent to the axillary artery.

The suprascapular artery, a branch of the thyrocervical trunk, runs laterally deep to the clavicle. When it reaches the scapular notch, it turns posteriorly into the supraspinous fossa, where it runs deep to the supraspinatus muscle. It then passes lateral to the spine of the scapula and runs deep to the infraspinatus muscle (Fig. 2-2).

THE SHOULDER

AXIAL
    Cryomicrotomes..........................FIGS. 2–3 to 2–7
    MR Images.............................FIGS. 2–8 to 2–13

SAGITTAL
    Cryomicrotomes..........................FIGS. 2–14 to 2–19
    MR Images.............................FIGS. 2–20 to 2–23

CORONAL
    Cryomicrotomes..........................FIGS. 2–24 to 2–28
    MR Images.............................FIGS. 2–29 to 2–33

Anatomy and MRI of the Joints

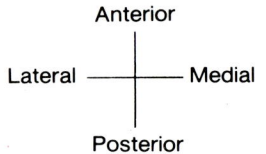

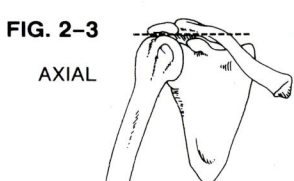

FIG. 2-3
AXIAL

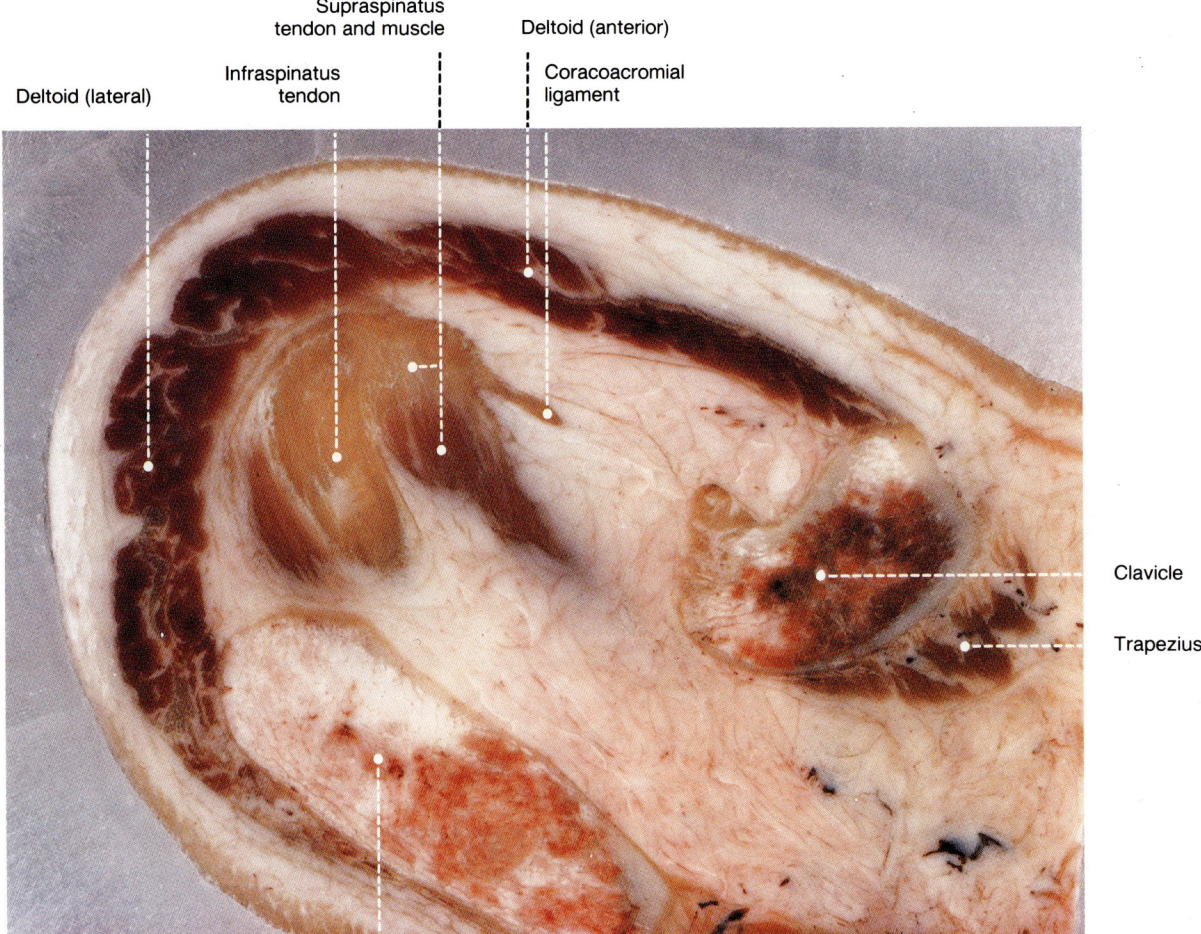

Deltoid (lateral) — Infraspinatus tendon — Supraspinatus tendon and muscle — Deltoid (anterior) — Coracoacromial ligament — Clavicle — Trapezius — Spine of scapula

THE SHOULDER

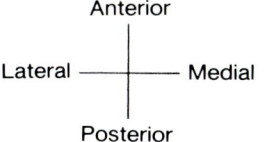

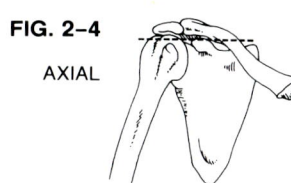

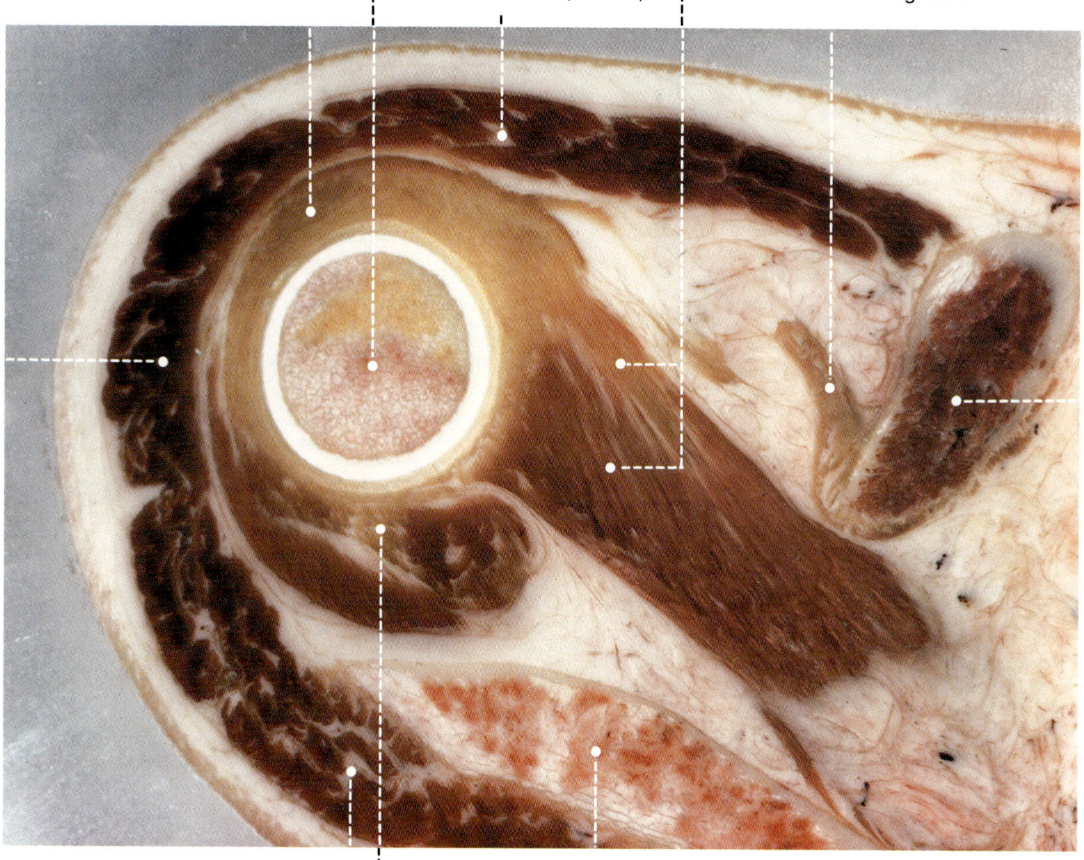

FIG. 2-4
AXIAL

Anatomy and MRI of the Joints   20

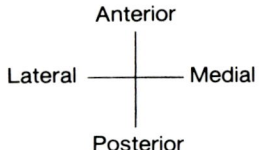

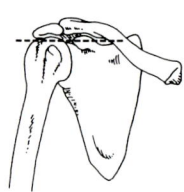
FIG. 2-5
AXIAL

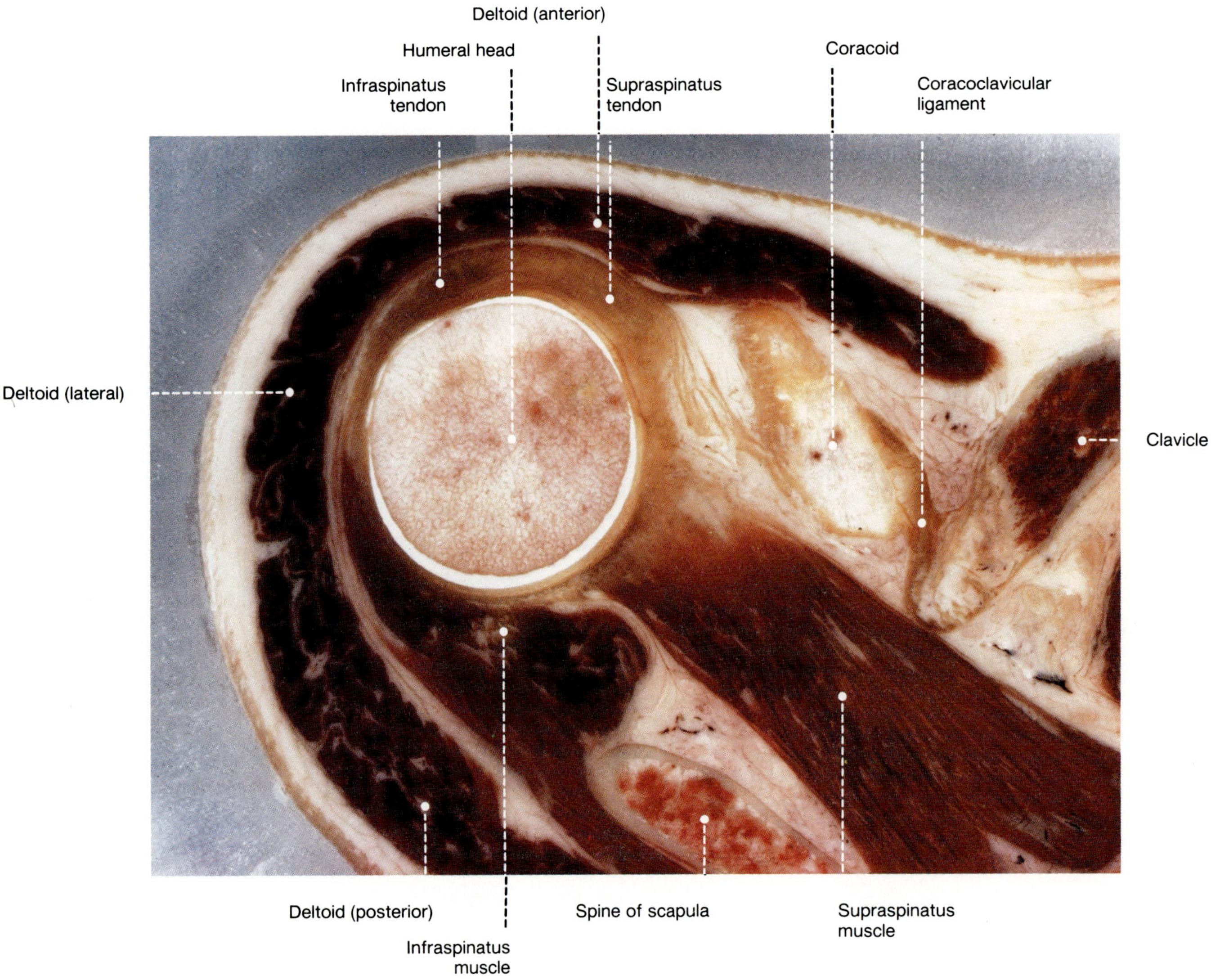

Deltoid (anterior)
Humeral head
Infraspinatus tendon
Supraspinatus tendon
Coracoid
Coracoclavicular ligament

Deltoid (lateral)

Clavicle

Deltoid (posterior)
Infraspinatus muscle
Spine of scapula
Supraspinatus muscle

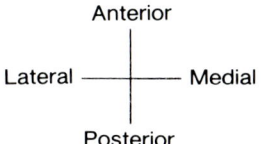

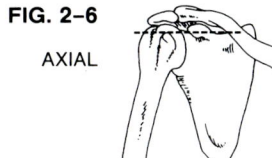

Anterior

Lateral — Medial

Posterior

FIG. 2–6

AXIAL

Supraspinatus tendon
Humeral head
Infraspinatus tendon
Deltoid (anterior)
Coracoid process
Clavicle
Subclavius muscle
Deltoid (lateral)
Infraspinatus muscle
Superior glenoid labrum
Spine of scapula
Supraspinatus muscle

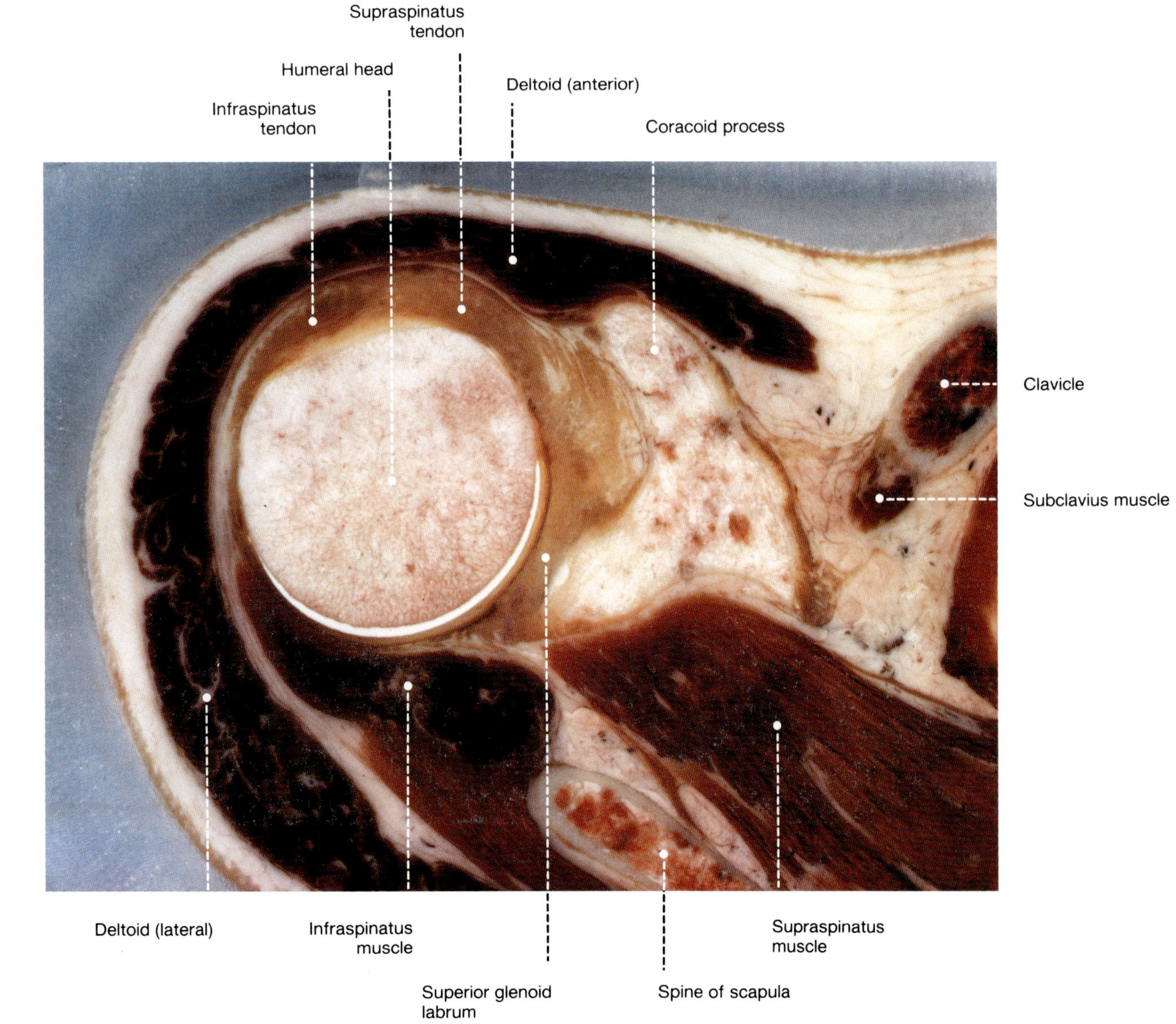

Anatomy and MRI of the Joints   22

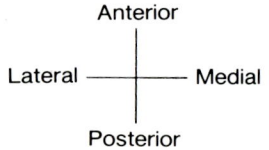

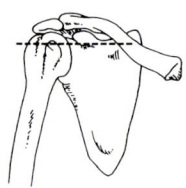

FIG. 2-7
AXIAL

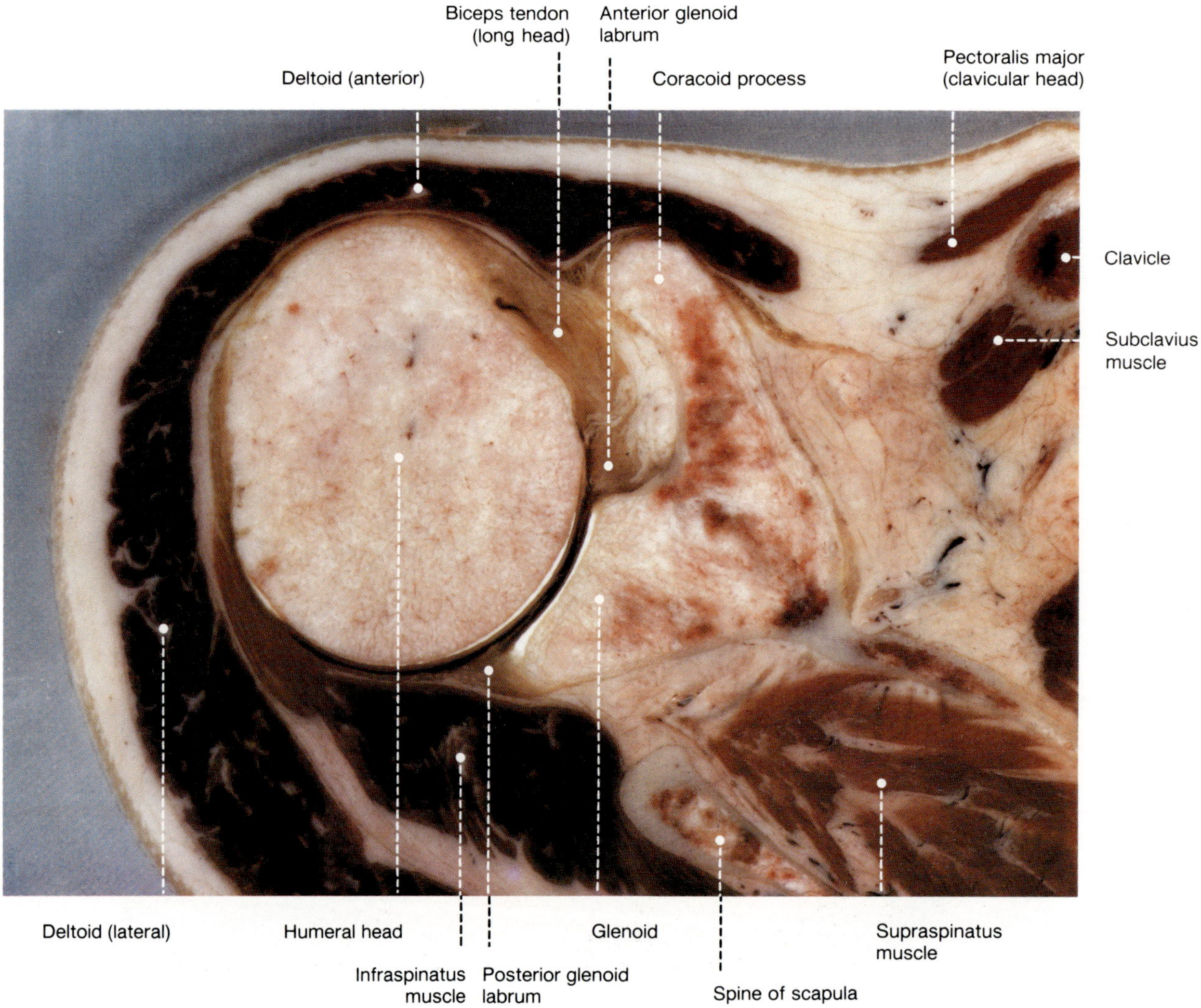

Deltoid (anterior) — Biceps tendon (long head) — Anterior glenoid labrum — Coracoid process — Pectoralis major (clavicular head) — Clavicle — Subclavius muscle

Deltoid (lateral) — Humeral head — Infraspinatus muscle — Posterior glenoid labrum — Glenoid — Spine of scapula — Supraspinatus muscle

THE SHOULDER

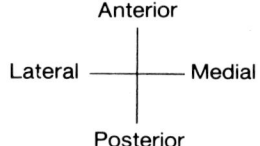

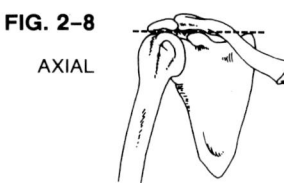

FIG. 2-8
AXIAL

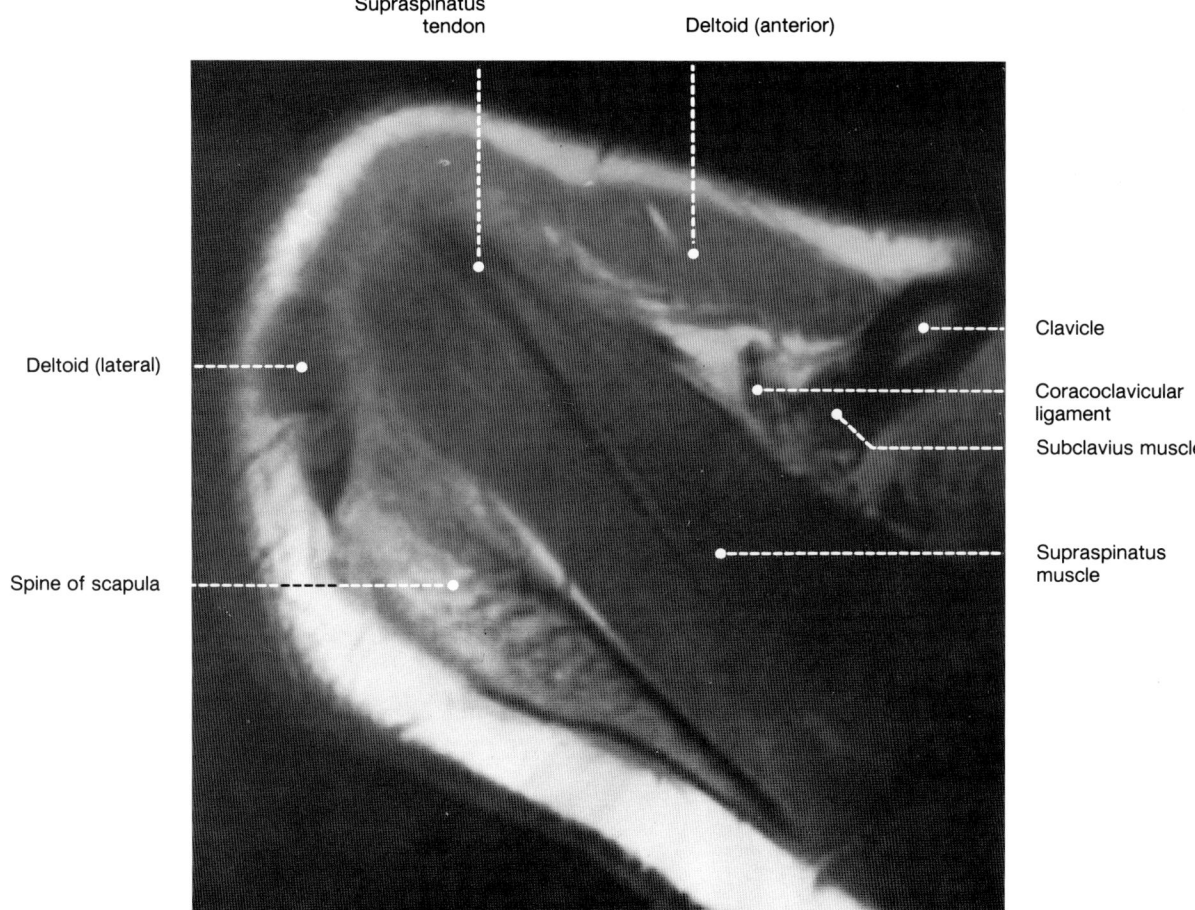

Anatomy and MRI of the Joints

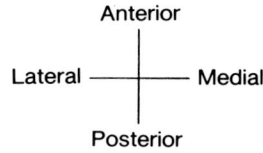

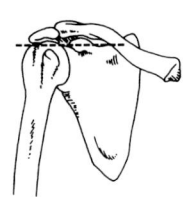

FIG. 2-9
AXIAL

THE SHOLDER

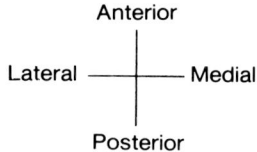

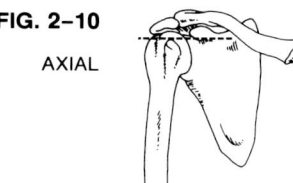

FIG. 2-10

AXIAL

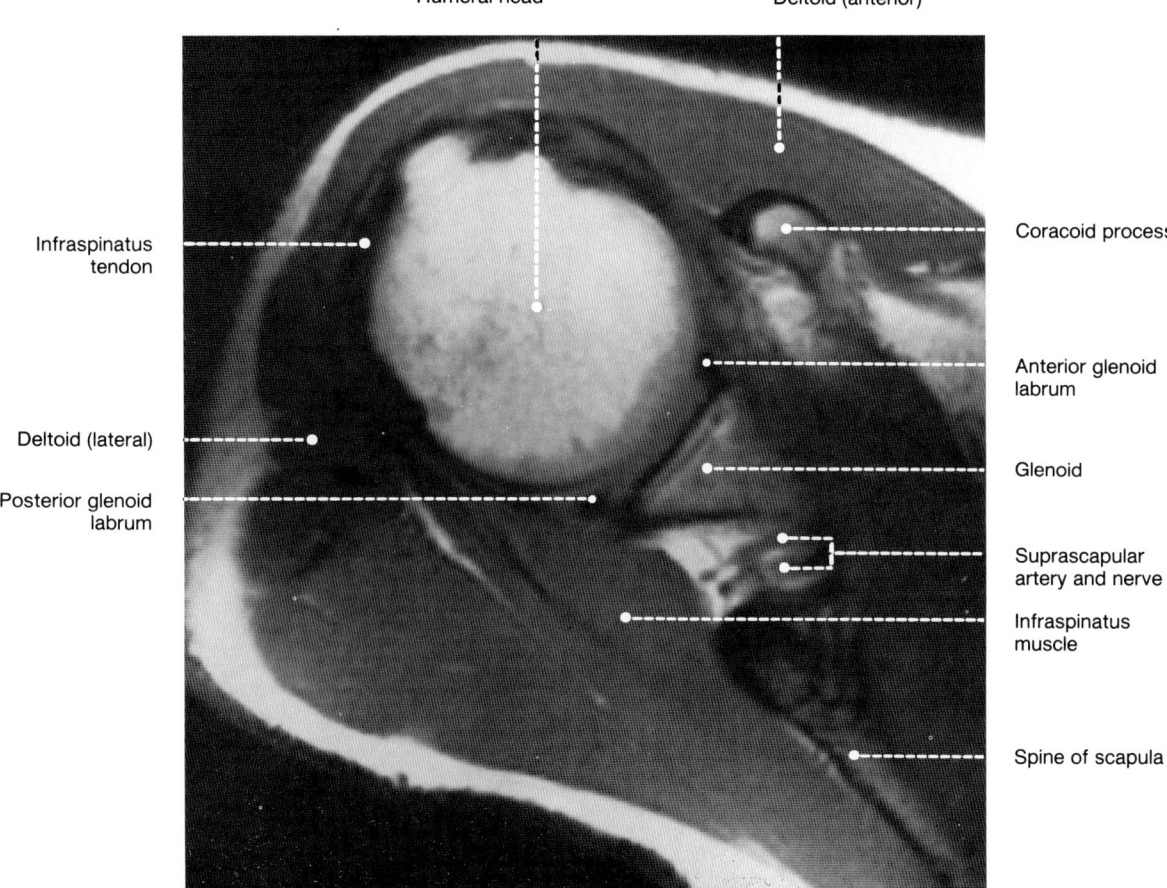

Anatomy and MRI of the Joints

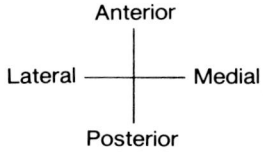

FIG. 2-11
AXIAL
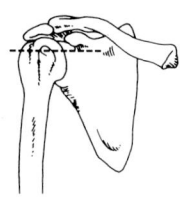

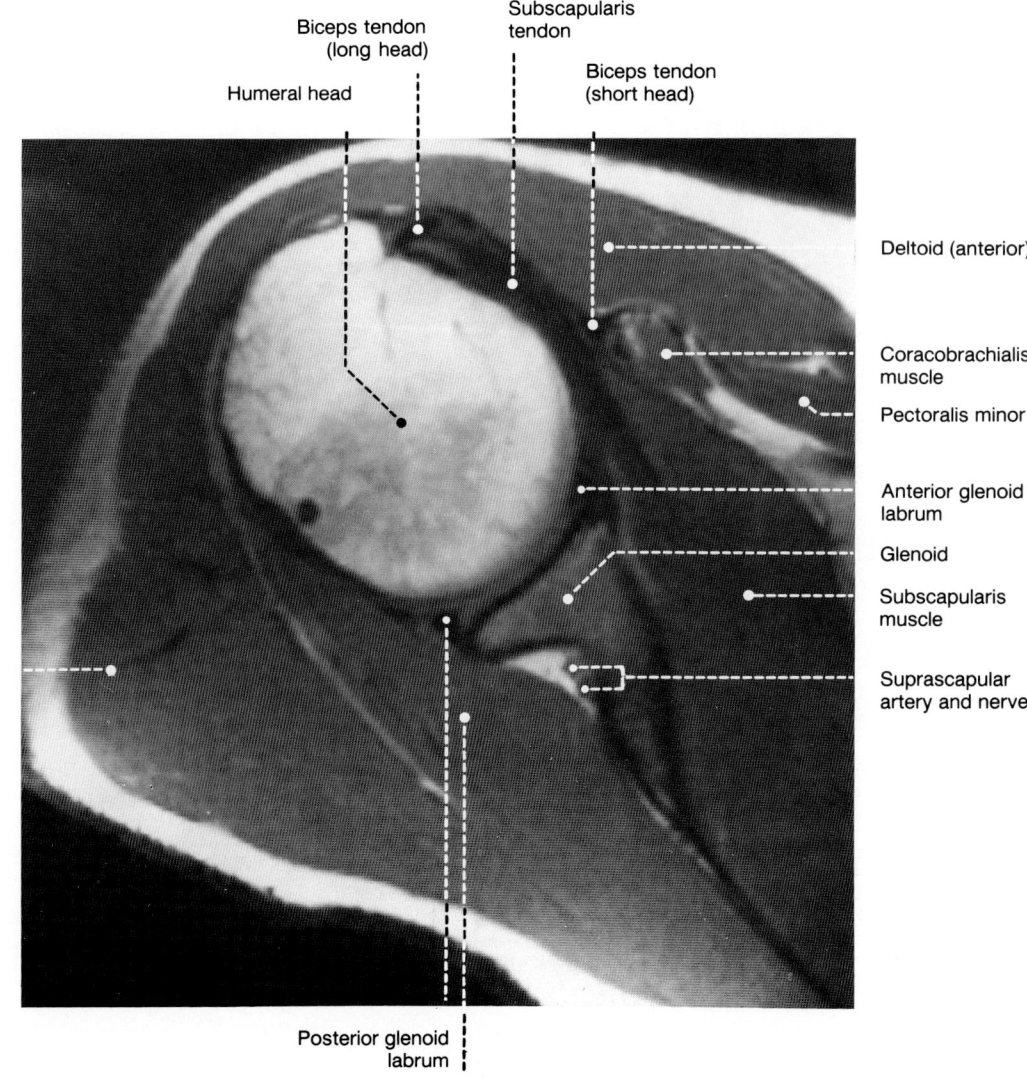

Anterior
Lateral
Medial
Posterior

FIG. 2-12

AXIAL

Deltoid (anterior)
Subscapularis tendon
Biceps tendon (short head)
Biceps tendon (long head)
Coracobrachialis
Humeral head
Pectoralis minor
Anterior glenoid labrum
Glenoid
Posterior glenoid labrum
Subscapularis muscle
Deltoid (lateral)
Infraspinatus muscle
Suprascapular artery and nerve

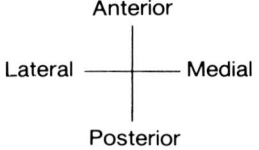

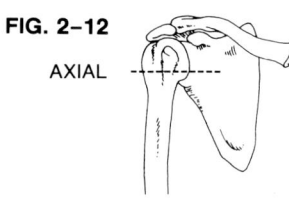

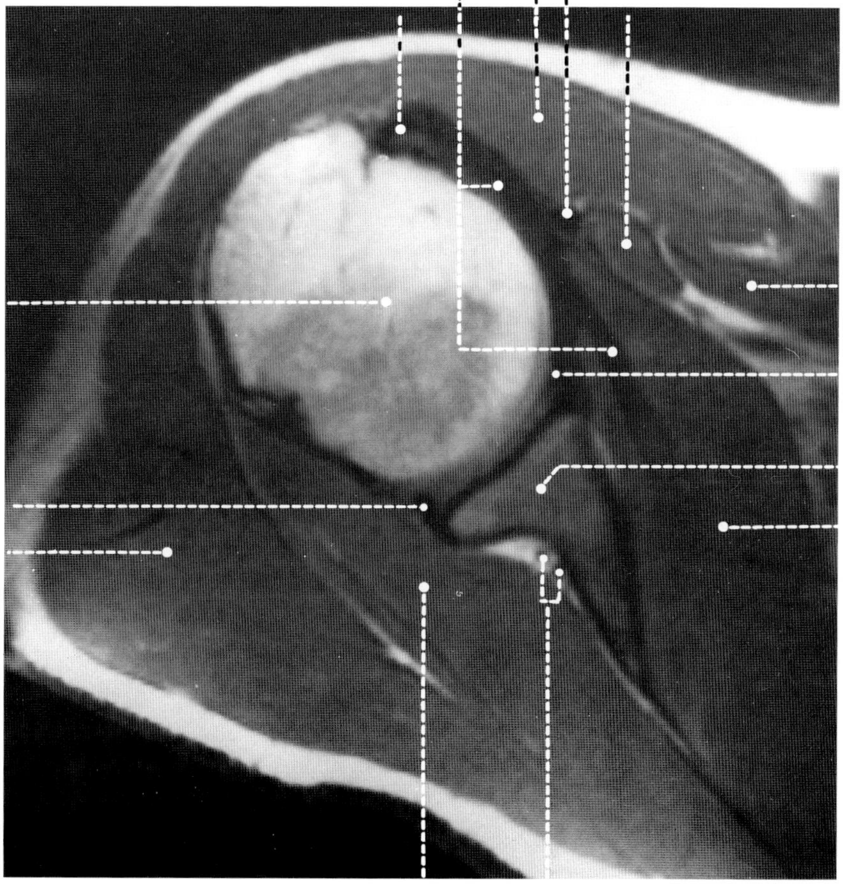

Anatomy and MRI of the Joints

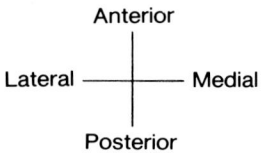

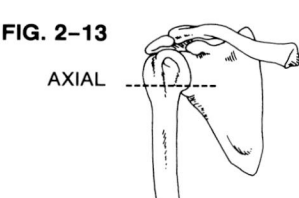

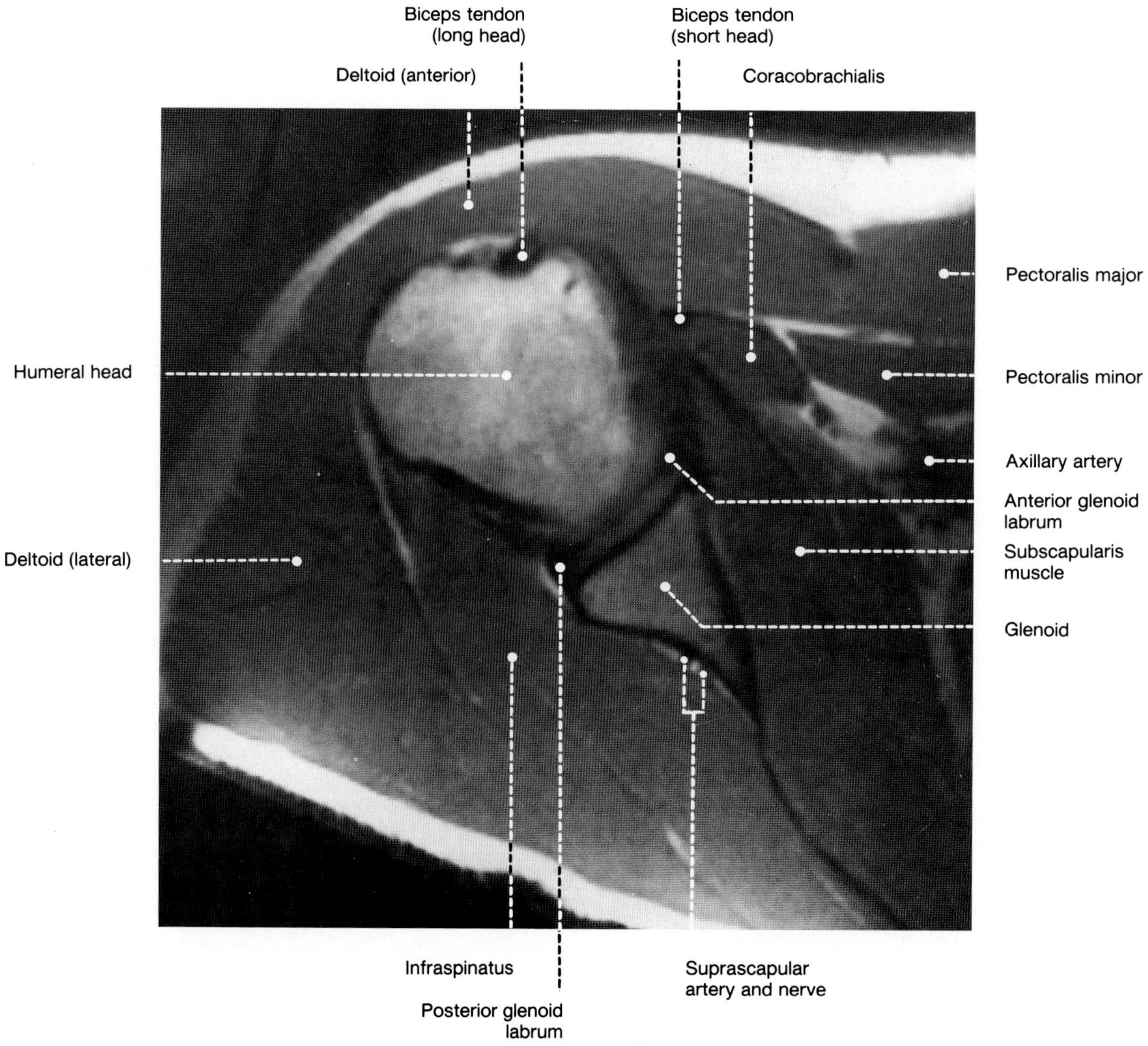

FIG. 2-13

Superior
Anterior
Posterior
Inferior

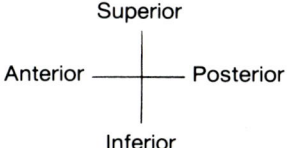

FIG. 2–14

SAGITTAL

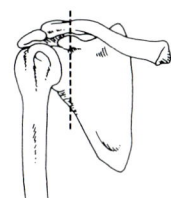

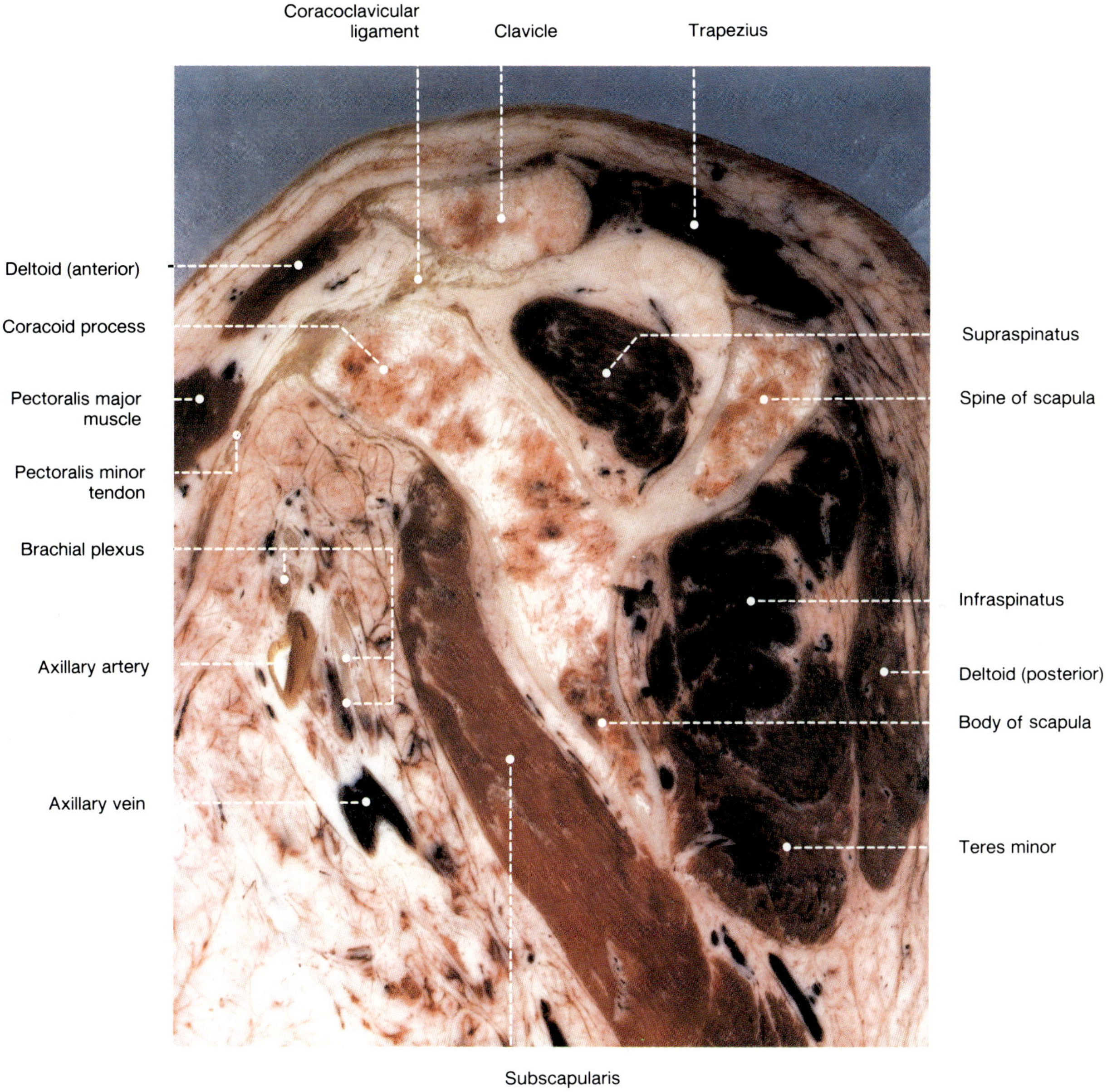

Coracoclavicular ligament
Clavicle
Trapezius
Deltoid (anterior)
Coracoid process
Pectoralis major muscle
Pectoralis minor tendon
Brachial plexus
Axillary artery
Axillary vein
Supraspinatus
Spine of scapula
Infraspinatus
Deltoid (posterior)
Body of scapula
Teres minor
Subscapularis

Anatomy and MRI of the Joints　　30

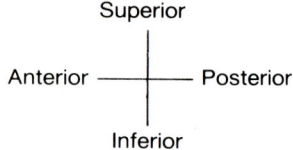

FIG. 2–15
SAGITTAL

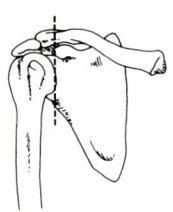

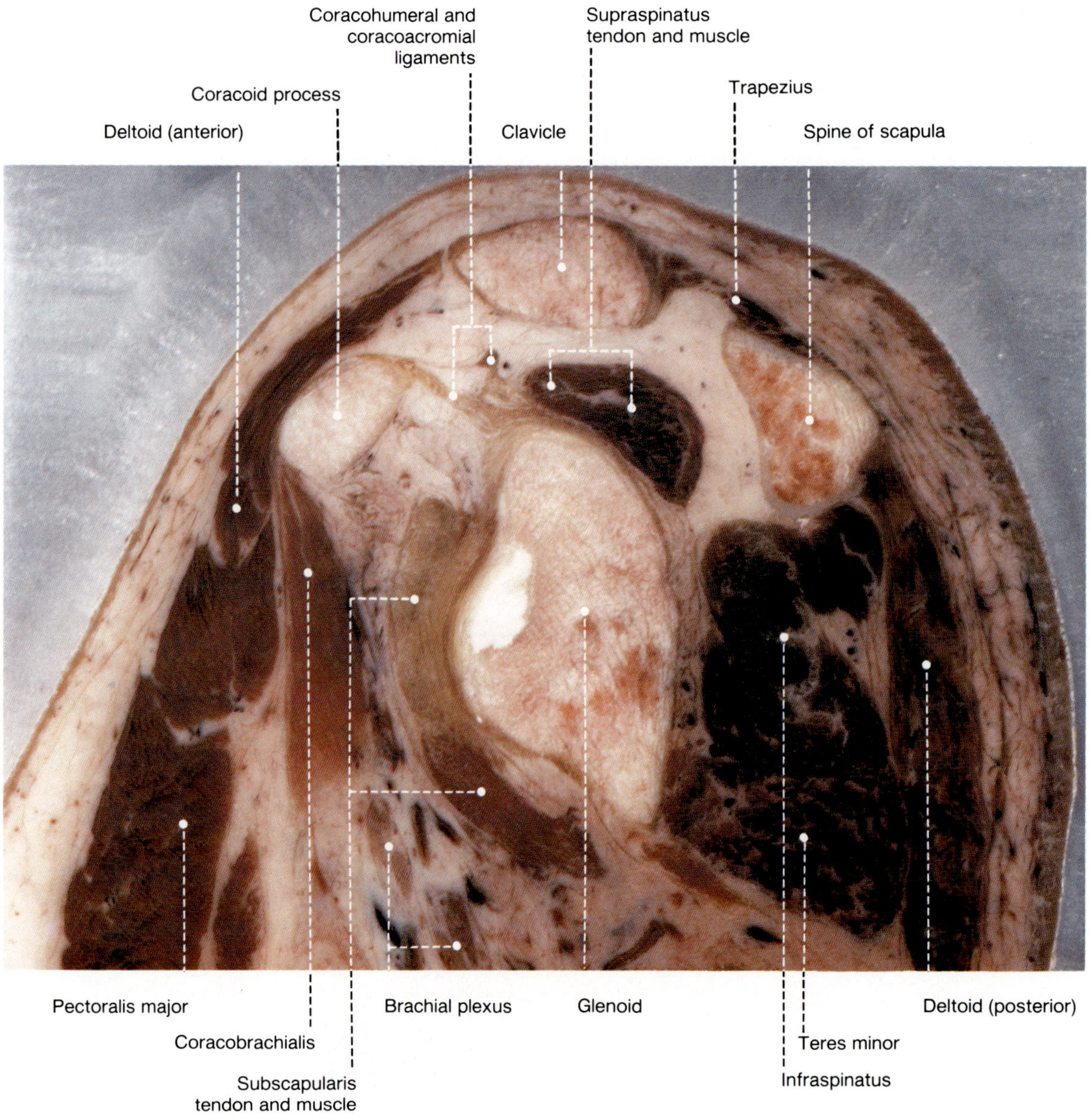

Deltoid (anterior) — Coracoid process — Coracohumeral and coracoacromial ligaments — Clavicle — Supraspinatus tendon and muscle — Trapezius — Spine of scapula

Pectoralis major — Coracobrachialis — Subscapularis tendon and muscle — Brachial plexus — Glenoid — Infraspinatus — Teres minor — Deltoid (posterior)

Superior
Anterior
Posterior
Inferior

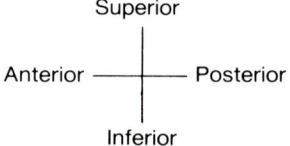

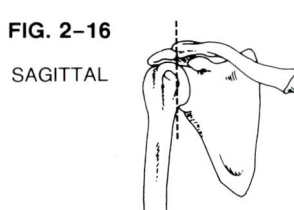

FIG. 2–16

SAGITTAL

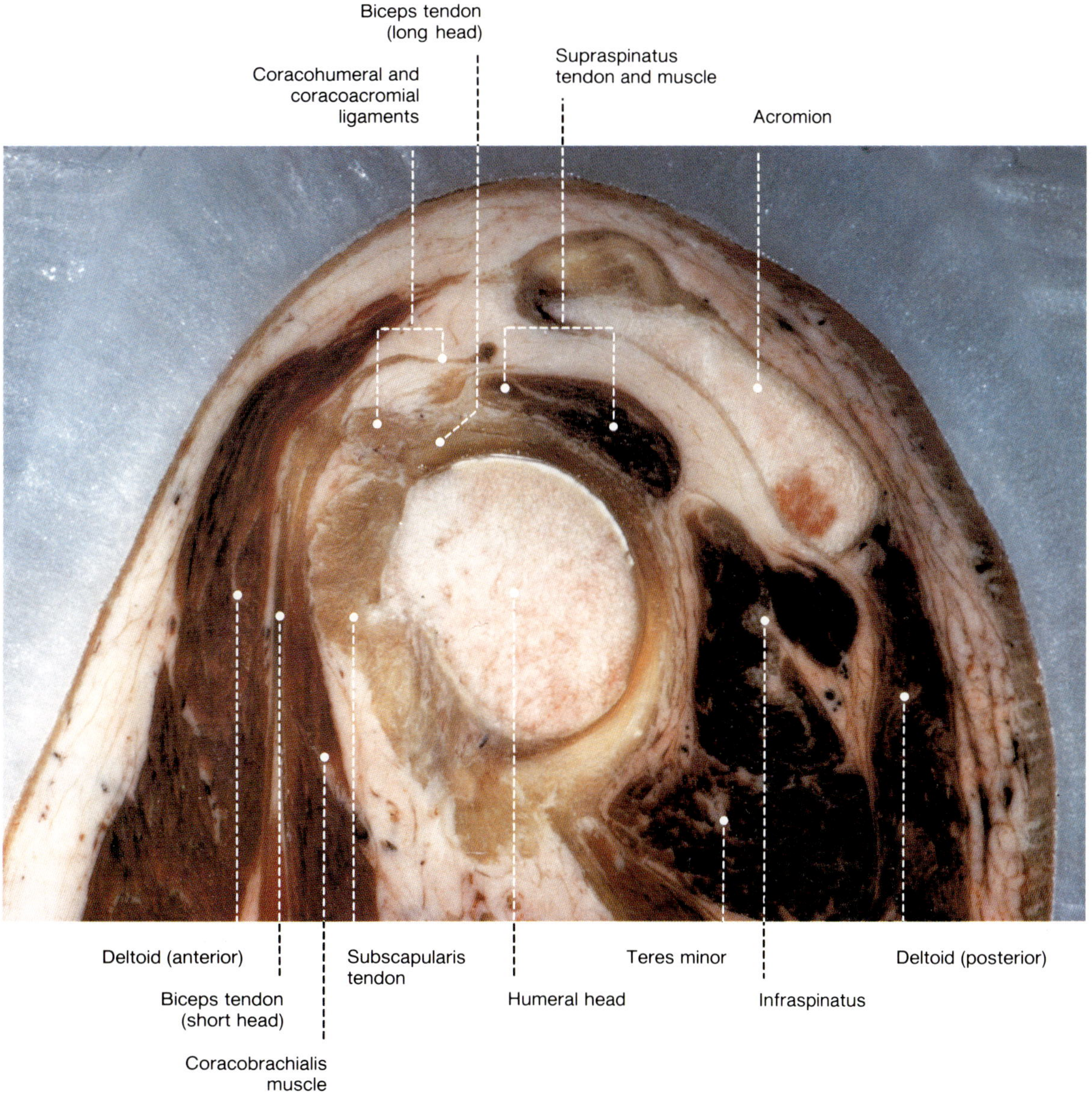

Biceps tendon (long head)
Coracohumeral and coracoacromial ligaments
Supraspinatus tendon and muscle
Acromion
Deltoid (anterior)
Biceps tendon (short head)
Coracobrachialis muscle
Subscapularis tendon
Humeral head
Teres minor
Infraspinatus
Deltoid (posterior)

Anatomy and MRI of the Joints

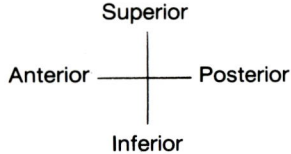

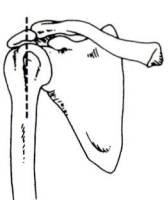

FIG. 2-17

SAGITTAL

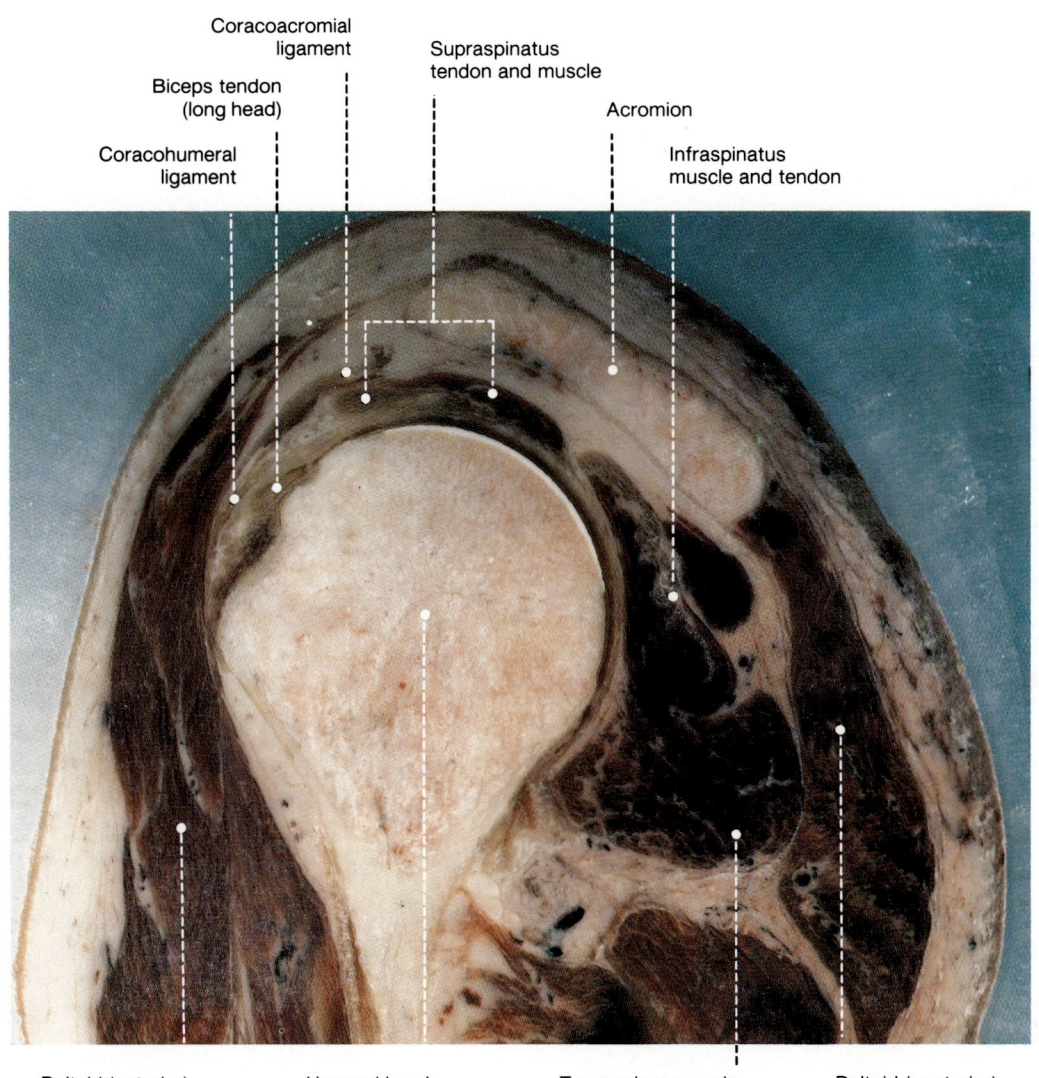

Coracoacromial ligament · Biceps tendon (long head) · Coracohumeral ligament · Supraspinatus tendon and muscle · Acromion · Infraspinatus muscle and tendon · Deltoid (anterior) · Humeral head · Teres minor muscle · Deltoid (posterior)

FIG. 2-18
SAGITTAL

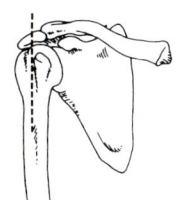

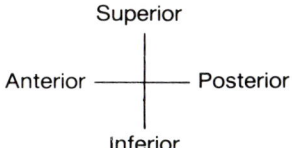

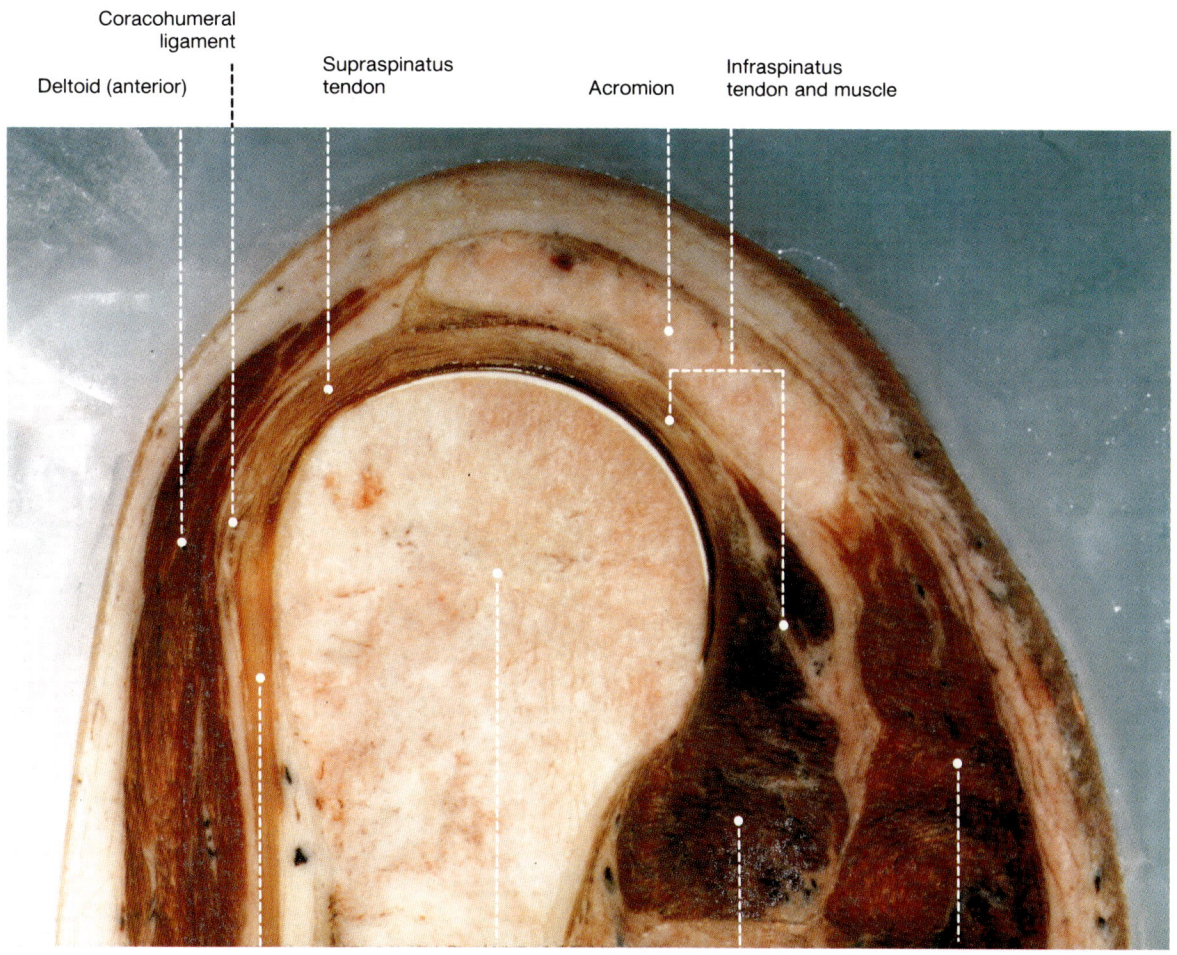

Deltoid (anterior) | Coracohumeral ligament | Supraspinatus tendon | Acromion | Infraspinatus tendon and muscle

Biceps tendon (long head) | Humeral head | Teres minor muscle | Deltoid (posterior)

Anatomy and MRI of the Joints 34

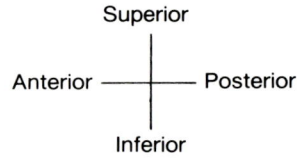

FIG. 2-19
SAGITTAL

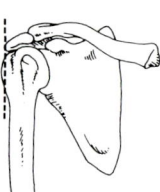

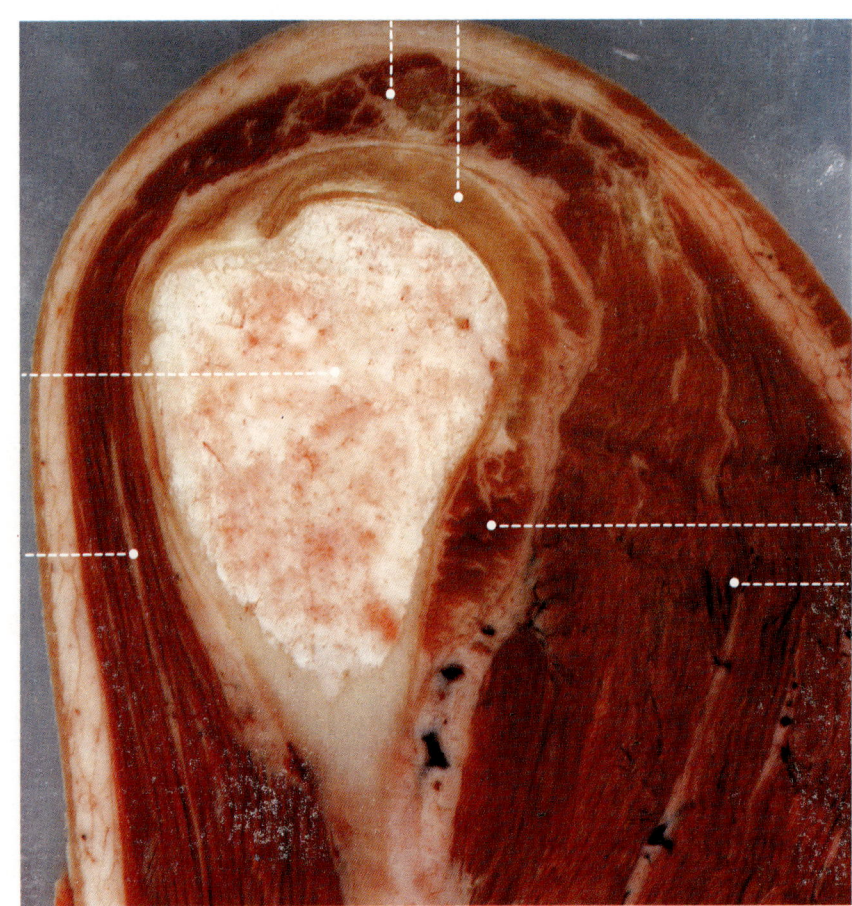

35 THE SHOULDER

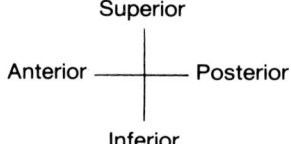

FIG. 2-20
SAGITTAL

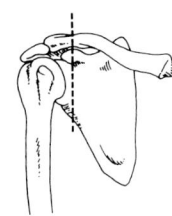

- Clavicle
- Trapezius
- Coracoclavicular ligament
- Deltoid (anterior)
- Coracoid process
- Brachial plexus
- Axillary artery
- Pectoralis major
- Pectoralis minor
- Axillary vein
- Subscapularis muscle
- Supraspinatus muscle
- Spine of scapula
- Suprascapular artery
- Infraspinatus muscle

Anatomy and MRI of the Joints

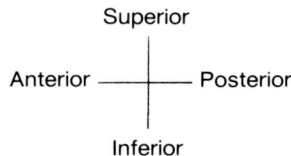

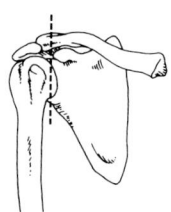

FIG. 2-21
SAGITTAL

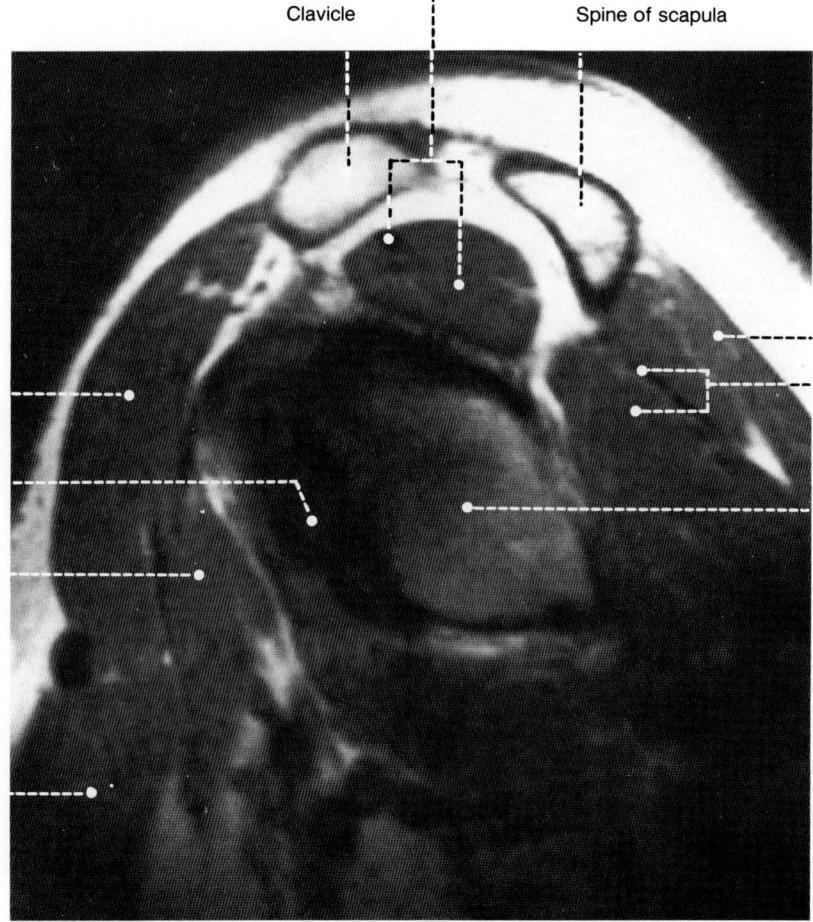

Superior

Anterior — Posterior

Inferior

FIG. 2–22

SAGITTAL

Supraspinatus tendon and muscle
Coracoacromial ligament
Acromion
Biceps tendon (long head)
Deltoid (anterior)
Subscapularis tendon
Infraspinatus tendon and muscle
Deltoid (posterior)
Humeral head
Teres minor

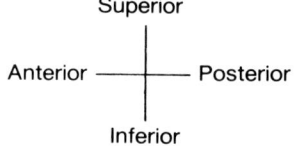

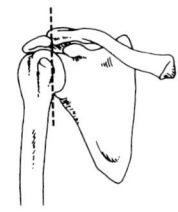

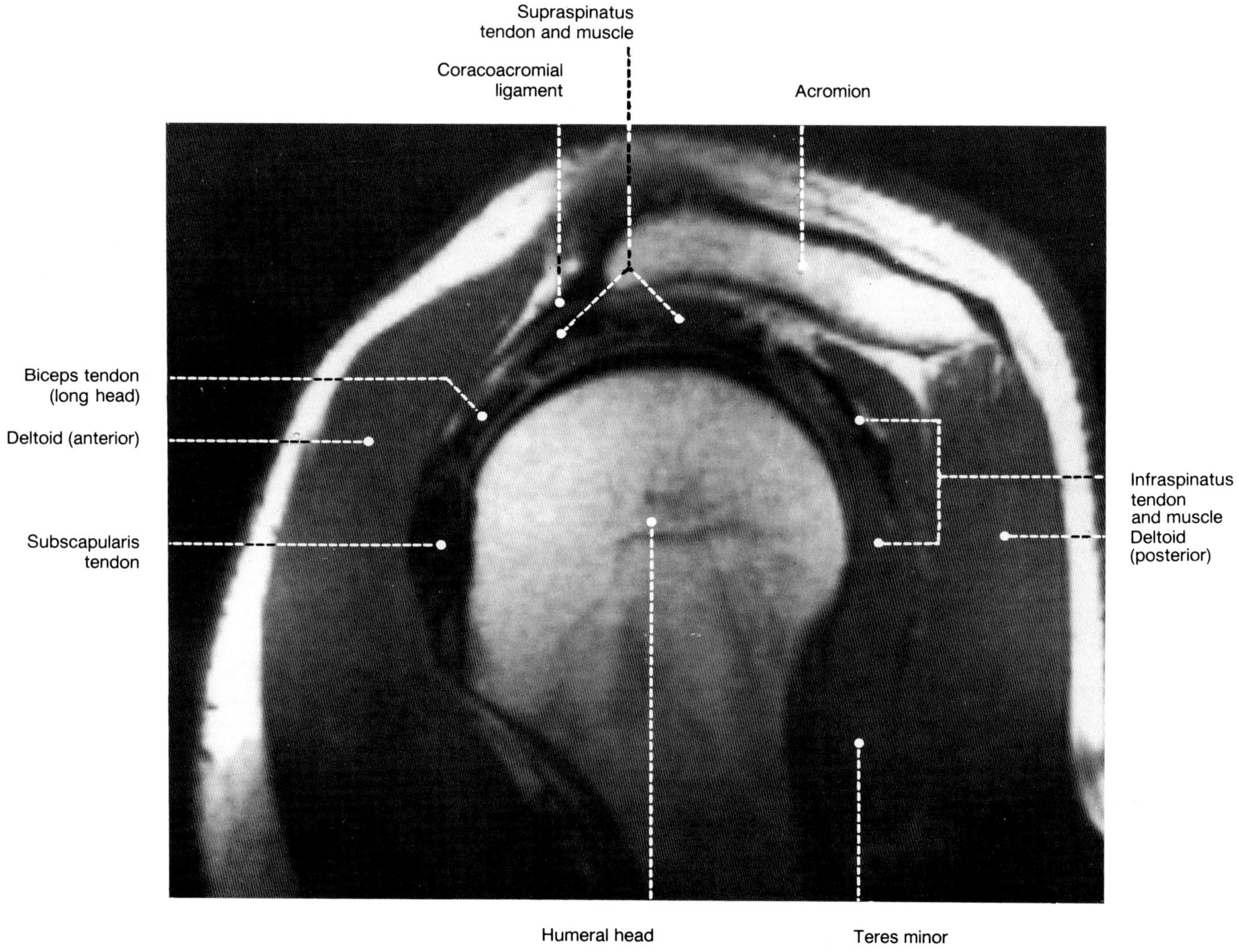

Anatomy and MRI of the Joints

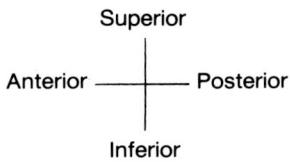

FIG. 2-23
SAGITTAL

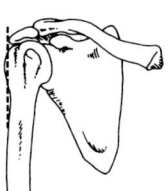

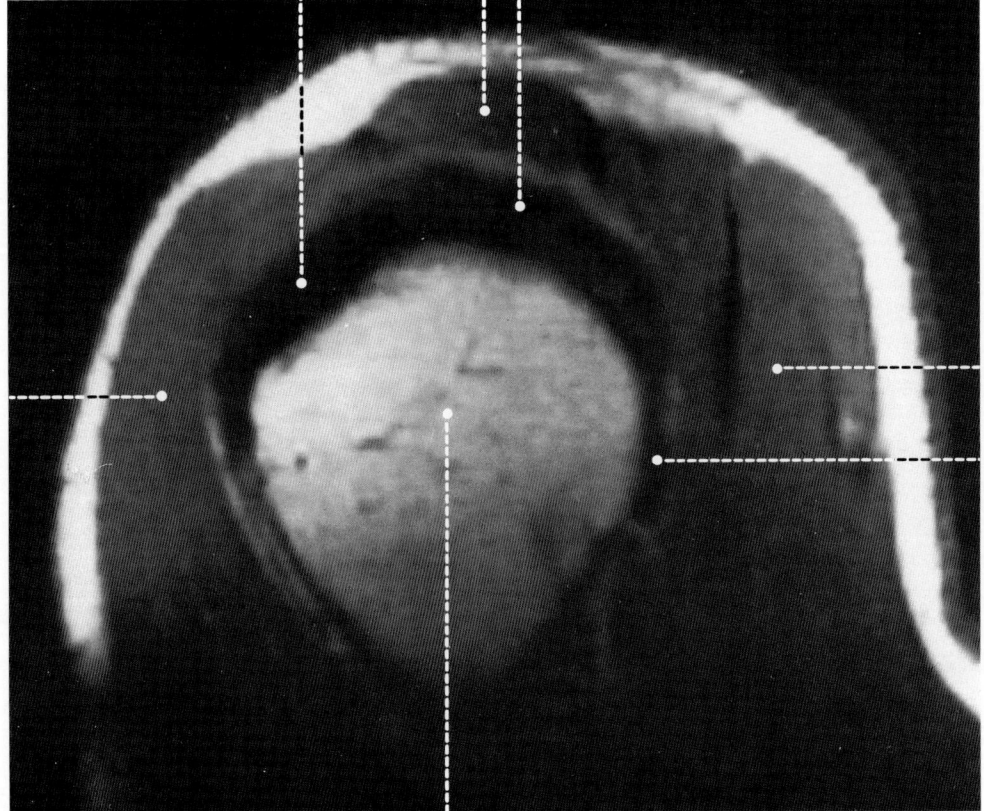

THE SHOULDER

FIG. 2-24

CORONAL

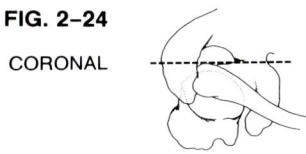

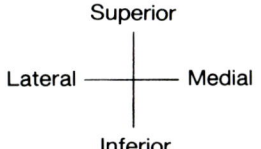

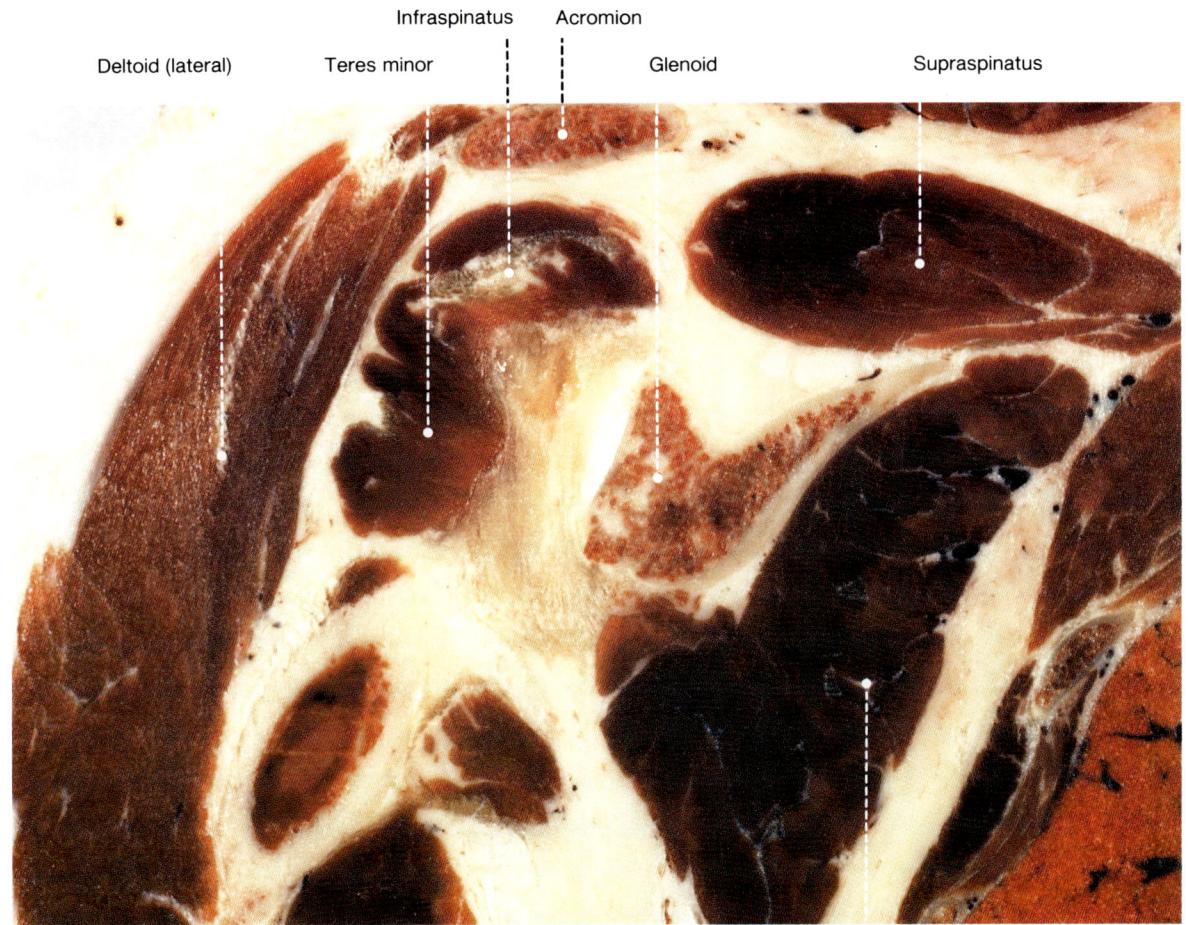

Anatomy and MRI of the Joints

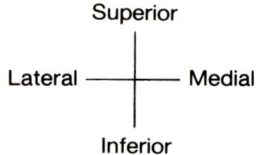

FIG. 2-25
CORONAL

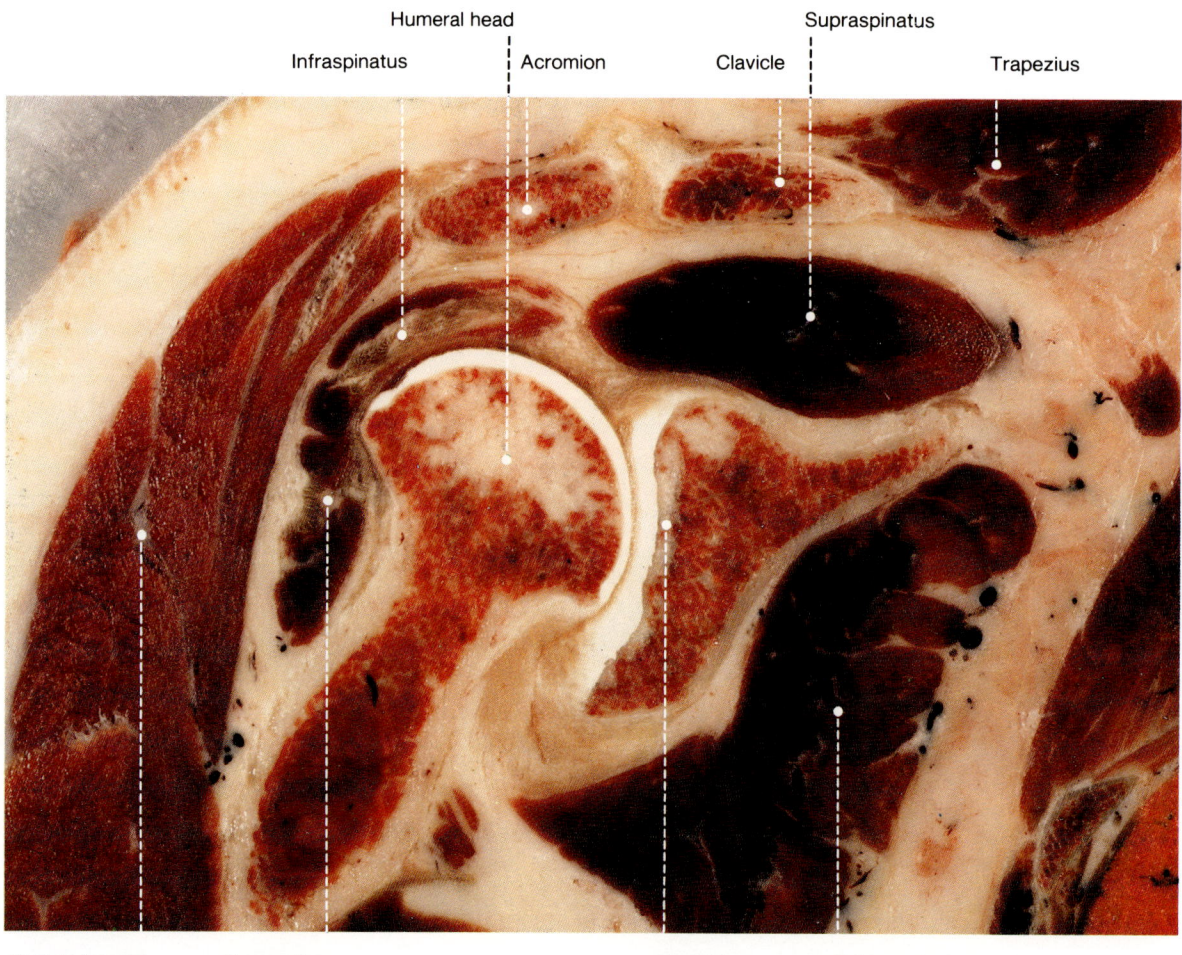

THE SHOULDER

FIG. 2-26
CORONAL

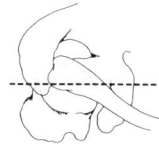

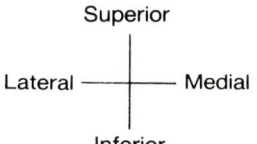

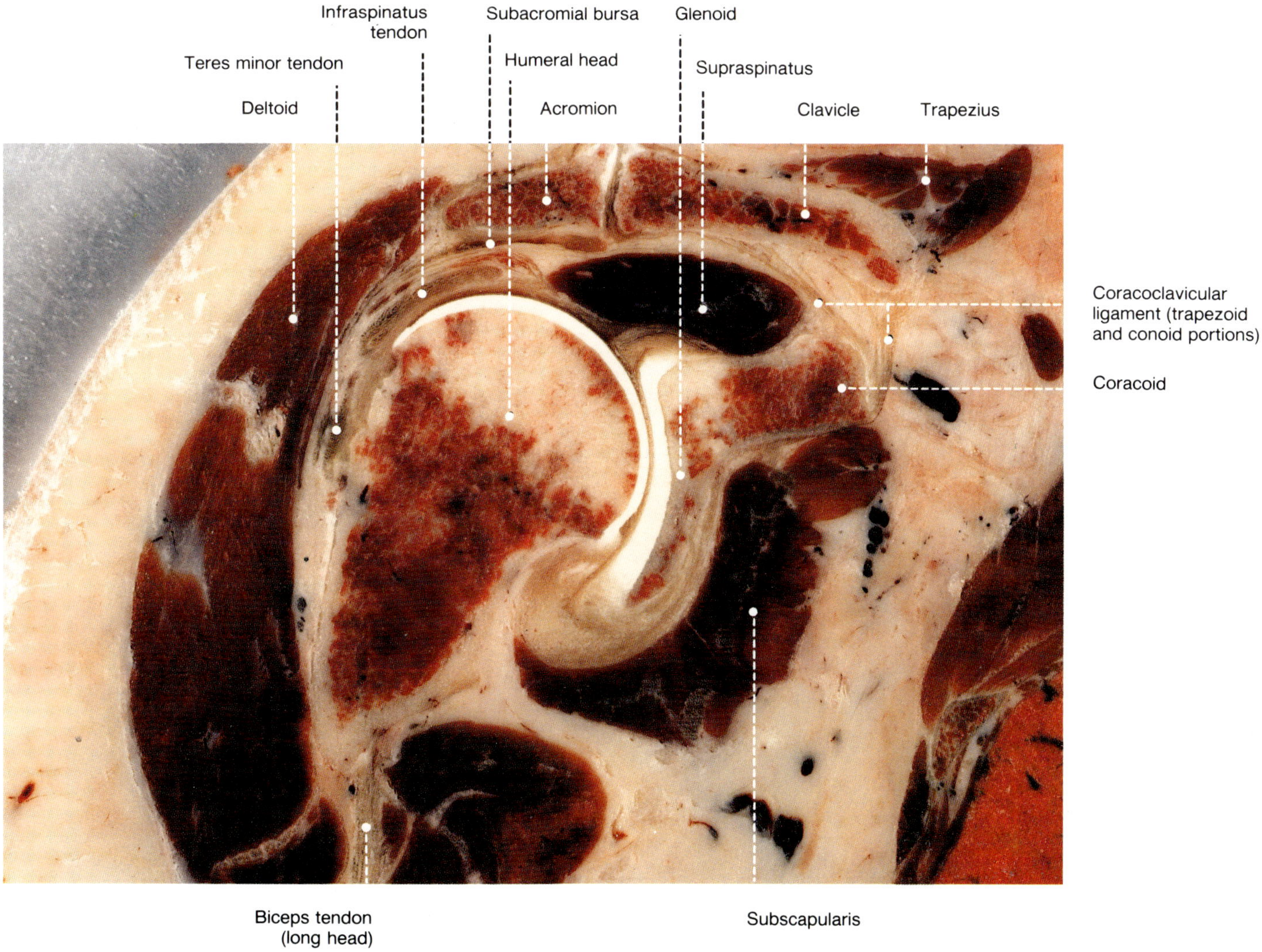

Superior — Inferior; Lateral — Medial

Labels: Teres minor tendon, Deltoid, Infraspinatus tendon, Subacromial bursa, Humeral head, Acromion, Glenoid, Supraspinatus, Clavicle, Trapezius, Coracoclavicular ligament (trapezoid and conoid portions), Coracoid, Biceps tendon (long head), Subscapularis

Anatomy and MRI of the Joints 42

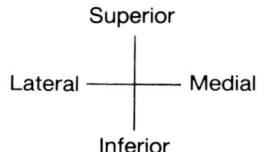

FIG. 2–27

CORONAL

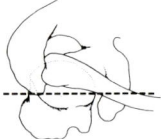

Teres minor tendon — Infraspinatus tendon — Humeral head — Coracoacromial ligament — Acromion — Suprapinatus muscle and tendon — Biceps tendon (long head) — Coracoid process — Clavicle — Subclavius muscle — Brachial plexus

Deltoid (lateral)

Biceps tendon (long head) — Subscapularis tendon — Axillary artery and vein

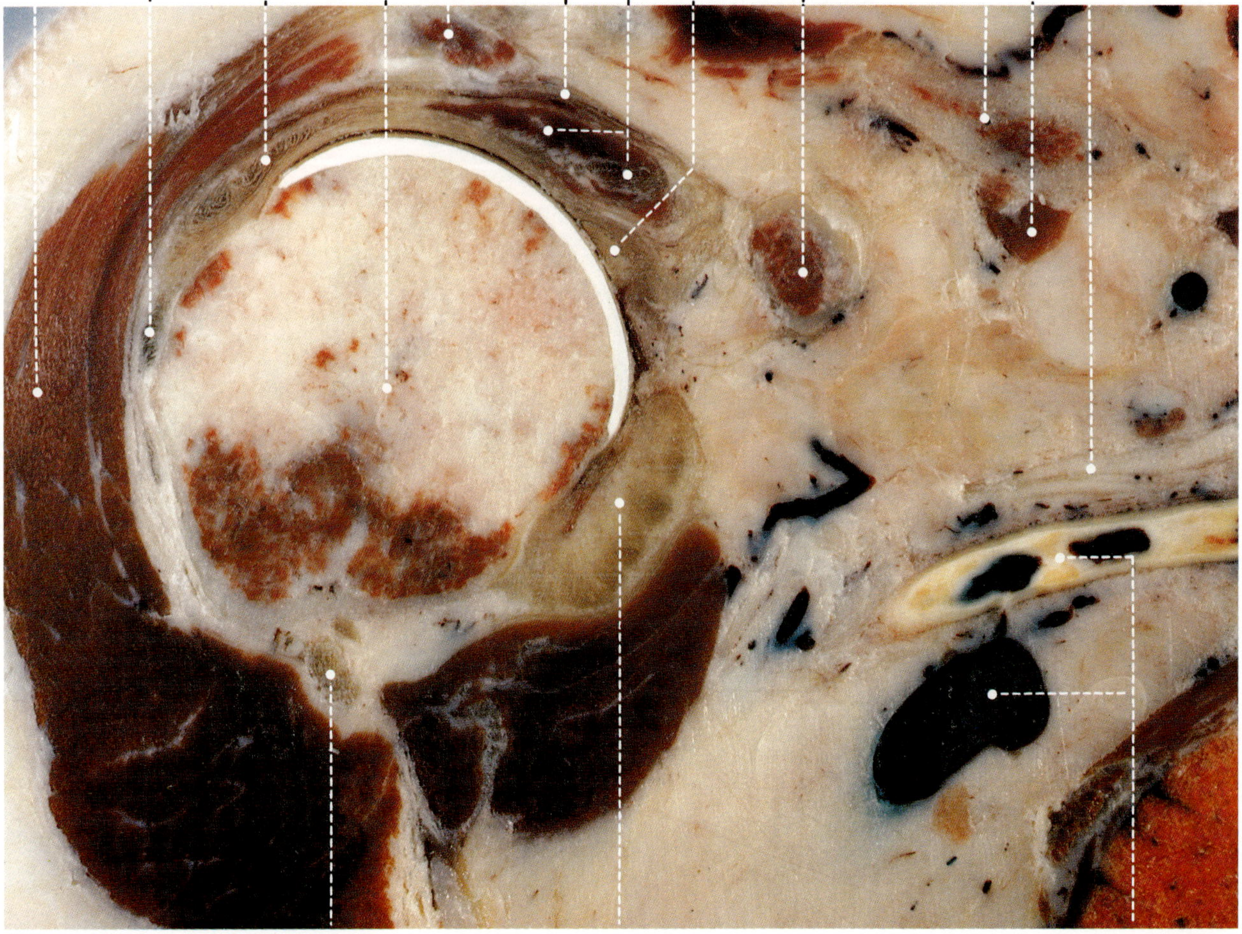

Superior

Lateral — Medial

Inferior

FIG. 2–28

CORONAL

Biceps tendon (long head)
Infraspinatus tendon
Supraspinatus tendon
Coracohumeral ligament
Subclavius muscle
Deltoid (lateral)
Humeral head
Coracoid
Clavicle
Biceps tendon (long head)
Subscapularis tendon
Subclavian vein
Deltoid (anterior)

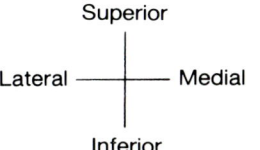

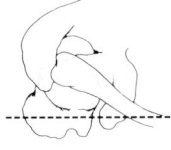

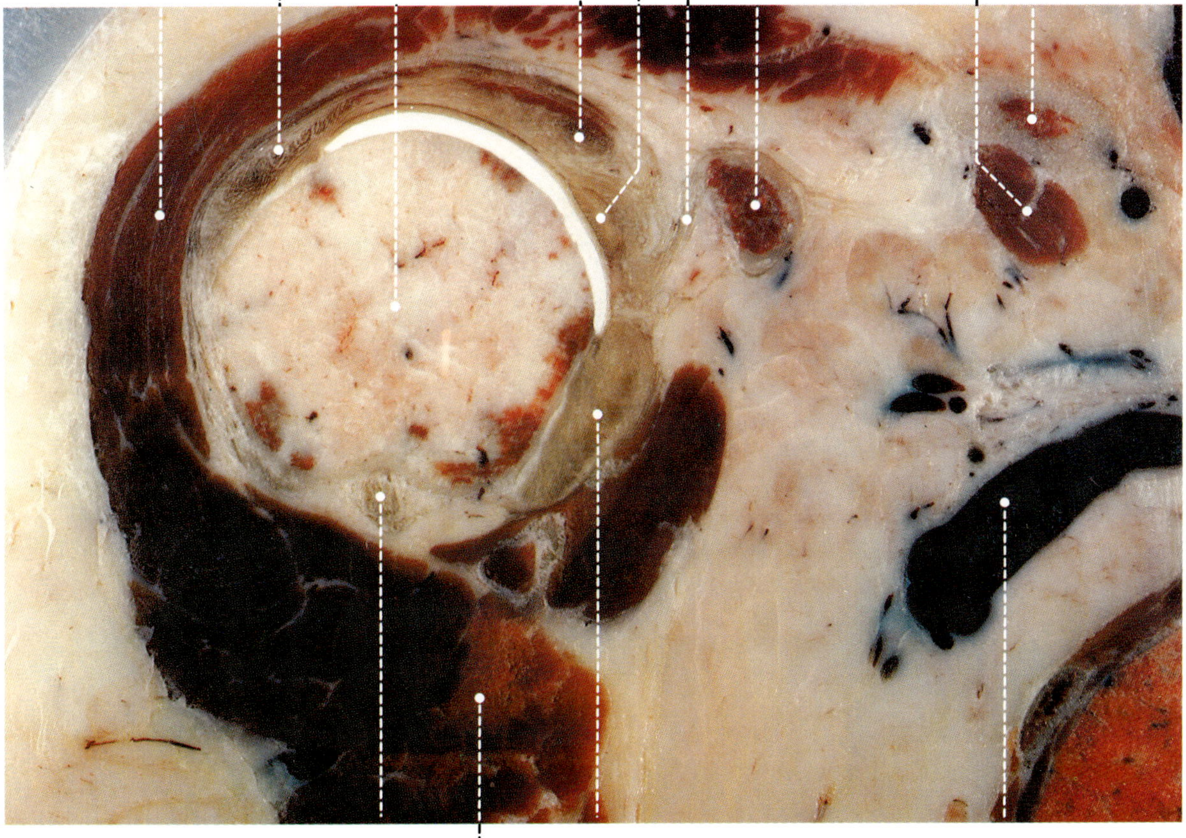

Anatomy and MRI of the Joints

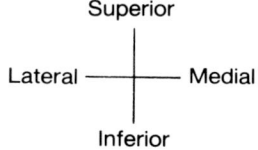

FIG. 2-29
CORONAL
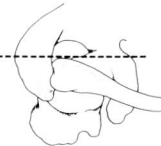

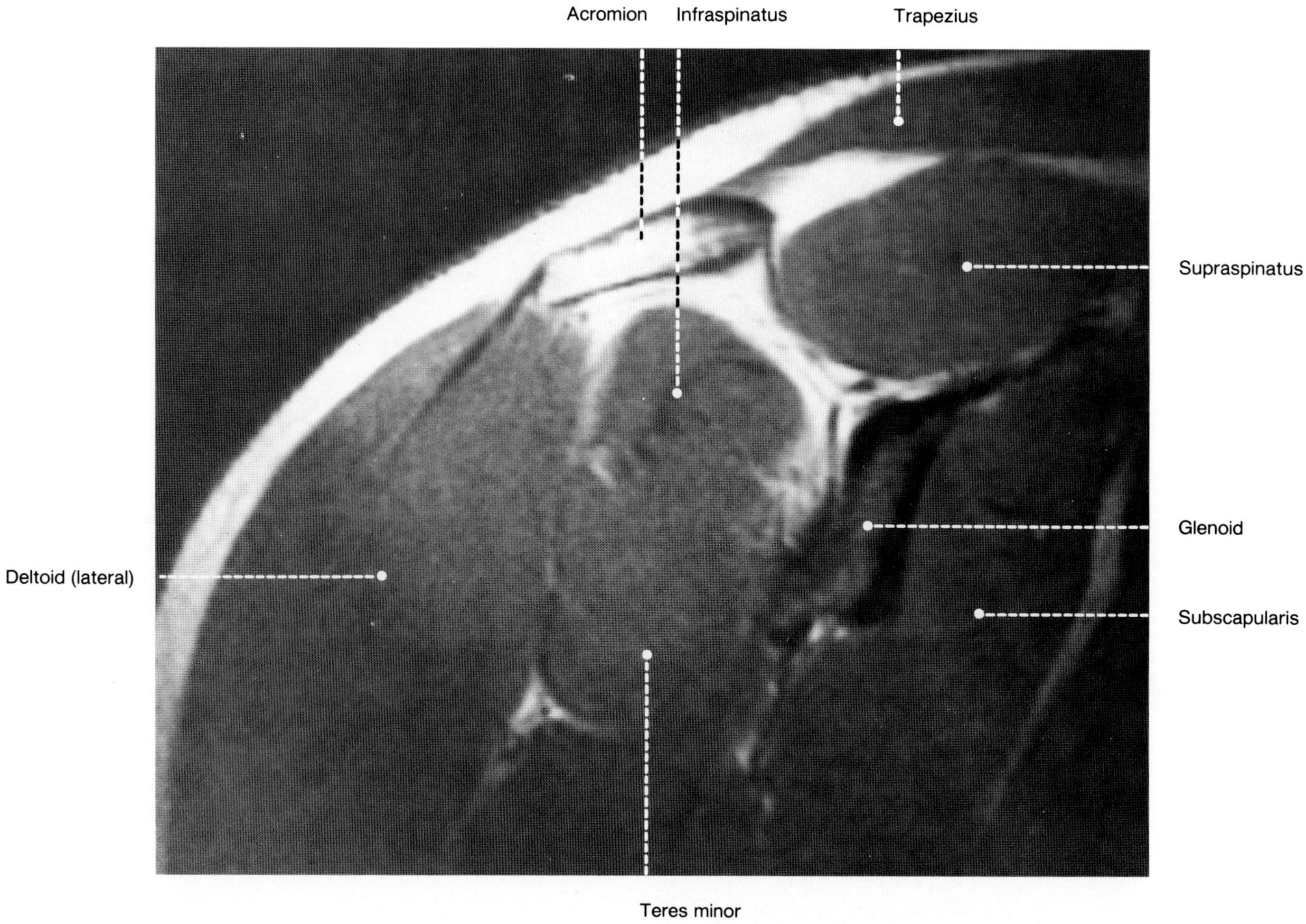

Acromion — Infraspinatus — Trapezius — Supraspinatus — Glenoid — Subscapularis — Deltoid (lateral) — Teres minor

THE SHOULDER

FIG. 2-30

CORONAL

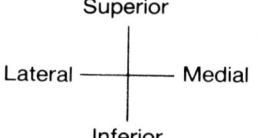

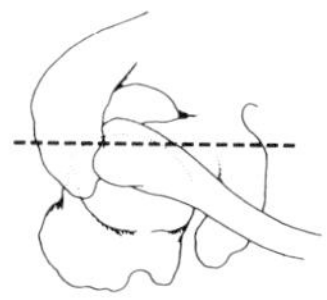

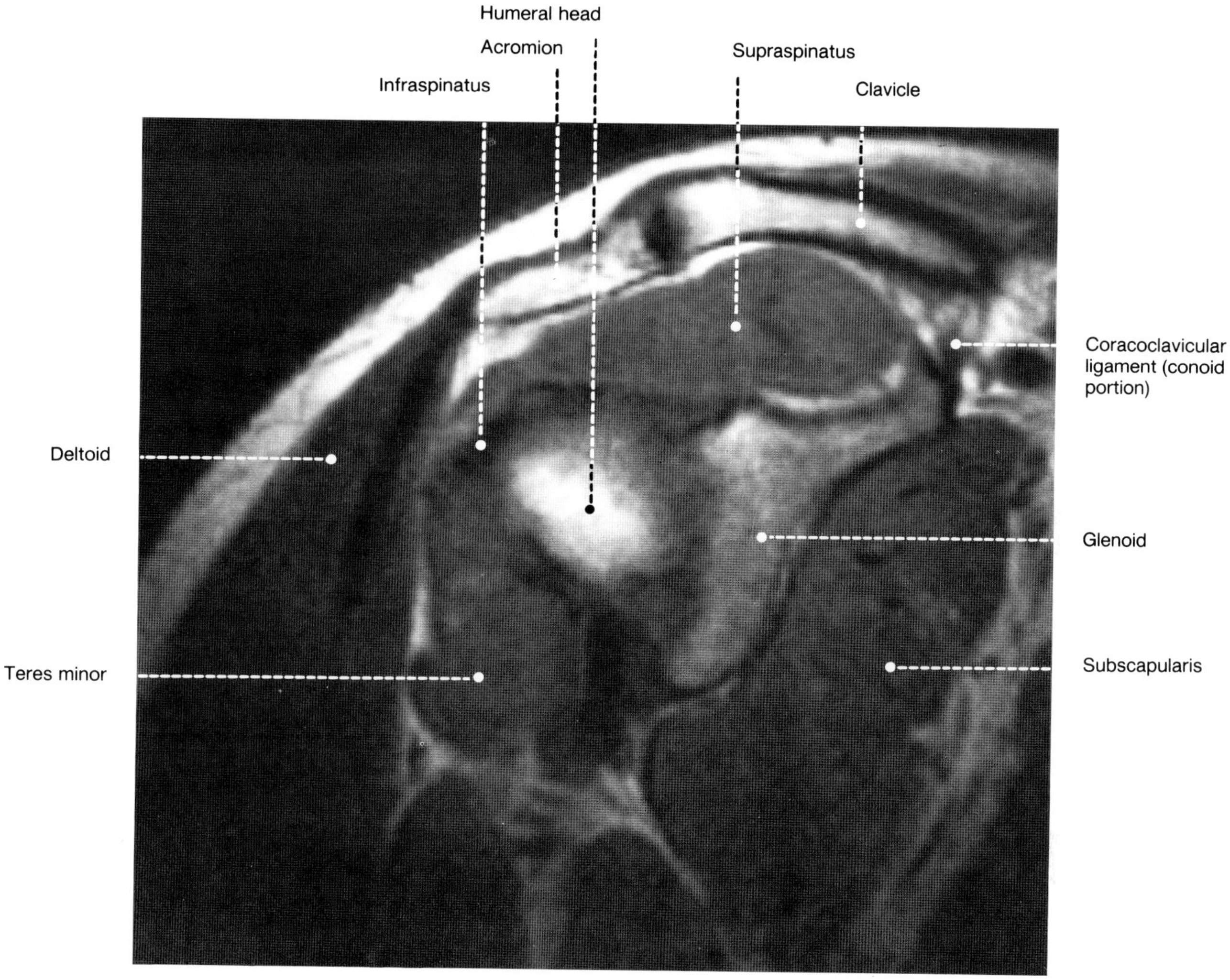

Superior — Lateral — Medial — Inferior

- Infraspinatus
- Acromion
- Humeral head
- Supraspinatus
- Clavicle
- Deltoid
- Teres minor
- Coracoclavicular ligament (conoid portion)
- Glenoid
- Subscapularis

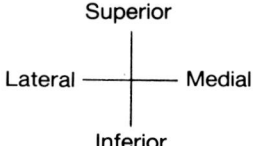

FIG. 2-31
CORONAL

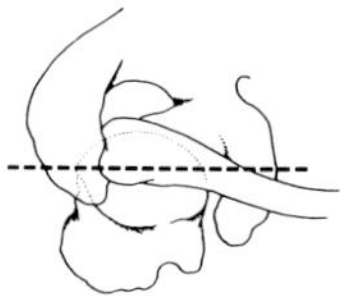

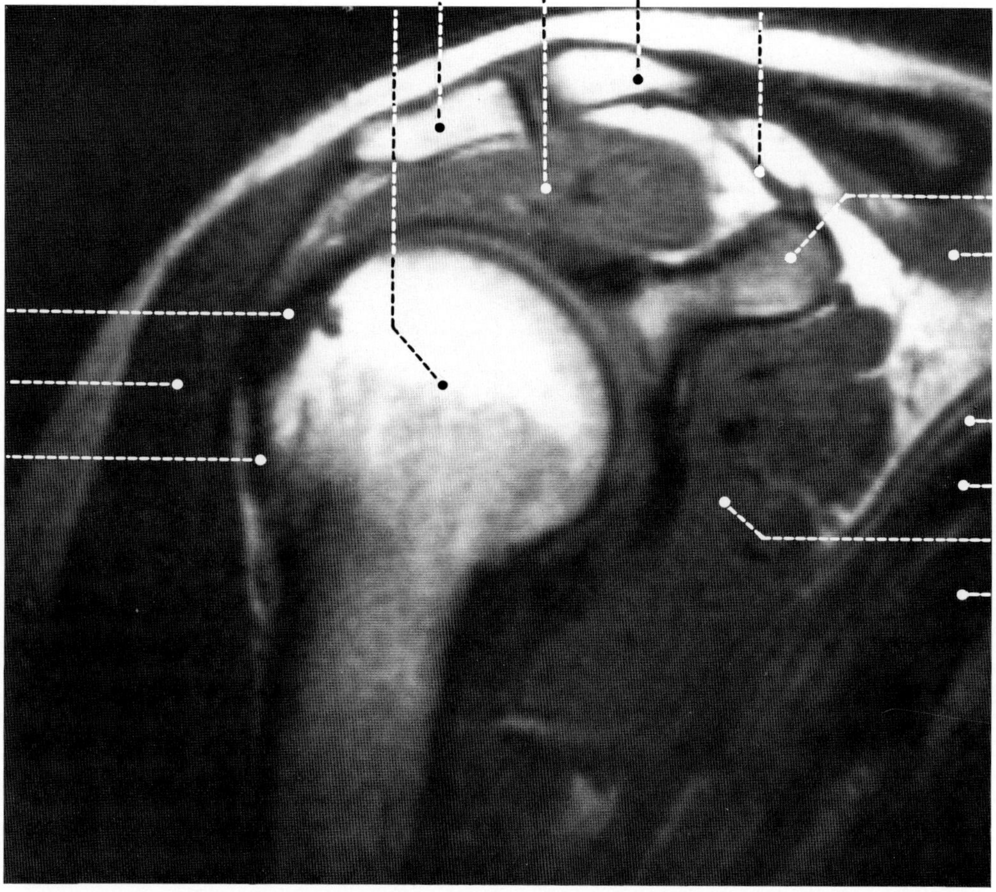

THE SHOULDER

FIG. 2-32

CORONAL

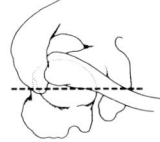

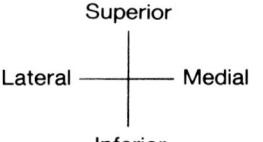

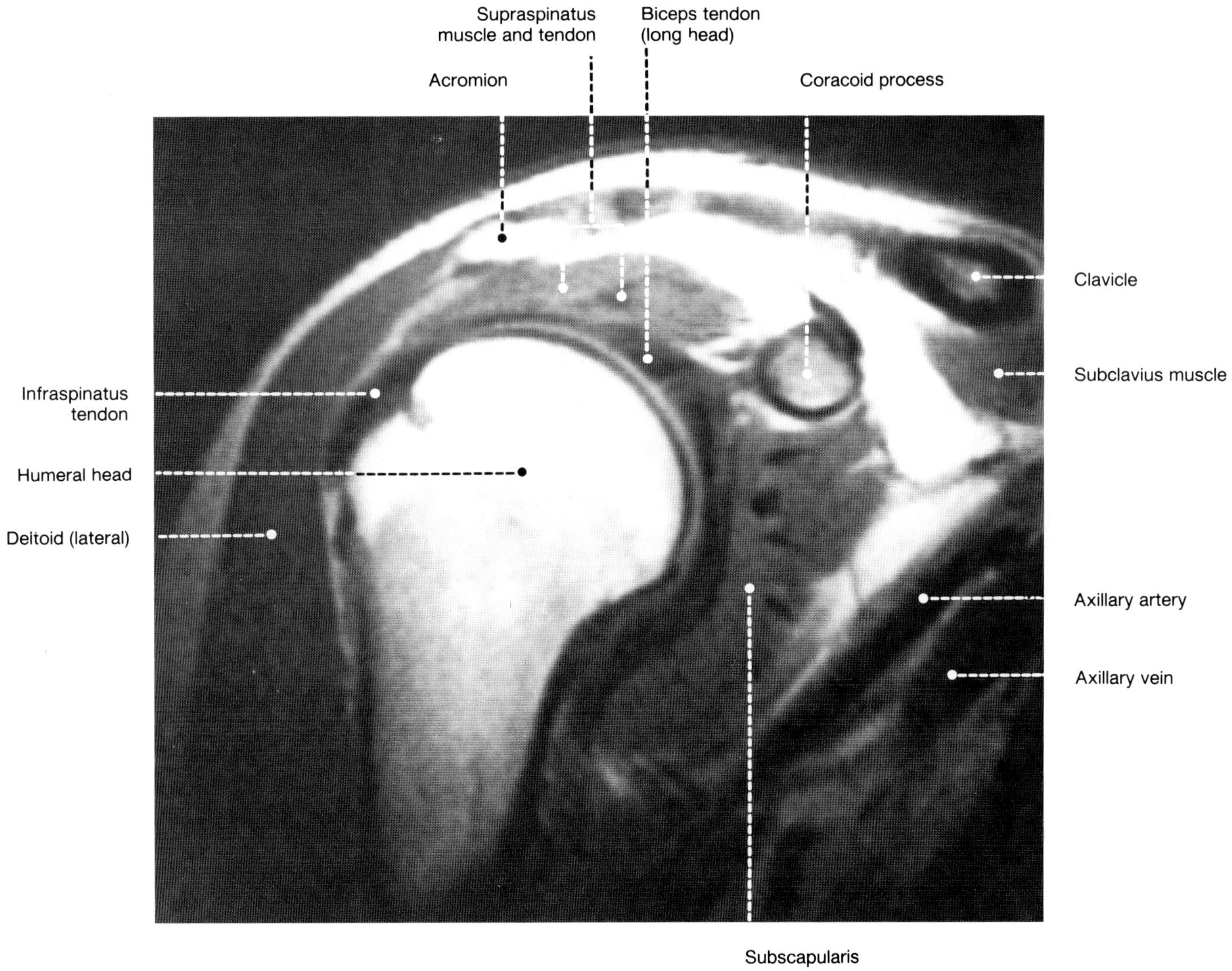

Anatomy and MRI of the Joints

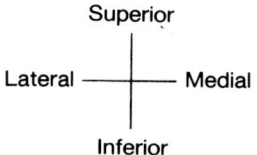

FIG. 2-33
CORONAL

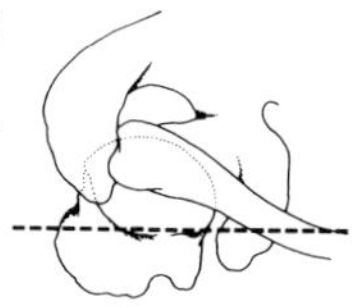

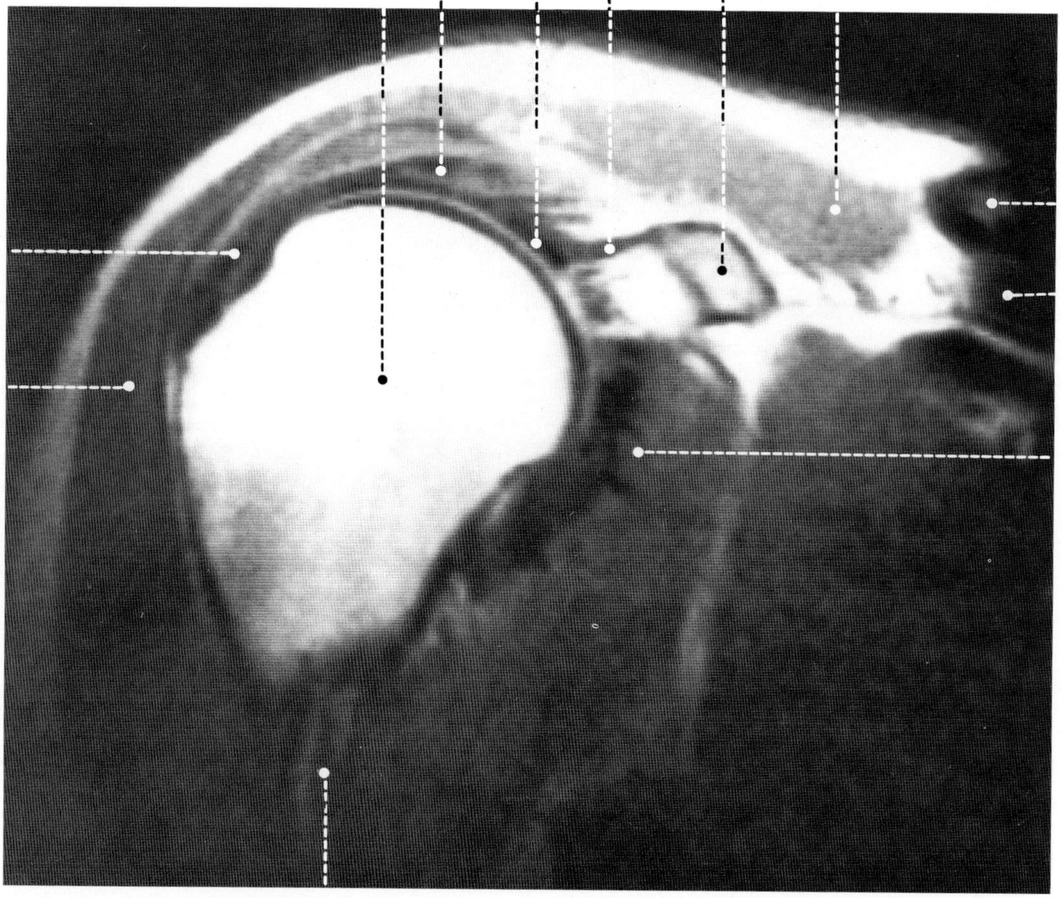

CHAPTER 3

THE ELBOW

Stephan J. Macrander, M.D.

The elbow is a hinged joint joining the distal humerus to the proximal radius and ulna. Intimately associated with the elbow joint proper is the superior radial ulnar joint. These two joints share a common joint capsule and both will be discussed in this chapter. In addition, all of the supporting ligaments, musculotendinous structures, and neurovascular structures will be described and illustrated.

Bones and articulations (Figs. 3-1 and 3-2):
The distal articular surface of the humerus is contoured into two components to accommodate the proximal ulna and radial head. The medial surface articulating with the ulna is the trochlea, which is shaped similar to an hourglass laid on its side. The lateral surface is the capitellum that articulates with the fovea of the radial head. The capitellum has a rounded convex surface.

Important non-articulating processes of the distal humerus are the medial and lateral epicondyles. The medial epicondyle is the most prominent of the two. It provides the surface of origin for the pronator teres and common tendon of origin for the flexor muscles of the forearm. The lateral epicondyle affords the surface of attachment for the supinator and the common tendon of origin for the forearm extensor muscles.

The olecranon fossa is a prominent concavity on the posterior surface of the distal humerus, just proximal to the trochlea. It accommodates the olecranon process when the elbow is extended. The coronoid fossa is a similar, but shallower depression located anteriorly that accommodates the coronoid process of the ulna during elbow flexion. A small radial fossa is also present above the capitellum.

The articular surface of the proximal ulna is composed of trochlear and radial notches. The trochlear notch is a rounded concavity situated between the olecranon and coronoid process. The radial notch is a concavity articulating with the radial head.

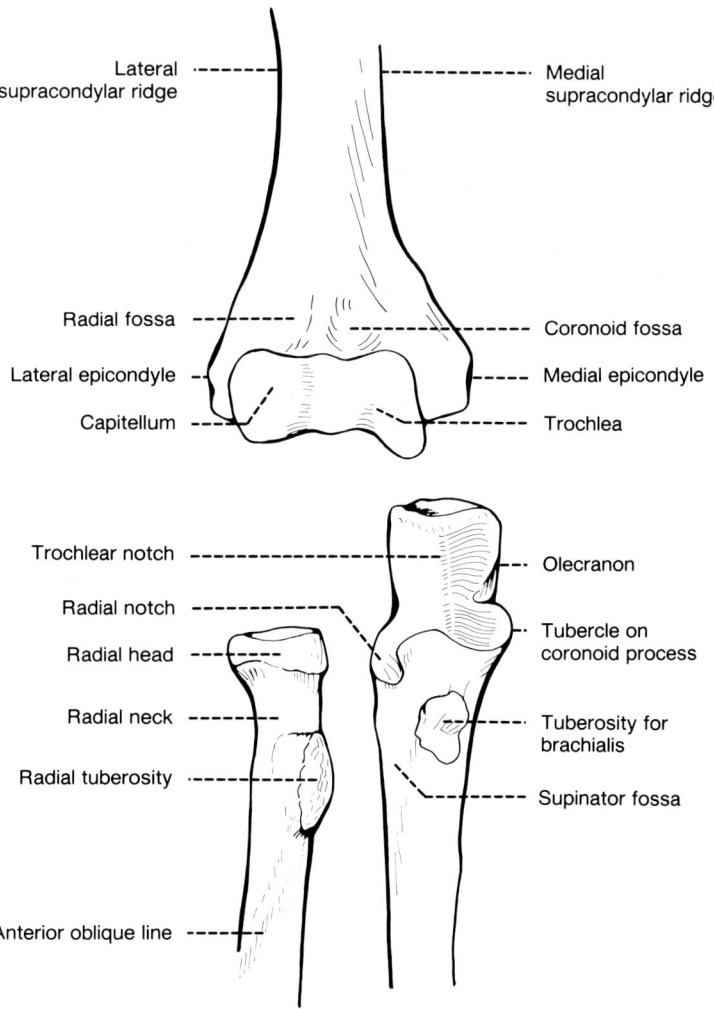

FIG. 3-1

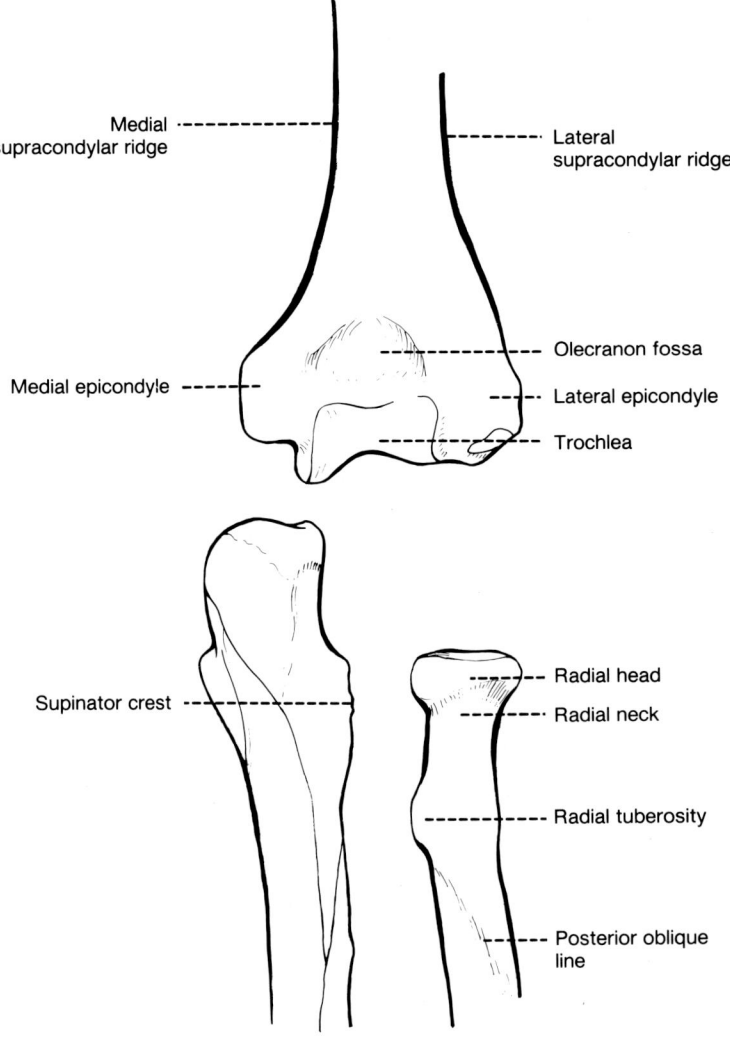

FIG. 3-2

The radial head is the round pill-shaped portion of the proximal radius. It has a proximal concave surface called the fovea that articulates with the capitellum and a circumferential portion that articulates with the radial notch.

Ligaments (Figs. 3-3 and 3-4): The entire joint is surrounded by a loose articular capsule allowing for flexion and extension. Medial and lateral thickening of this capsule represent the collateral ligaments. The ulnar collateral ligament originates from the medial epicondyle and fans out to attach to the medial aspect of the trochlear notch. The anterior and oblique portions are thicker than the intermediate posterior fanlike portion.

The radial collateral ligament is triangular shaped with the apex arising from the lateral epicondyle and the base attaching to the annular ligament.

The annular ligament surrounds the circumference of the radial head and secures it in the radial notch. The ligament is attached to the anterior and posterior aspect of the radial notch.

Muscles and tendons (Figs. 3-5 and 3-6): A large number of muscles and tendons originate and insert at the elbow. This makes the cross-sectional anatomy of the muscles and tendons of the elbow rather confusing. Understanding the spatial relations of the musculotendinous structures is best accomplished by dividing them into posterior, anterior, lateral, and medial groups. These groups are best identified on axial images.

The lateral muscle group includes the brachioradialis, the extensors of the fingers and wrist, and the supinator.

The most superficial and anterior muscle of this group is the brachioradialis. It originates from the lateral supracondylar ridge of the distal humerus and extends to insert on the lateral aspect of the radial styloid. Just posterior and deep to the brachioradialis is the extensor carpi radialis longus. The extensor carpi radialis longus originates from the supracondylar ridge inferior to the brachioradialis and inserts on the base of the second metacarpal. The extensor carpi radialis brevis, extensor digitorum, ex-

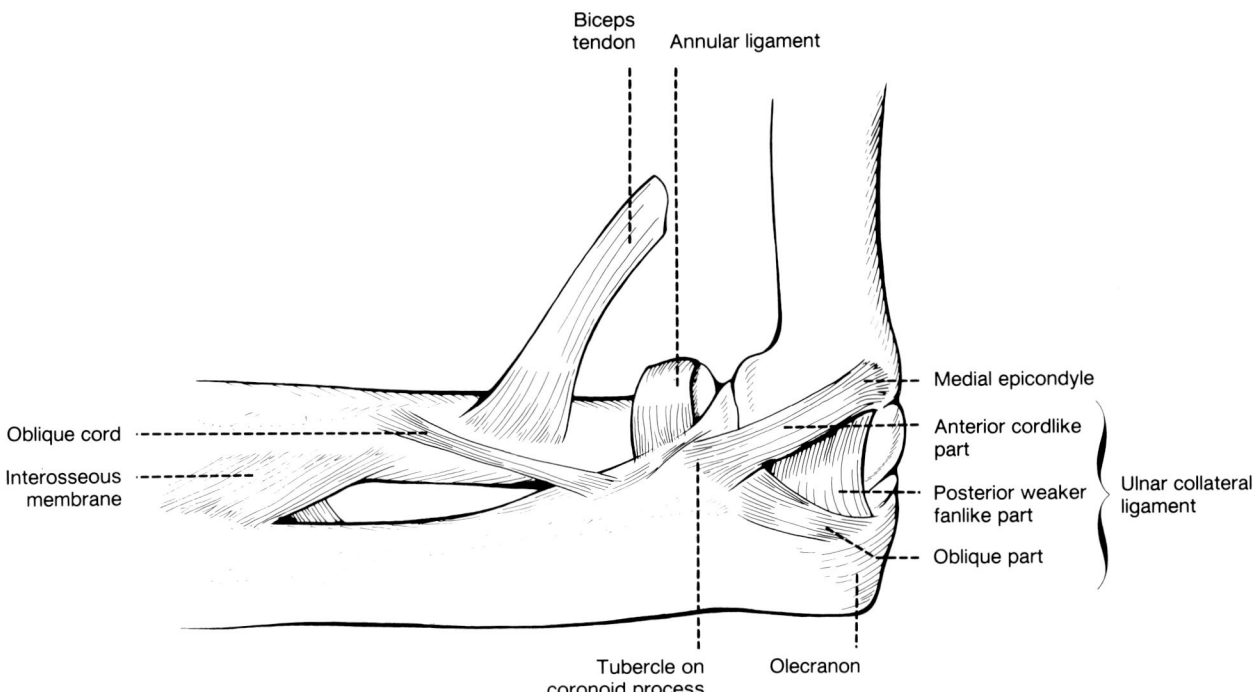

FIG. 3-3

tensor carpi ulnaris, and extensor digiti minimi all arise from a common extensor tendon originating on the lateral epicondyle. Because of their common origin, these latter four muscles are difficult to separate from each other in the region of the elbow. They become progressively more distinct distally.

The supinator is the deepest of the lateral muscle group. It arises primarily from the posterolateral aspect of the ulna. However, portions of the muscle arise from the lateral epicondyle. It runs inferiorly and laterally to insert on the lateral aspect of the proximal radius. With the arm pronated, the supinator completely surrounds the radius.

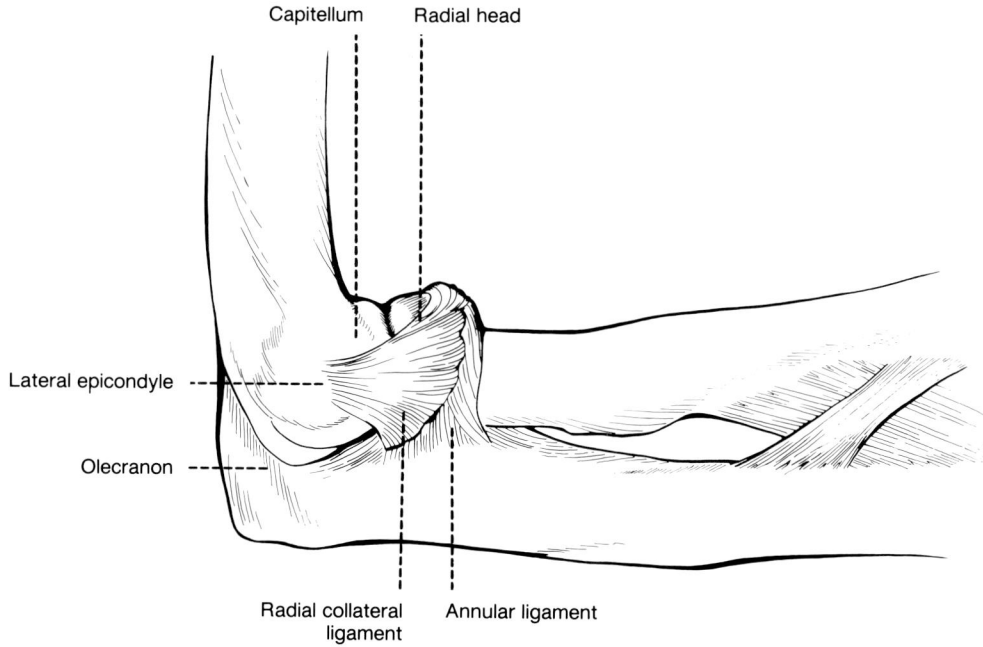

FIG. 3-4

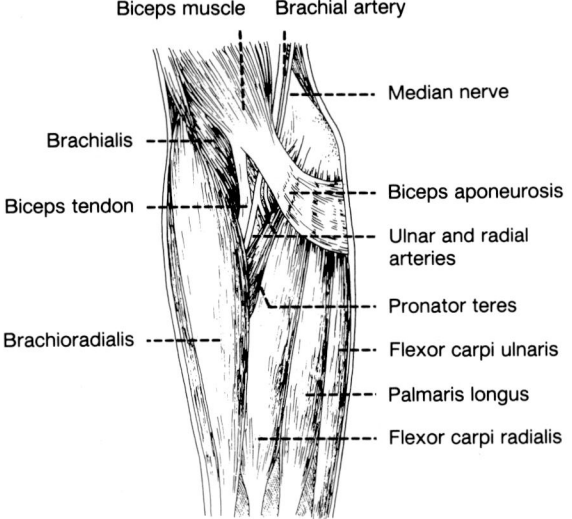

FIG. 3-5

The medial muscle group includes the pronator teres, the flexors of the fingers and wrist, and the palmaris longus. These muscles are arranged in an arc along the anterior and medial aspect of the elbow. The pronator teres is the most anterior and lateral of the group. It has a superficial and deep portion arising respectively from the distal humerus just proximal to the medial epicondyle and from the proximal ulna just medial to the ulnar tuberosity. The median nerve runs between the smaller deep portion and the larger superficial portion of the pronator teres. The other muscles of the medial group arise as a group from a common flexor tendon originating on the medial epicondyle. They are arranged from anterior to posterior as the flexor carpi radialis, palmaris longus, flexor digitorum superficialis, flexor carpi ulnaris, and flexor digitorum profundus. These muscles become progressively more distinct distally. The flexor carpi ulnaris also has a head originating from the proximal ulna and the flexor digitorum superficialis has a second and third head originating from the proximal ulna and the proximal to mid radius.

The anterior muscle group consists of the brachialis and biceps. The brachialis originates from the anterior surface of the distal humerus and crosses the elbow joint to insert on the ulnar tuberosity. The brachialis remains muscular with its central tendon embedded within the muscle belly as it inserts on the tuberosity.

The biceps muscle originates as two heads, but before reaching the elbow, these separate muscle bellies converge and become tendinous in the region of the elbow. The biceps tendon travels along the superficial surface of the brachialis, and inserts onto the radial tuberosity.

A prominent fascial band known as the biceps aponeurosis runs obliquely from the distal biceps tendon to the superficial surface of the pronator teres. The brachial artery, vein, and median nerve run under the biceps aponeurosis in a fibromuscular tunnel also bordered by the biceps tendon, the brachialis muscle, and the pronator teres muscle.

The posterior muscle group includes the triceps and anconeus muscles. The triceps muscle originates as three muscle bellies. These muscle bellies converge in the region of the elbow and fuse into a single musculotendinous unit. The central tendon of the triceps inserts onto the posterior and superior surface of the olecranon process. The anconeus is a small triangular shaped muscle which originates from the posterior aspect of the lateral epicondyle and crosses the elbow joint to insert on the posterior lateral aspect of the olecranon. It is felt by some to represent a detached portion of the triceps muscle.

Neurovascular structures: The brachial artery represents the only major arterial vessel in the region of the elbow. It runs along the superficial aspect of the brachialis muscle medial to the biceps muscle and tendon. In the region of the elbow it divides into the radial and ulnar arteries. The ulnar artery runs deep to the pronator teres whereas the radial artery runs between the brachioradialis and pronator teres. Recurrent branches arise from both the radial and ulnar arteries and travel superiorly adjacent to the radial and ulnar nerves. The brachial artery and its branches have corresponding venae comitantes which run adjacent to the arteries. The superficial veins include the medial basilic vein and the anterolateral cephalic vein.

Three major nerves are present in the region of the elbow. The radial nerve runs between the brachialis and brachioradialis. It divides into a deep and superficial branch at the elbow. These branches of the radial nerve can be distinguished from the recurrent radial artery be-

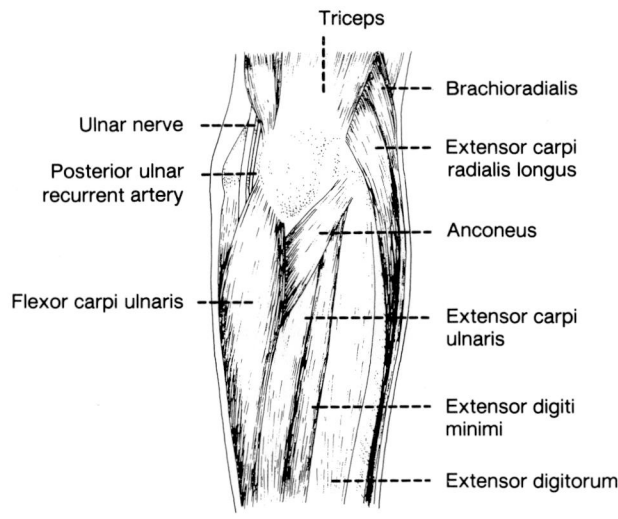

FIG. 3-6

cause they are more superficial in position. Identification of the nerves as well as the recurrent radial artery depends on the amount of fat separating these structures from the adjacent muscles. The ulnar nerve is identified just posterior to the medial epicondyle. On more distal sections, the ulnar nerve becomes difficult to identify as it runs in a triangular region formed between the flexor digitorum superficialis, the flexor digitorum profundis, and the flexor carpi ulnaris.

The median nerve runs medial to the brachial artery along the superficial surface of the brachialis muscle and goes on to pierce the pronator teres muscle between the superficial and deep heads. As with the other nerves, visualization depends on the amount of adjacent fat. Because of this, the median nerve is best identified on proximal sections. Distally as the nerve becomes surrounded by the brachioradialis and pronator teres muscles, it becomes progressively more difficult to identify.

THE ELBOW

AXIAL
    Cryomicrotomes..........................FIGS. 3–7 to 3–11
    MR Images..............................FIGS. 3–12 to 3–16

SAGITTAL
    Cryomicrotomes..........................FIGS. 3–17 to 3–20
    MR Images..............................FIGS. 3–21 to 3–24

CORONAL
    Cryomicrotomes..........................FIGS. 3–25 to 3–28
    MR Images..............................FIGS. 3–29 to 3–32

Anatomy and MRI of the Joints

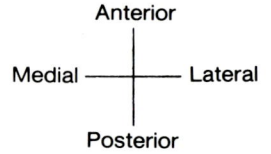

FIG. 3-7
AXIAL
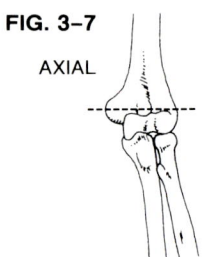

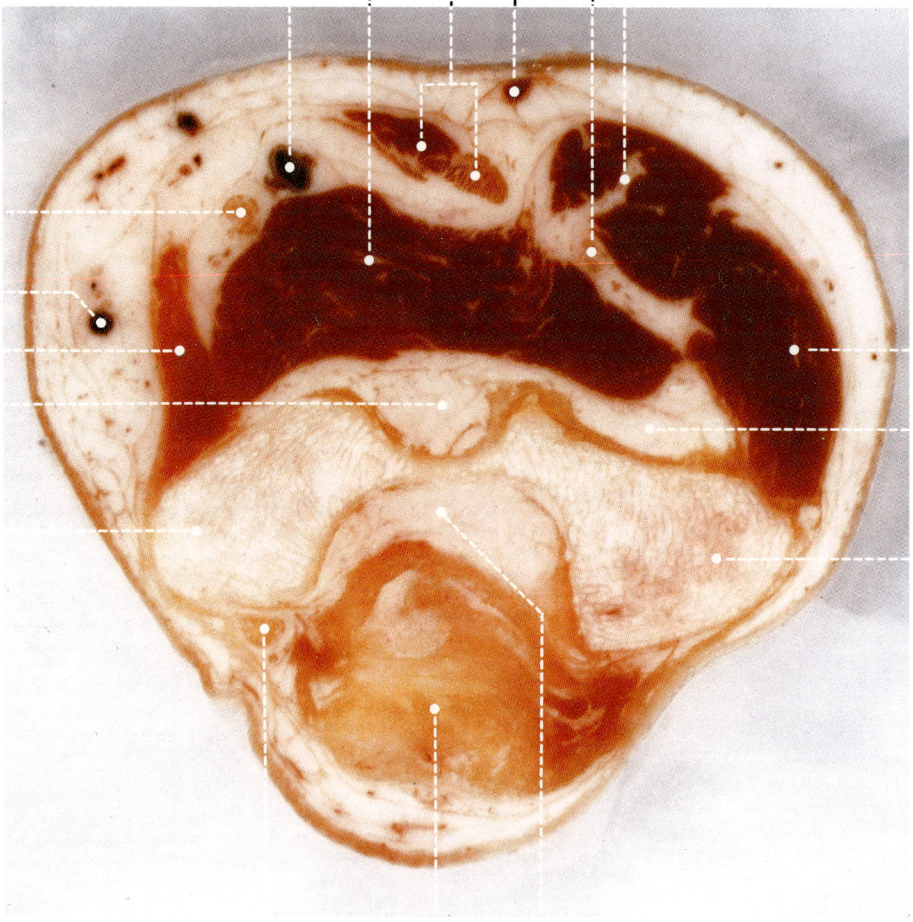

- Biceps muscle and tendon
- Brachialis
- Brachial artery
- Cephalic vein
- Radial nerve
- Brachioradialis
- Median nerve
- Basilic vein
- Pronator teres
- Coronoid fossa
- Medial epicondyle
- Extensor carpi radialis longus
- Radial fossa
- Lateral epicondyle
- Ulnar nerve
- Triceps tendon
- Olecranon fossa

THE ELBOW

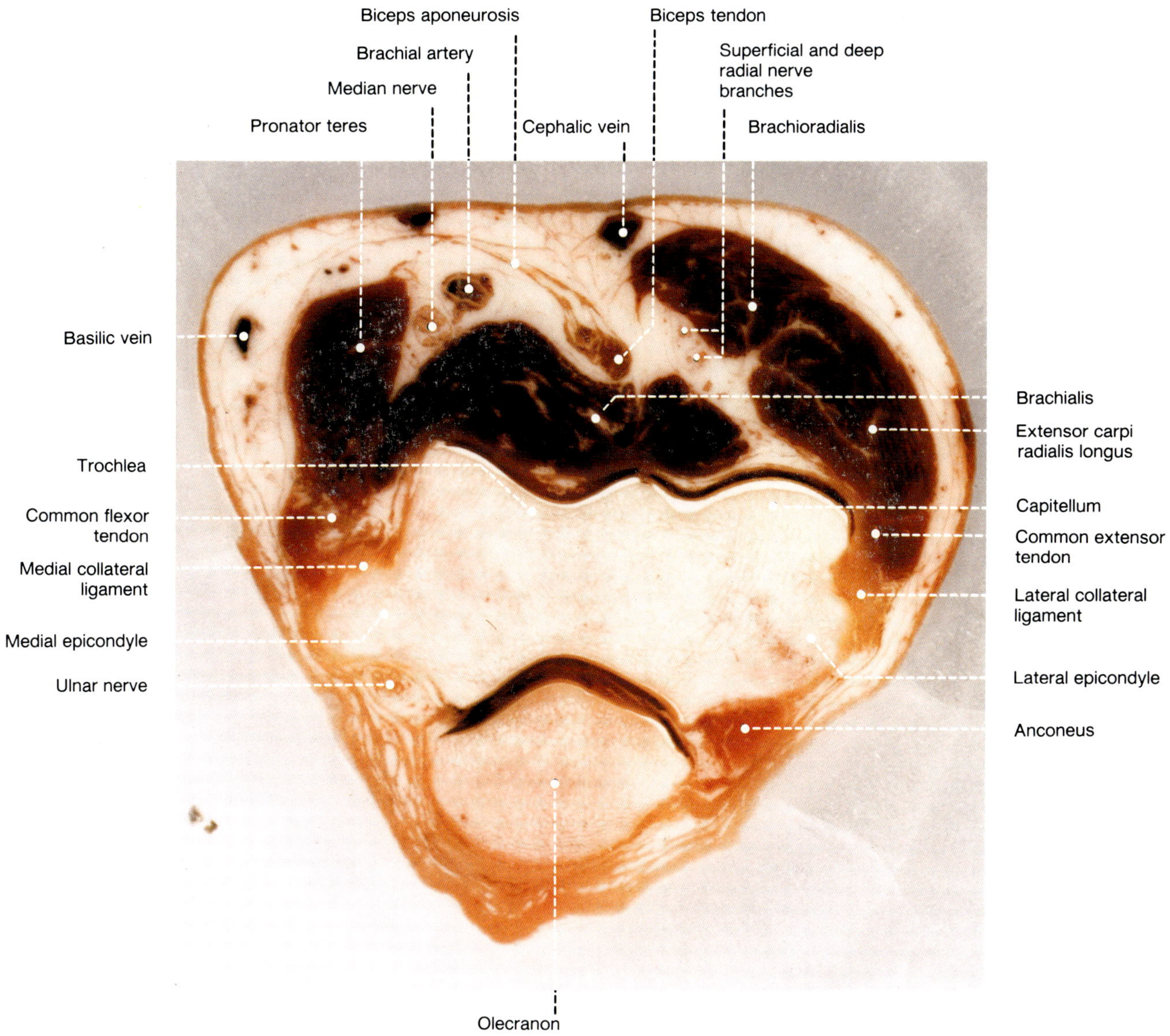

FIG. 3-8
AXIAL

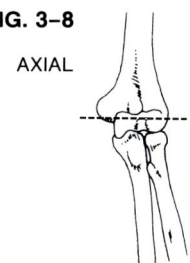

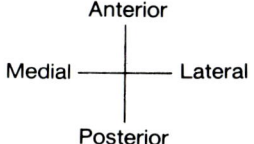

FIG. 3-8 AXIAL

Anatomy and MRI of the Joints 58

Anterior
Medial ─┼─ Lateral
Posterior

FIG. 3-9
AXIAL

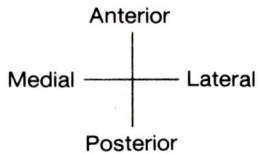

Labels (clockwise from top):
- Median nerve
- Brachial artery
- Biceps tendon
- Superficial and deep radial nerve branches
- Brachioradialis
- Radial recurrent artery
- Extensor carpi radialis longus and brevis
- Supinator
- Extensor digitorum
- Annular ligament
- Common extensor tendon
- Radial head
- Radial notch
- Anconeus
- Flexor digitorum profundus
- Flexor carpi ulnaris
- Ulnar recurrent artery
- Ulnar nerve
- Flexor digitorum superficialis
- Brachialis
- Flexor carpi radialis
- Pronator teres

THE ELBOW

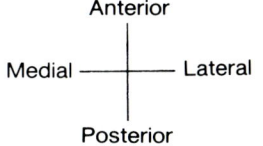

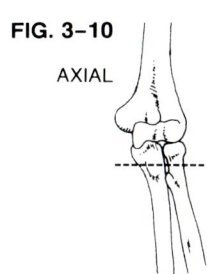

FIG. 3-10
AXIAL

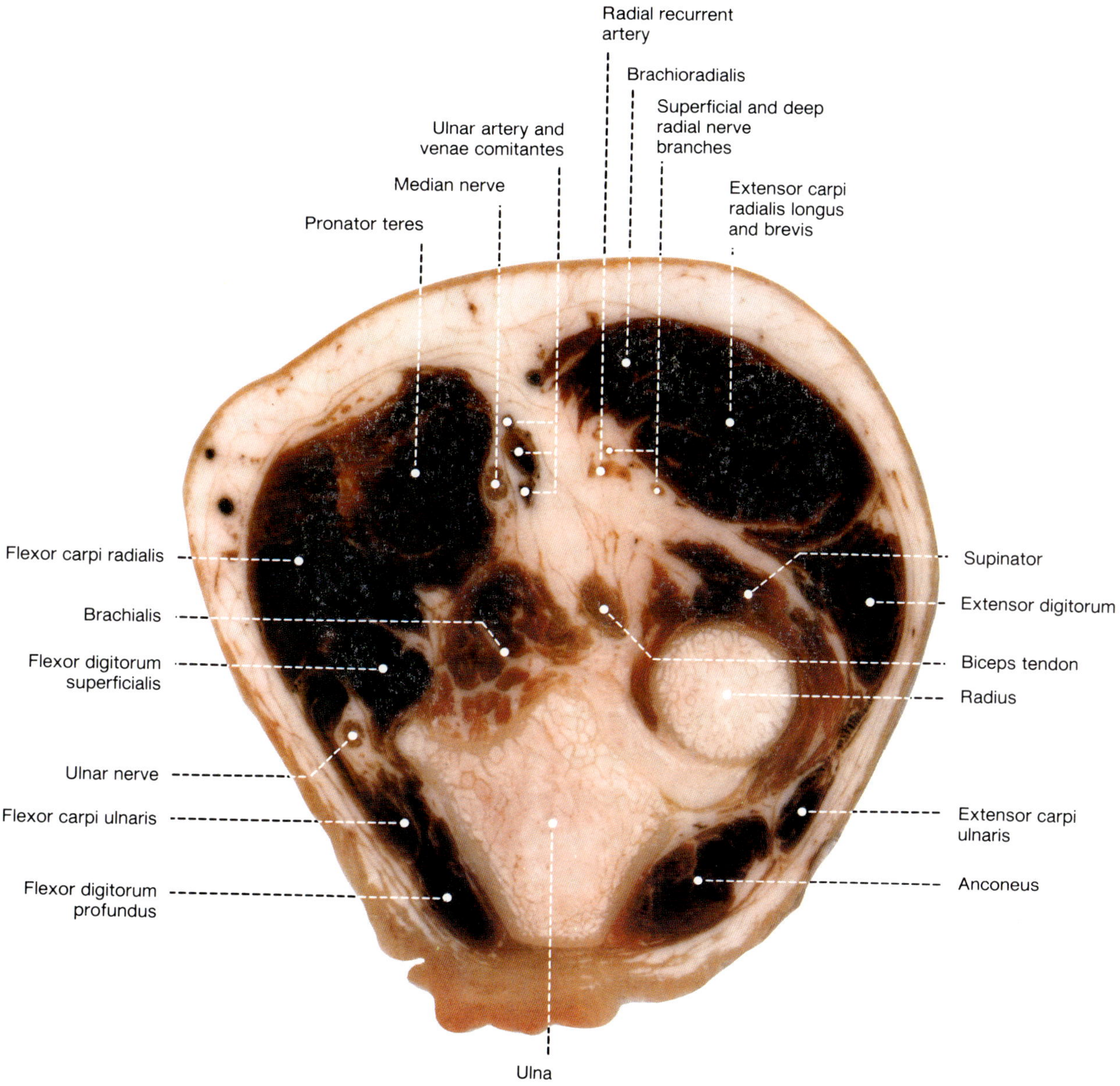

Anatomy and MRI of the Joints

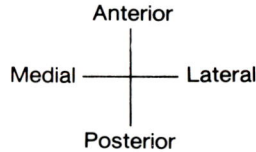

FIG. 3-11
AXIAL

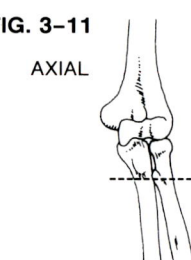

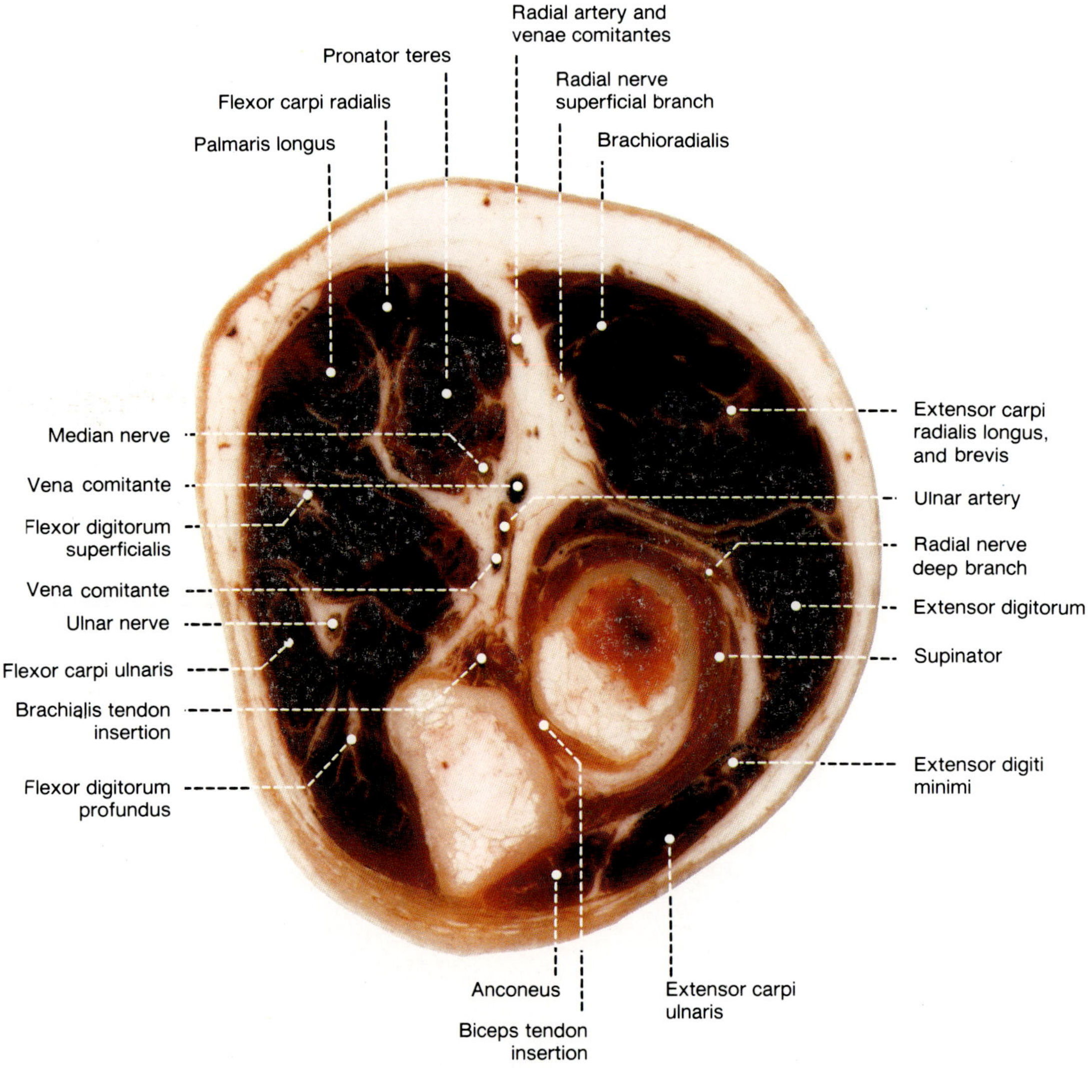

Labels:
- Palmaris longus
- Flexor carpi radialis
- Pronator teres
- Radial artery and venae comitantes
- Radial nerve superficial branch
- Brachioradialis
- Median nerve
- Vena comitante
- Flexor digitorum superficialis
- Vena comitante
- Ulnar nerve
- Flexor carpi ulnaris
- Brachialis tendon insertion
- Flexor digitorum profundus
- Anconeus
- Biceps tendon insertion
- Extensor carpi ulnaris
- Extensor digiti minimi
- Supinator
- Extensor digitorum
- Radial nerve deep branch
- Ulnar artery
- Extensor carpi radialis longus, and brevis

Anterior
Medial
Lateral
Posterior

FIG. 3–12

AXIAL

Biceps tendon
Brachialis
Cephalic vein
Brachial artery
Radial nerve
Median nerve
Brachioradialis
Pronator teres
Basilic vein
Coronoid fossa
Extensor carpi radialis longus
Medial epicondyle
Ulnar nerve
Triceps tendon
Lateral epicondyle
Olecranon fossa
Radial fossa

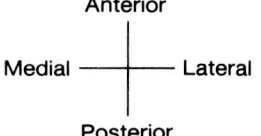

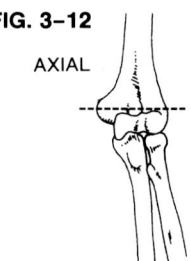

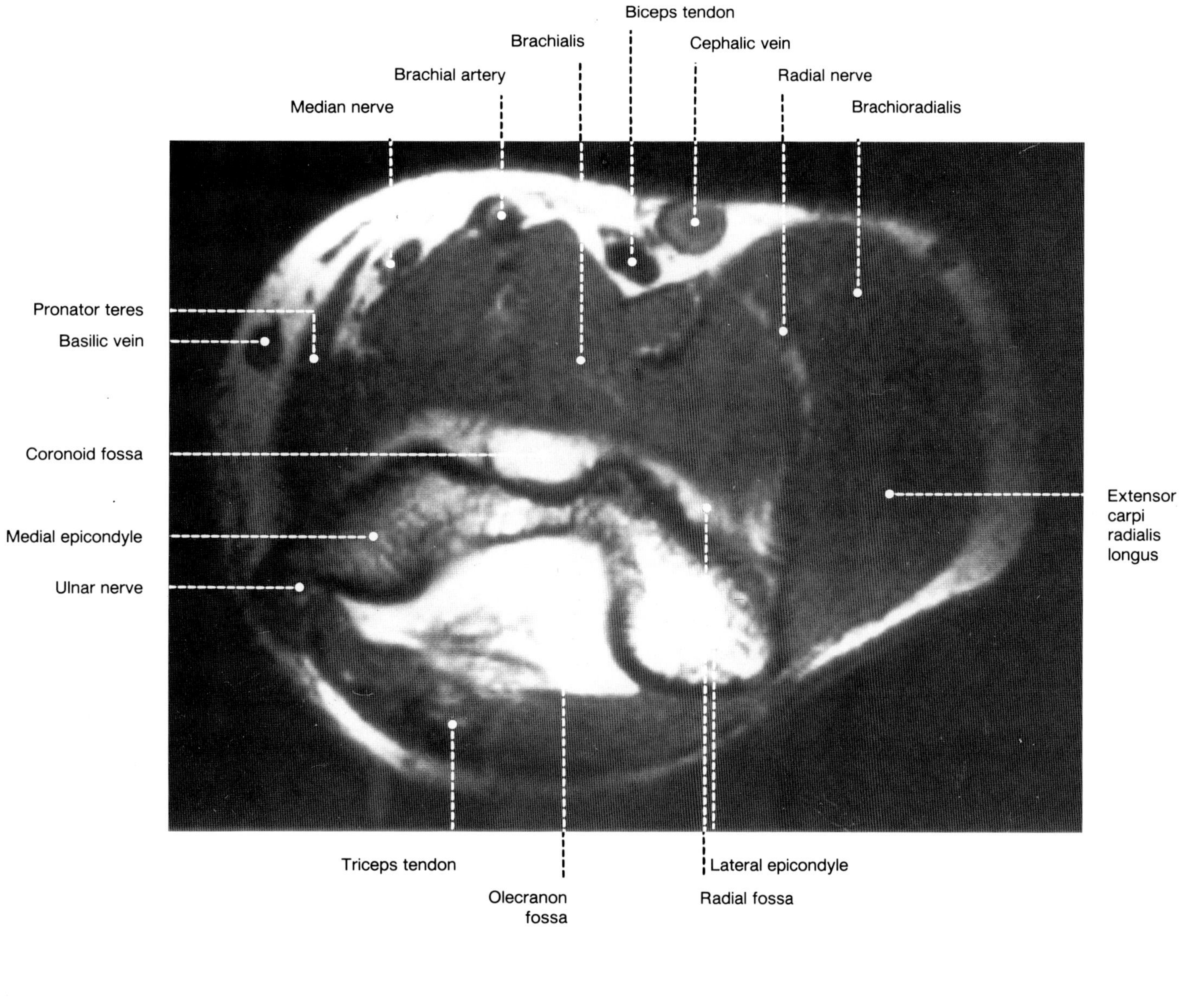

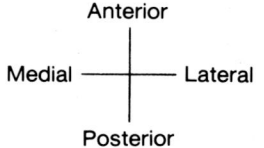
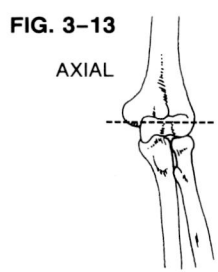

FIG. 3–13
AXIAL

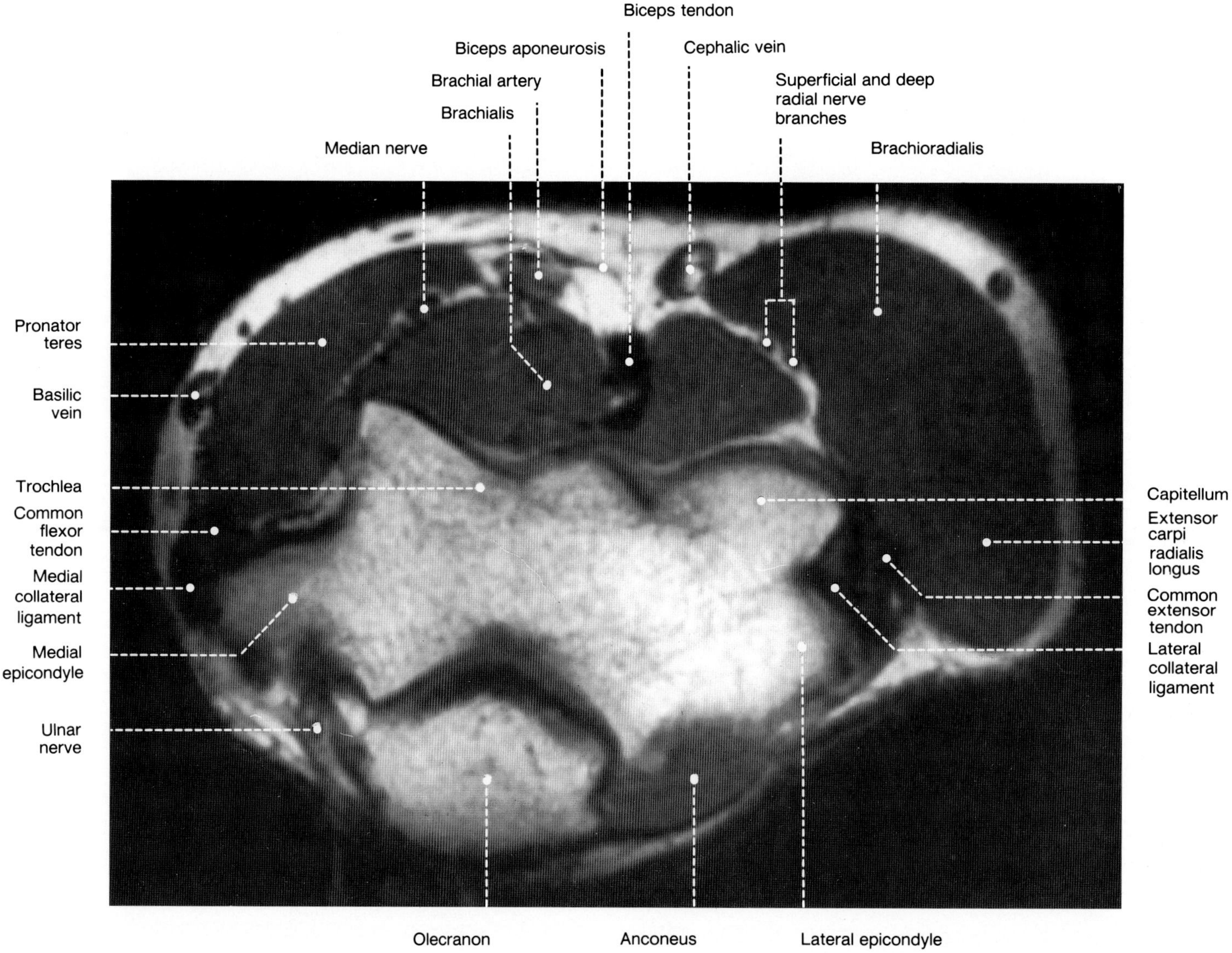

Anterior
Medial
Lateral
Posterior

FIG. 3–14

AXIAL

Biceps tendon
Radial recurrent artery
Venae comitantes
Brachial artery
Superficial and deep radial nerve branches
Median nerve
Pronator teres
Brachialis
Brachioradialis
Supinator
Flexor carpi radialis
Annular ligament
Flexor digitorum superficialis
Extensor carpi radialis longus and brevis
Ulnar nerve
Ulnar recurrent artery
Extensor digitorum
Common extensor tendon
Flexor carpi ulnaris
Radial notch
Radial head
Flexor digitorum profundus
Anconeus

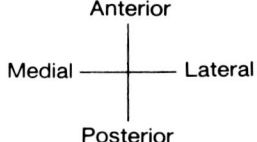

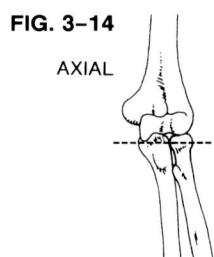

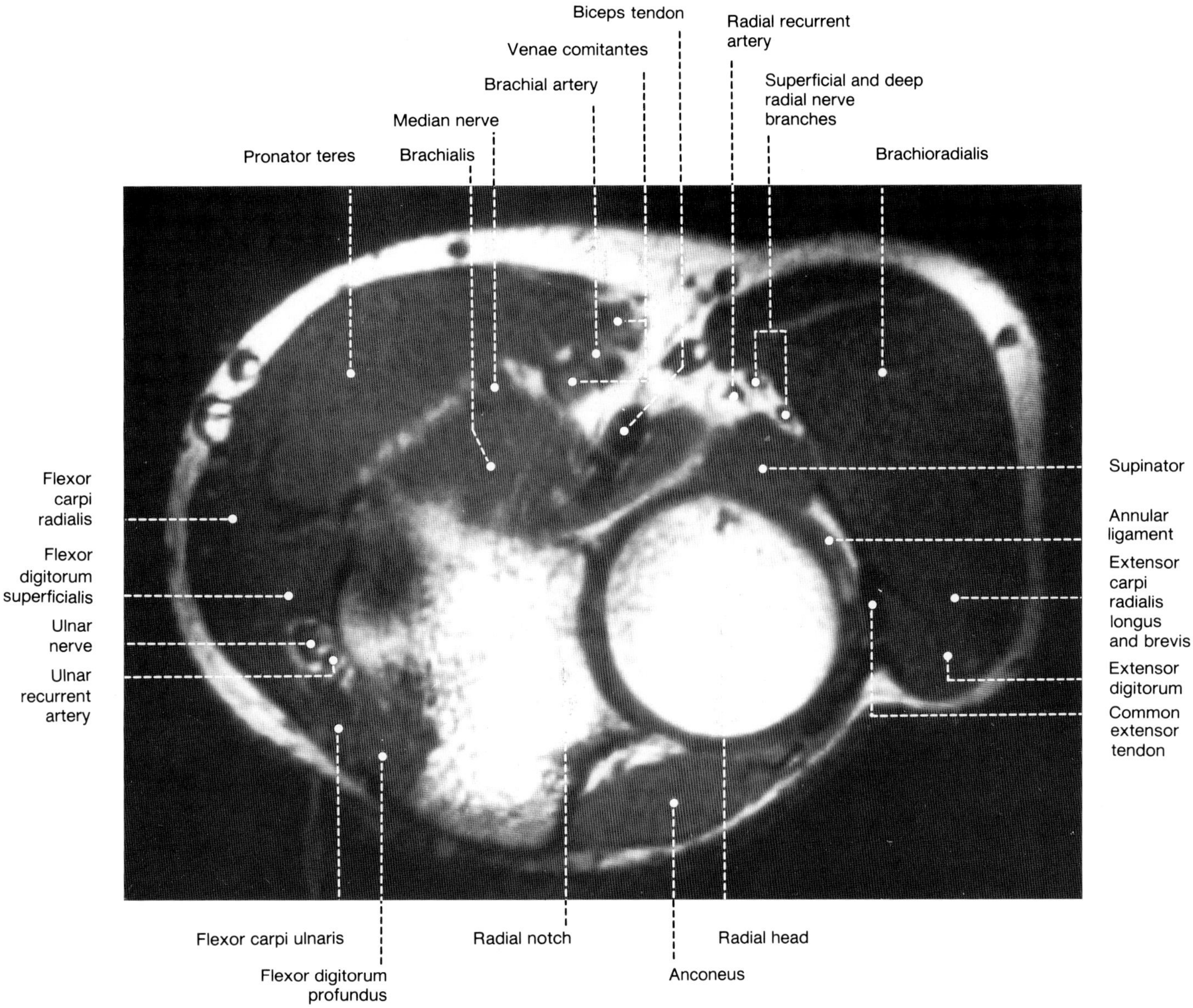

Anatomy and MRI of the Joints 64

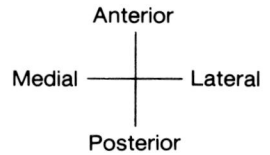

FIG. 3–15

AXIAL

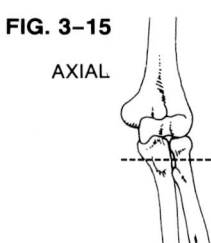

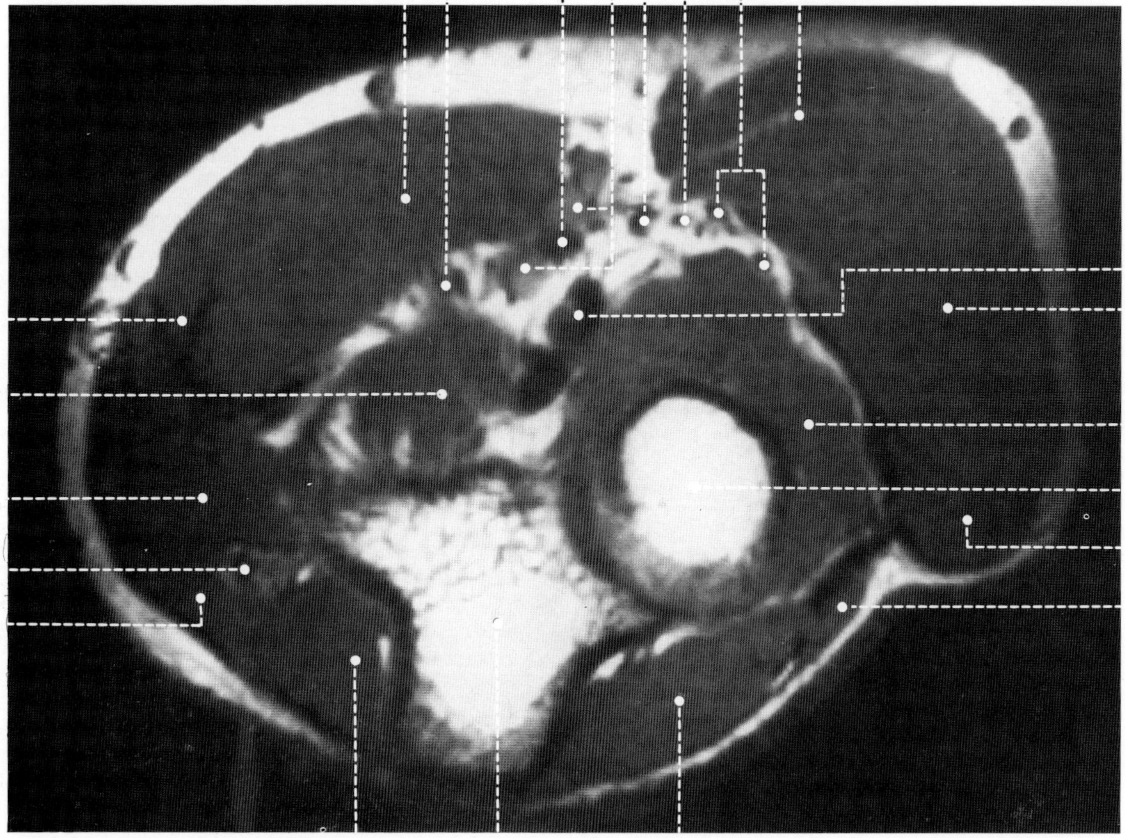

Pronator teres
Median nerve
Ulnar artery
Venae comitantes
Radial artery
Radial recurrent artery
Superficial and deep radial nerve branches
Brachioradialis

Flexor carpi radialis
Brachialis
Flexor digitorum superficialis
Ulnar nerve
Flexor carpi ulnaris

Biceps tendon
Extensor carpi radialis longus and brevis
Supinator
Radius
Extensor digitorum
Extensor carpi ulnaris

Flexor digitorum profundus
Ulna
Anconeus

Anterior
Medial
Lateral
Posterior

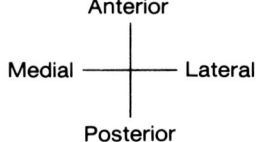

FIG. 3–16

AXIAL

Venae comitantes
Radial artery and venae comitantes
Ulnar artery
Radial nerve superficial branch
Flexor carpi radialis
Pronator teres
Brachioradialis
Radial nerve deep branch
Median nerve
Extensor carpi radialis longus and brevis
Flexor digitorum superficialis
Supinator
Ulnar nerve
Flexor carpi ulnaris
Flexor digitorum profundus
Anconeus
Extensor digitorum
Extensor digiti minimi
Brachialis tendon insertion
Extensor carpi ulnaris
Biceps tendon insertion

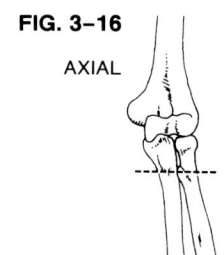

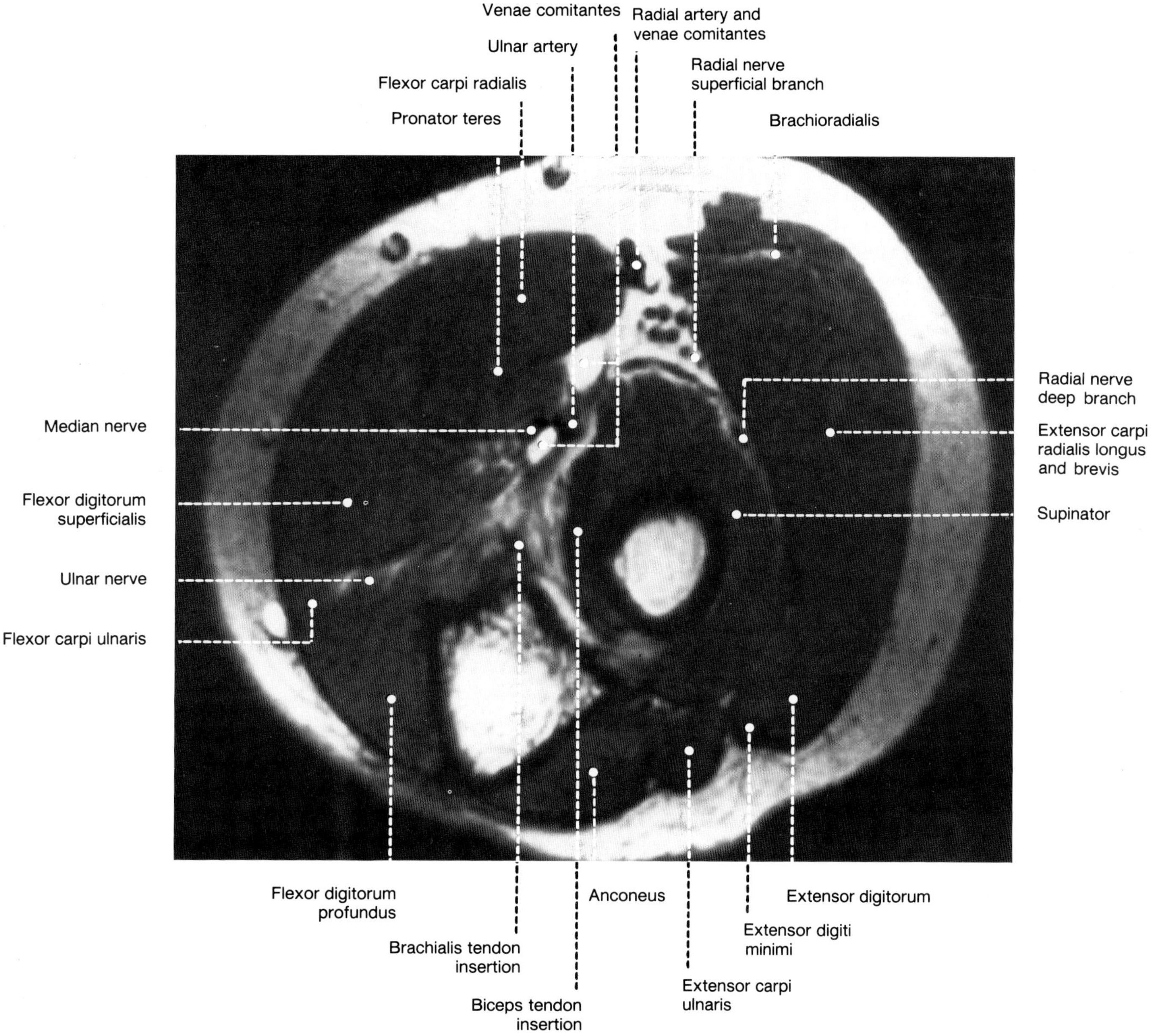

Anatomy and MRI of the Joints

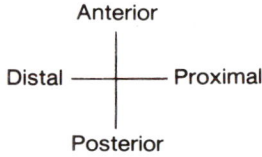

FIG. 3-17

SAGITTAL

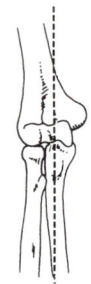

Labels (top): Radial artery · Pronator teres · Biceps tendon · Anterior fat pad · Brachialis · Biceps

Labels (left): Vena comitante · Ulnar artery · Vena comitante · Brachialis tendon insertion · Flexor digitorum profundus

Labels (bottom): Coronoid process · Trochlear notch · Trochlea · Olecranon · Posterior fat pad · Triceps tendon · Triceps

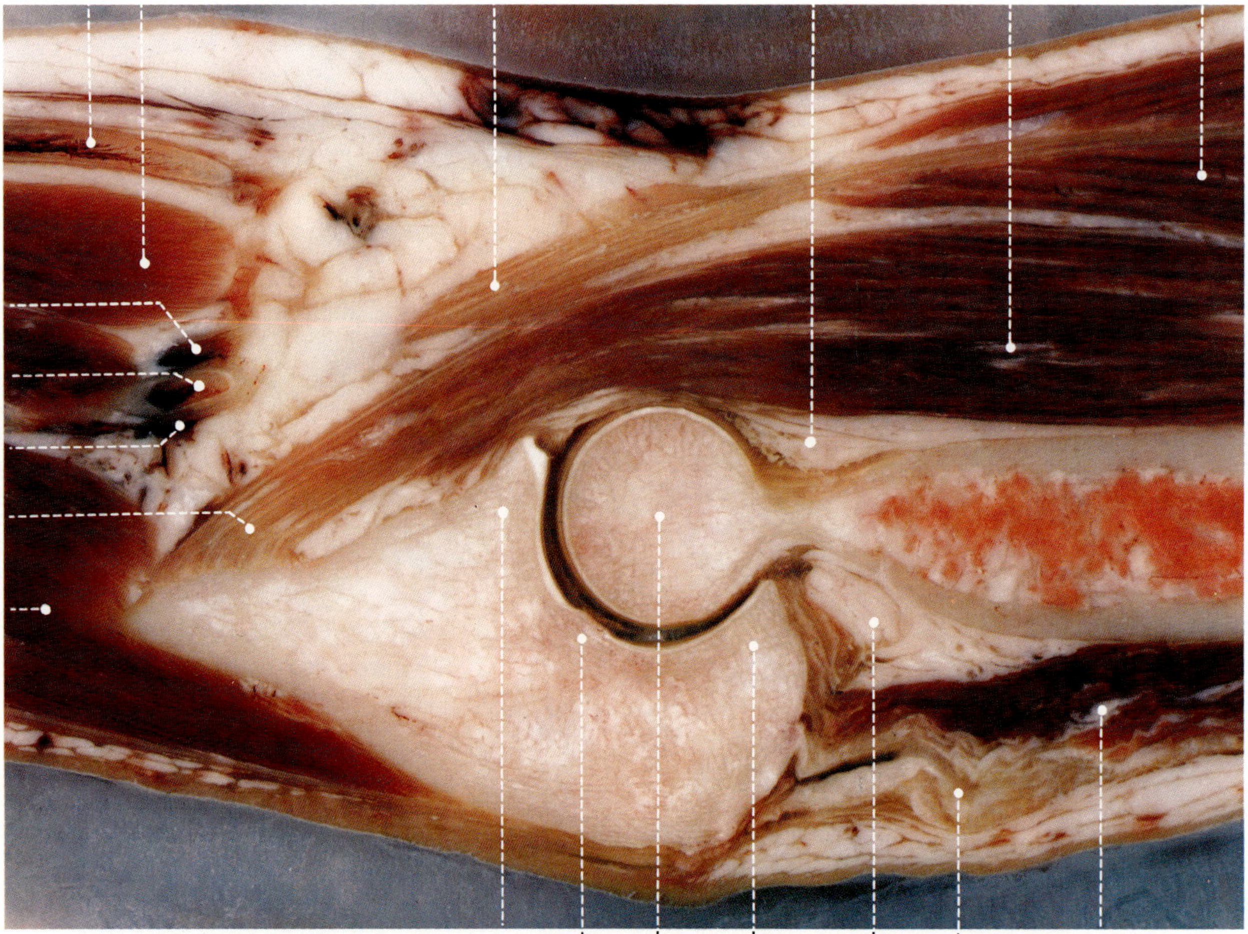

Anterior

Distal —— Proximal

Posterior

FIG. 3–18

SAGITTAL

Brachialis tendon
Brachioradialis
Anterior fat pad
Brachialis
Biceps tendon
Biceps
Pronator teres
Supinator
Ulnar artery
Biceps tendon insertion
Flexor digitorum profundus
Coronoid process
Trochlea
Olecranon
Posterior fat pad
Triceps

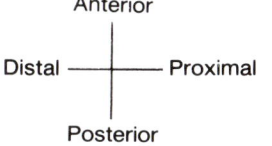

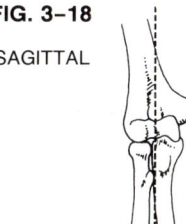

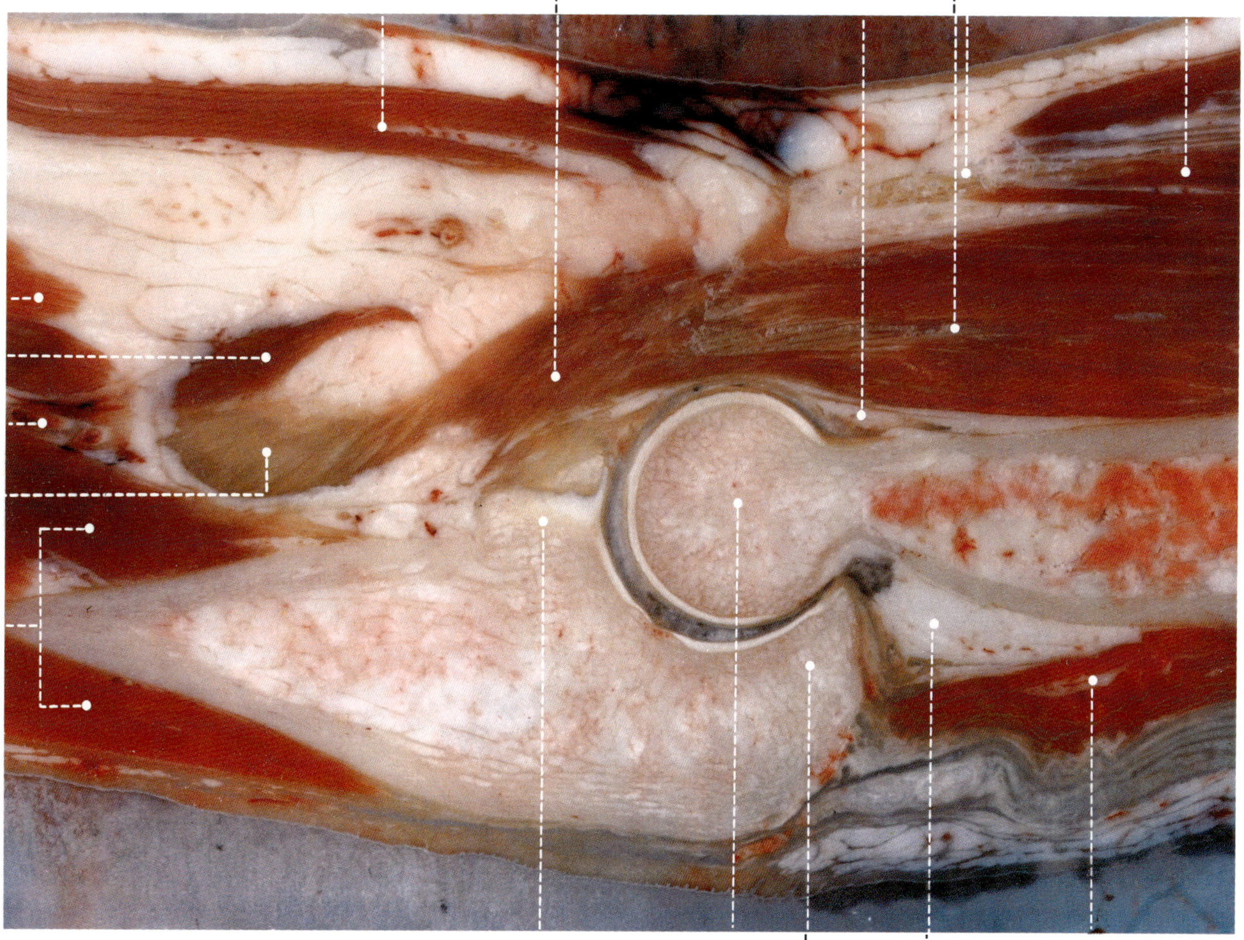

Anatomy and MRI of the Joints

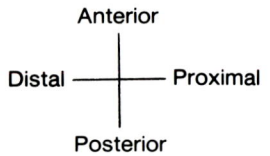

FIG. 3-19
SAGITTAL

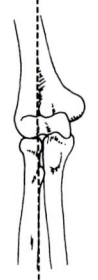

Brachioradialis
Extensor carpi radialis longus and brevis
Supinator
Capitellum
Radial nerve superficial branch
Brachialis

Radial tuberosity Ulna Radial neck Radial notch Anconeus Triceps tendon Triceps
Radial head

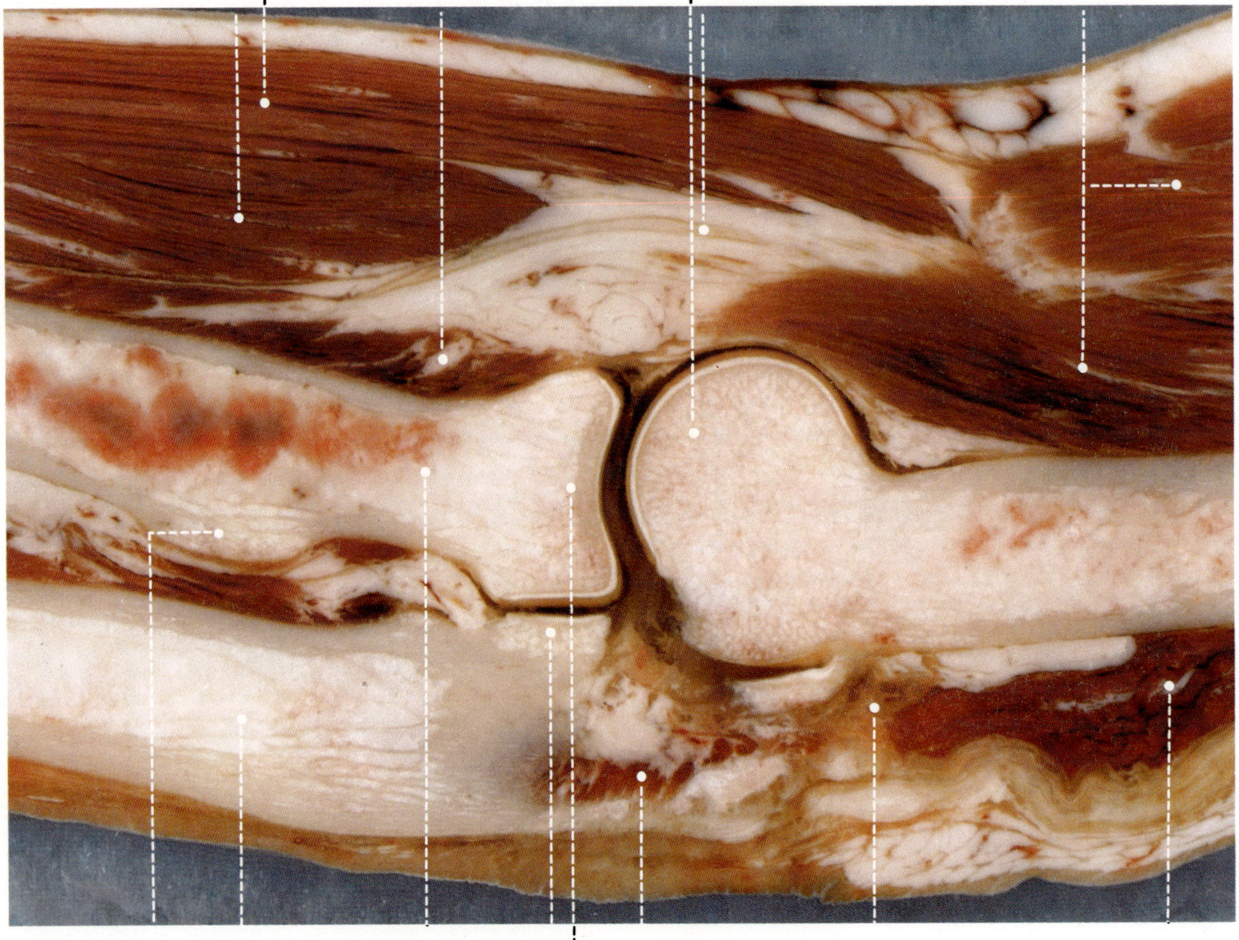

THE ELBOW

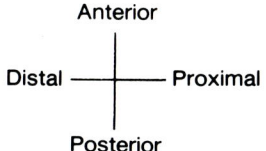

FIG. 3-20
SAGITTAL

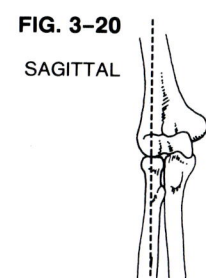

Extensor carpi radialis longus and brevis — Brachioradialis — Capitellum — Radial nerve

Supinator — Extensors — Radial head — Triceps — Brachialis

Anatomy and MRI of the Joints

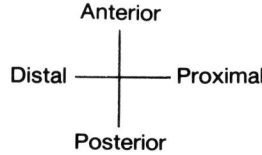

FIG. 3-21
SAGITTAL

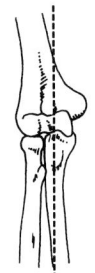

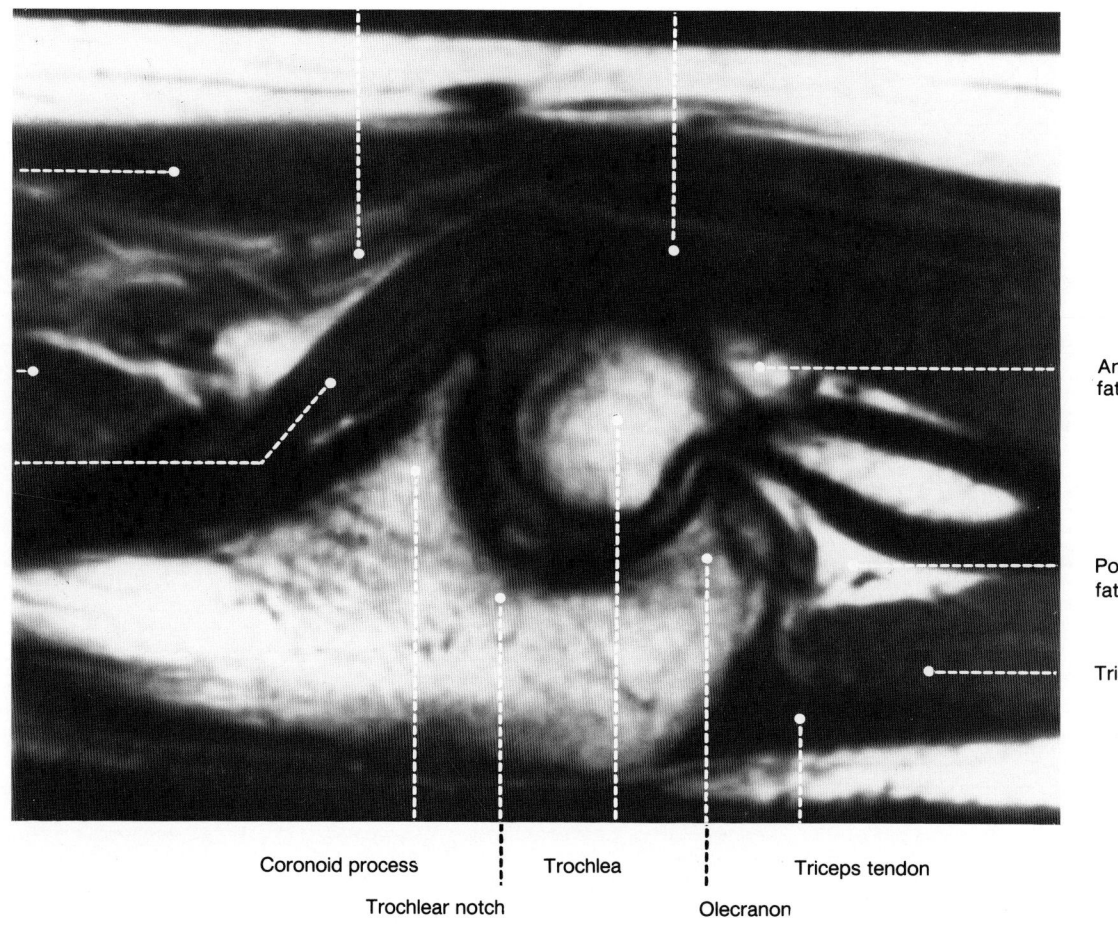

71 THE ELBOW

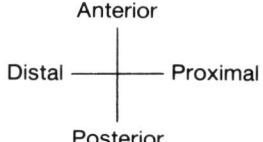

FIG. 3-22
SAGITTAL

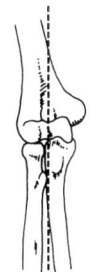

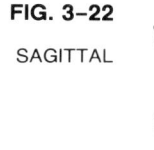

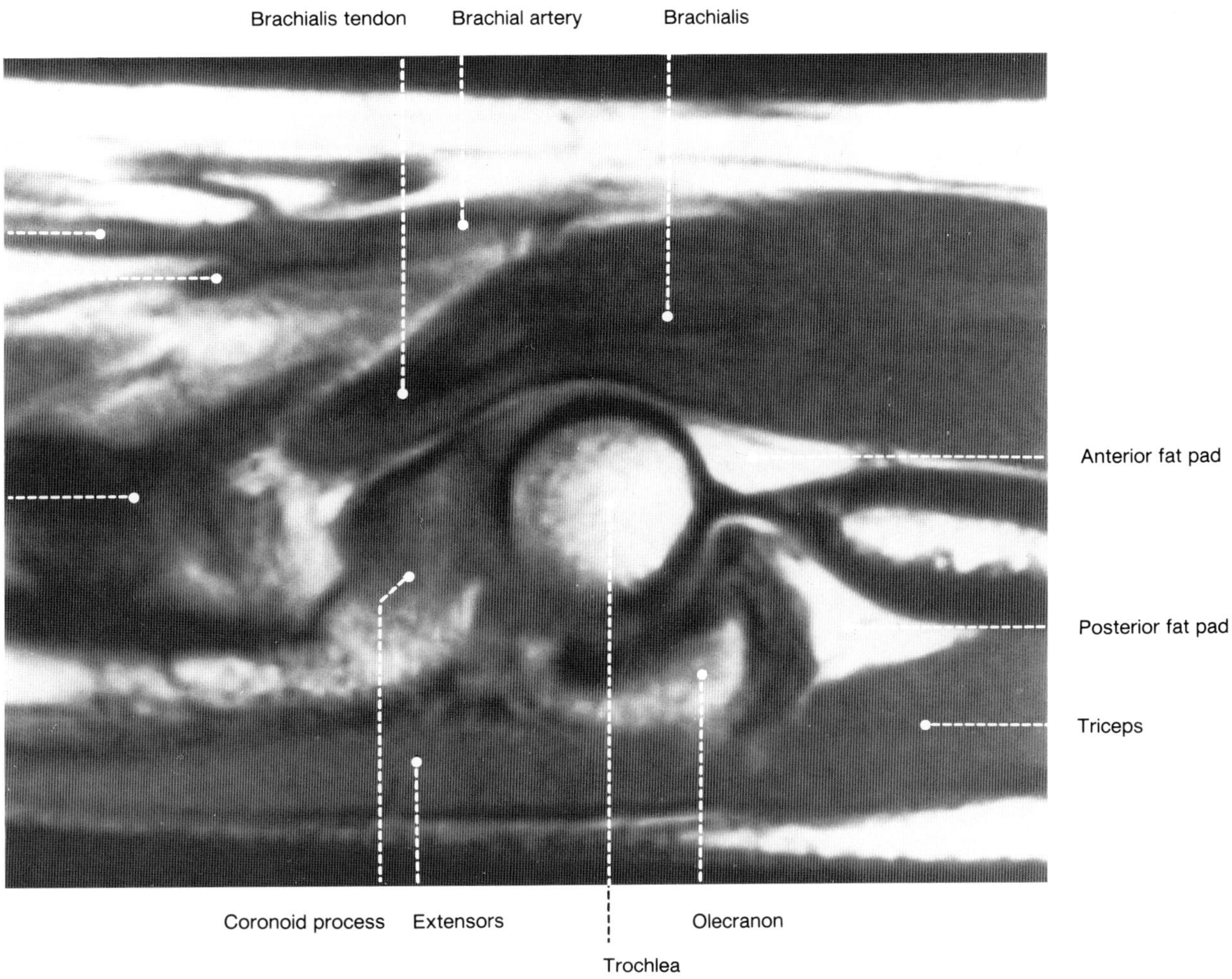

Anatomy and MRI of the Joints

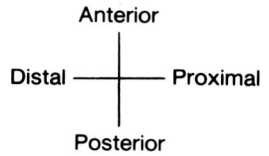

FIG. 3-23
SAGITTAL

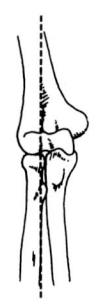

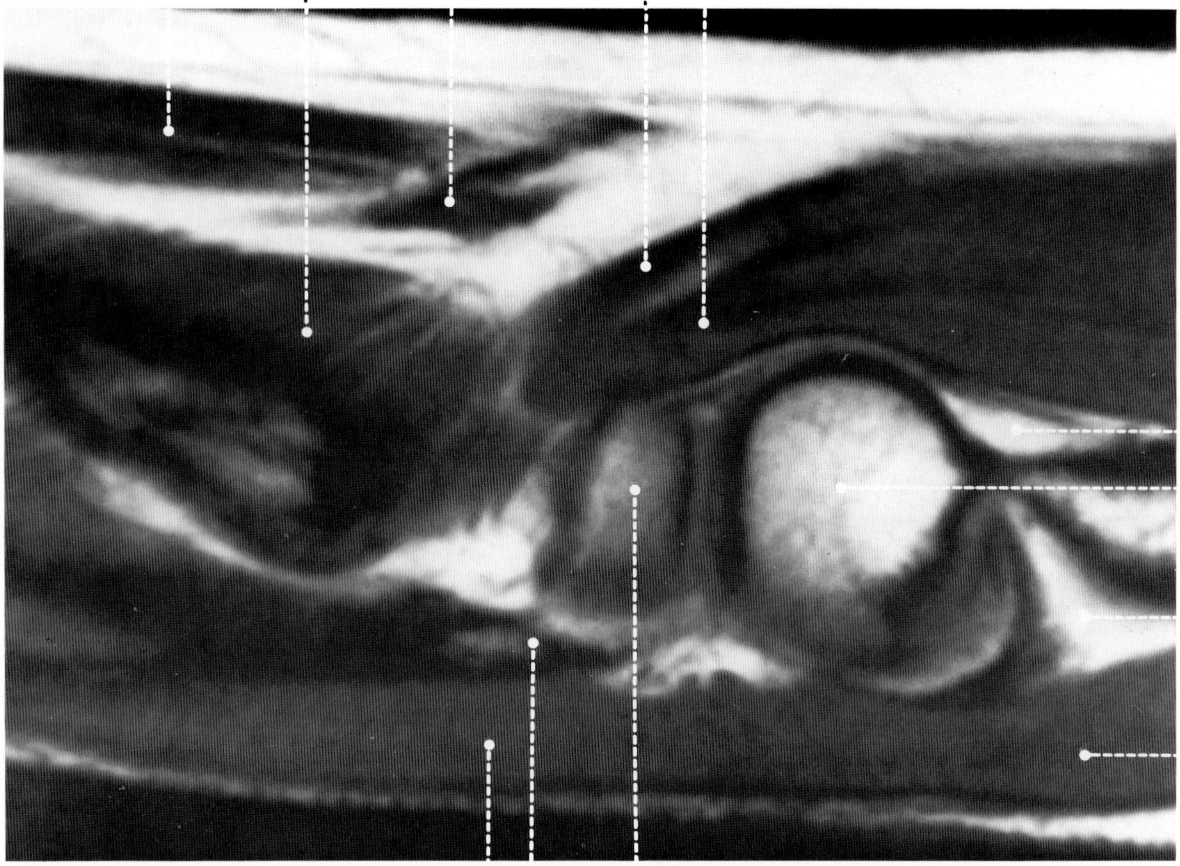

THE ELBOW

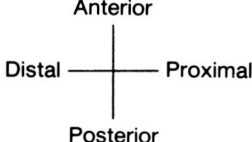

FIG. 3-24
SAGITTAL

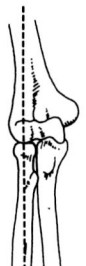

Extensor carpi radialis longus and brevis · Brachioradialis · Biceps tendon

Supinator

Radial tuberosity

Extensors · Radial neck · Radial head

Brachialis

Capitellum

Triceps

Anatomy and MRI of the Joints 74

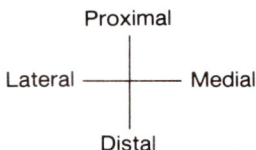

FIG. 3–25
CORONAL

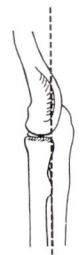

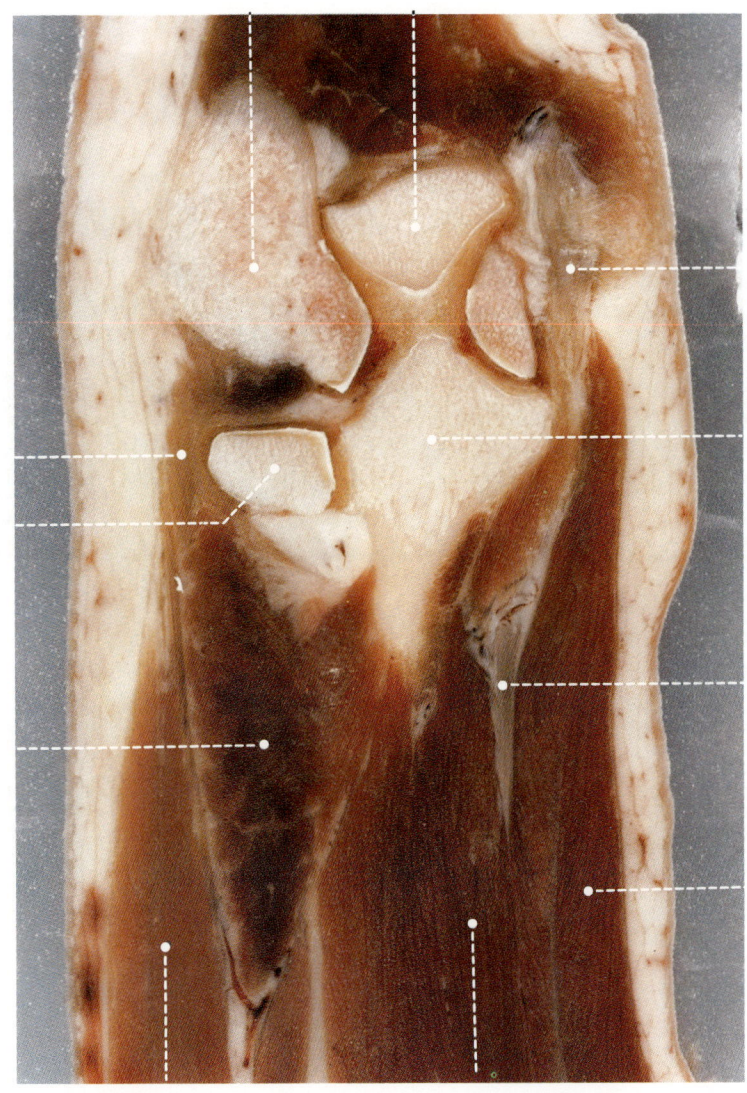

75 THE ELBOW

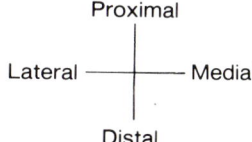

FIG. 3-26

CORONAL

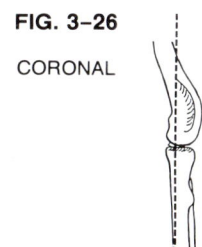

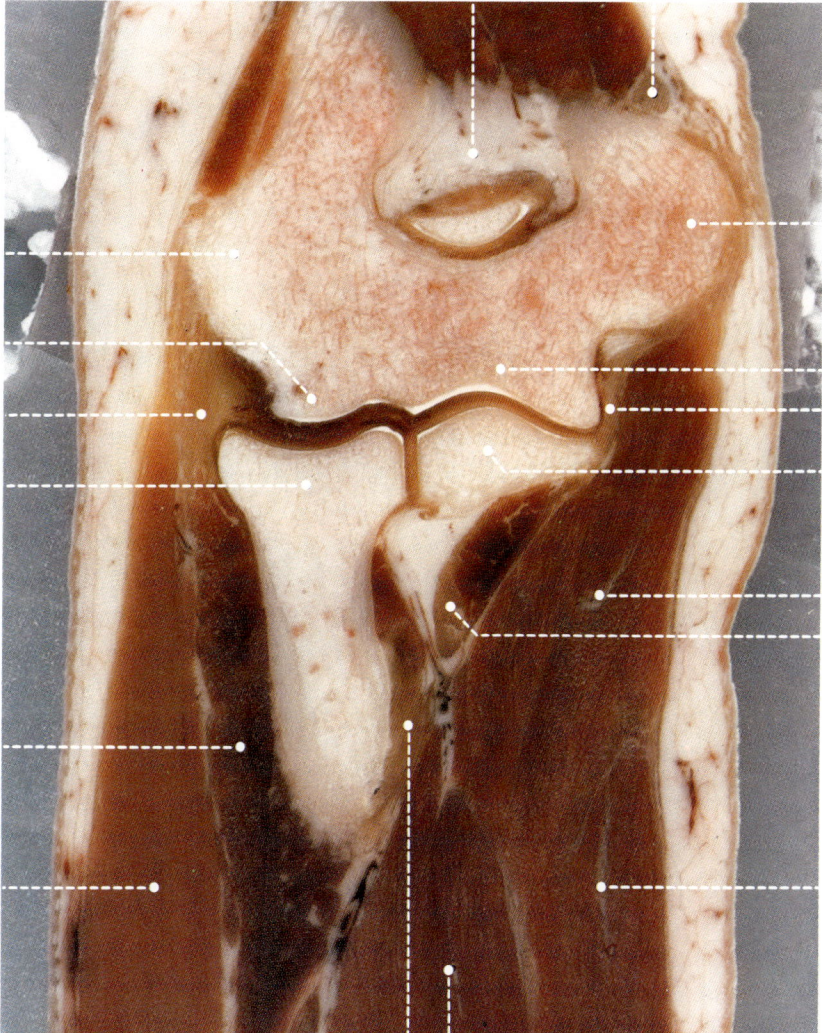

Biceps tendon insertion   Flexor digitorum profundus

Anatomy and MRI of the Joints

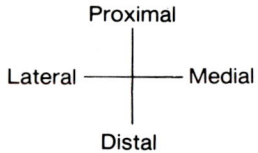

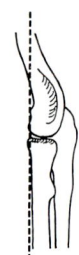

FIG. 3-27
CORONAL

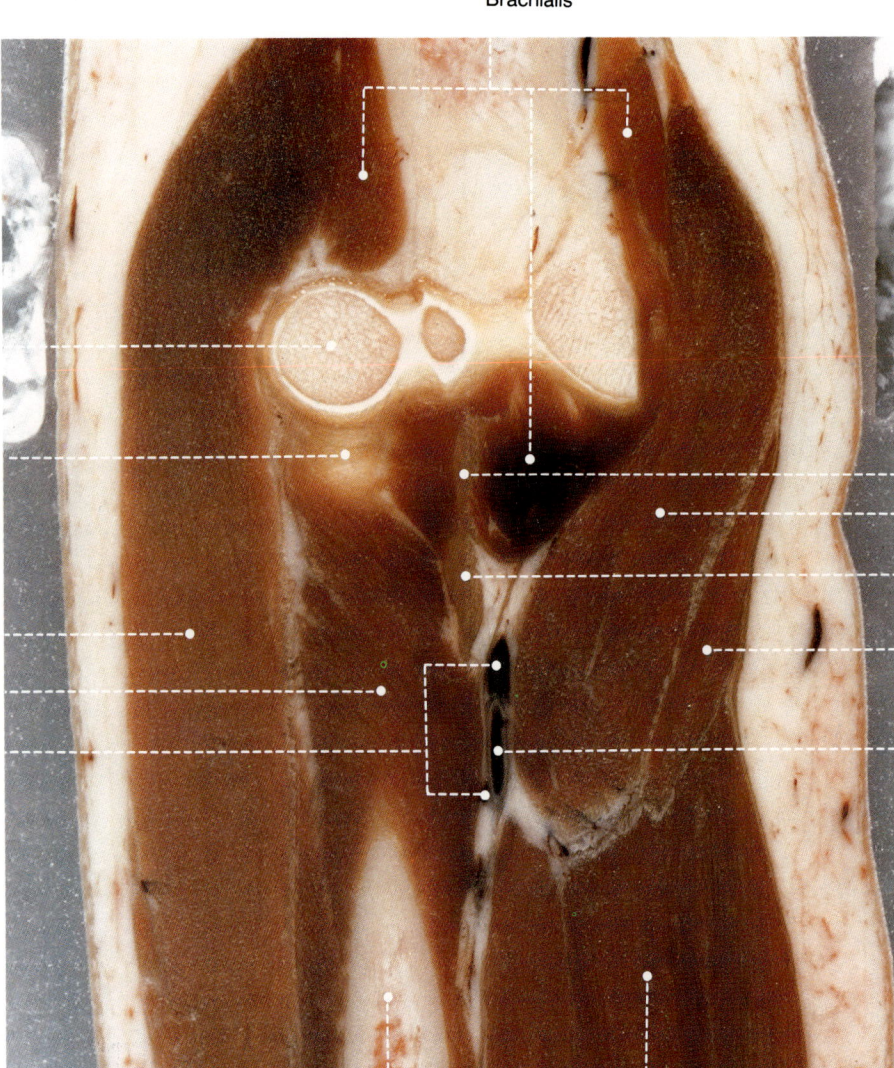

Proximal
Lateral
Medial
Distal

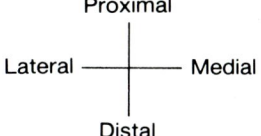

FIG. 3–28

CORONAL

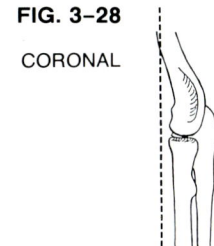

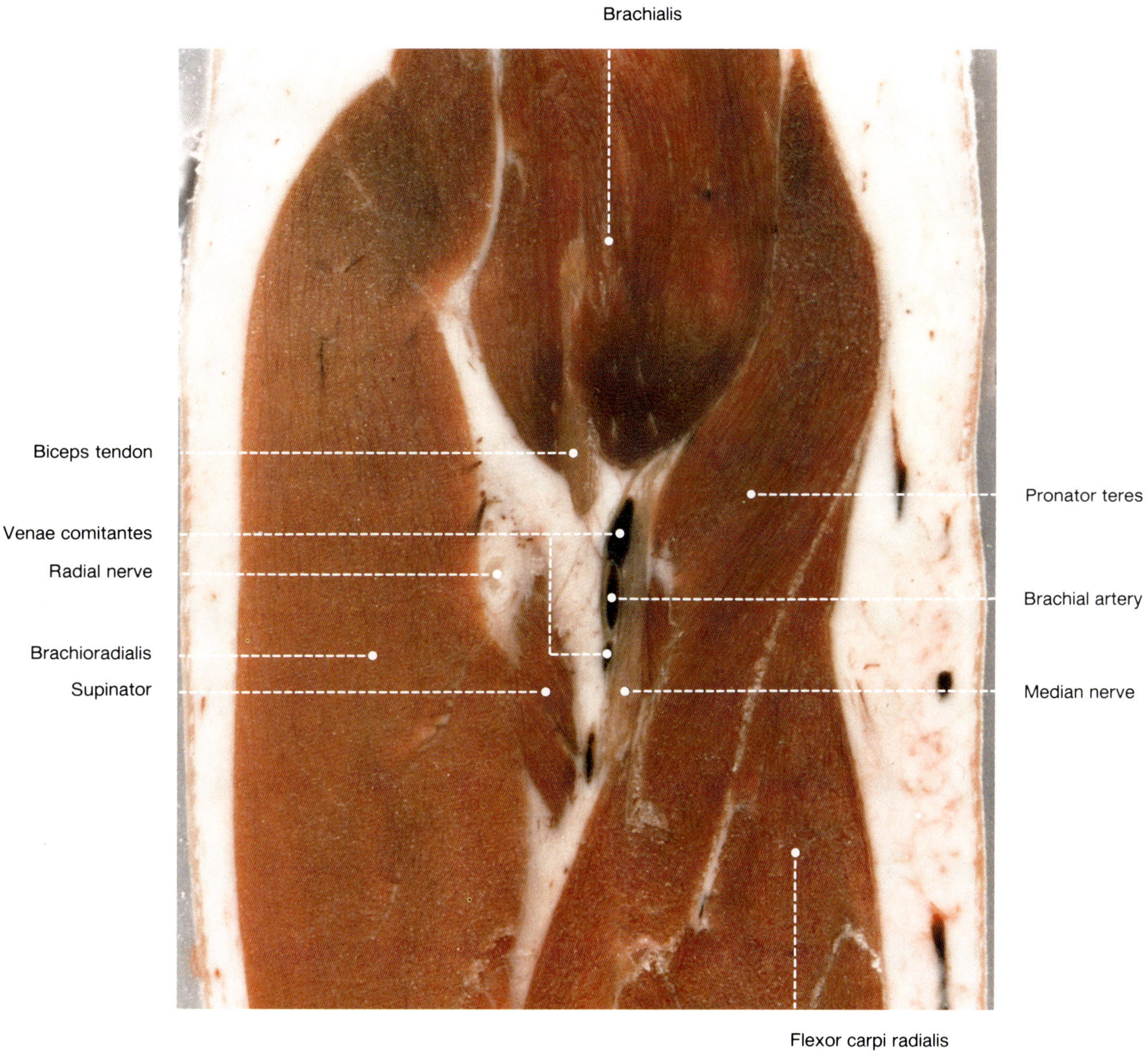

Brachialis
Biceps tendon
Venae comitantes
Radial nerve
Brachioradialis
Supinator
Pronator teres
Brachial artery
Median nerve
Flexor carpi radialis

Anatomy and MRI of the Joints

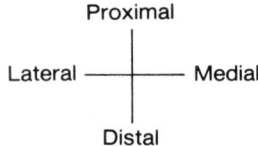

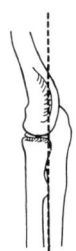

FIG. 3-29
CORONAL

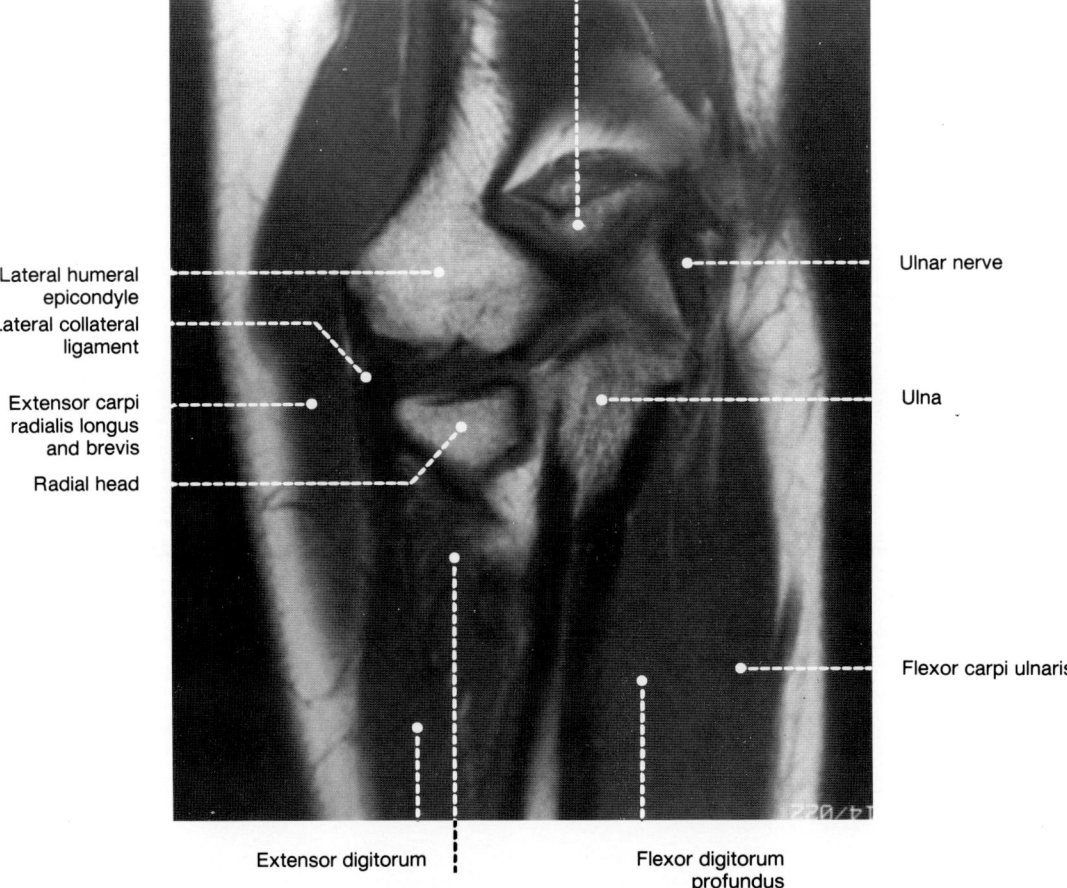

THE ELBOW

FIG. 3-30
CORONAL

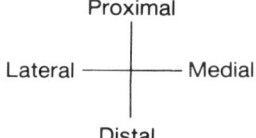
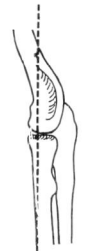
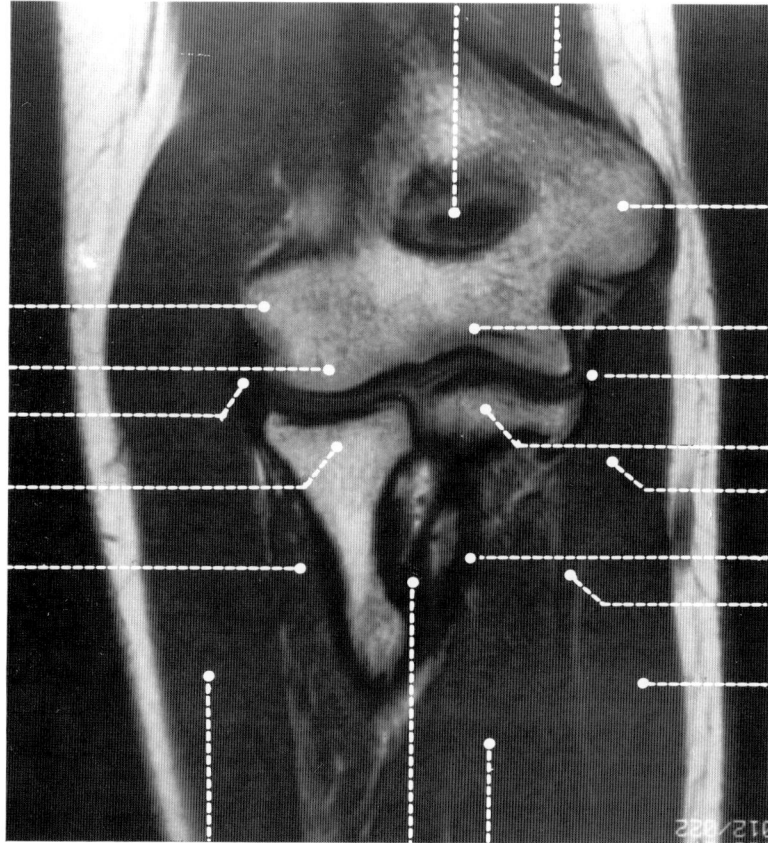

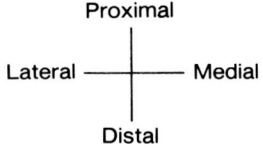

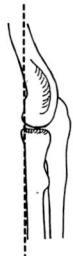

FIG. 3-31
CORONAL

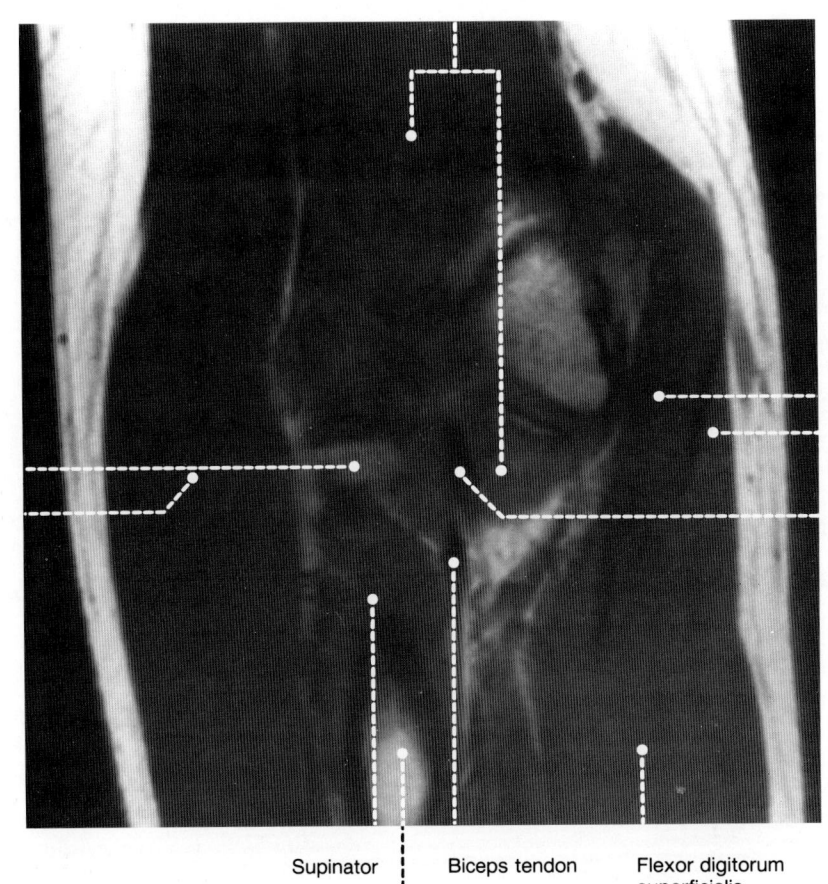

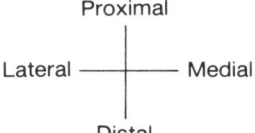

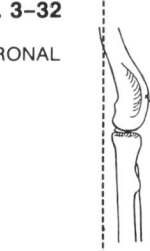

FIG. 3-32
CORONAL

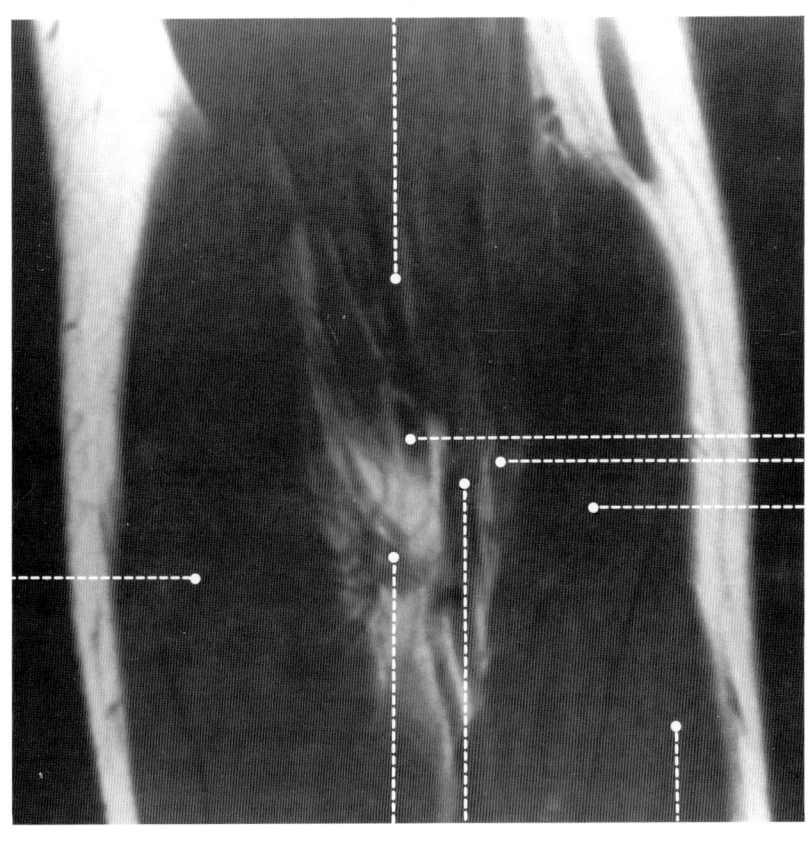

Brachialis

Brachioradialis

Biceps tendon
Median nerve
Pronator teres

Supinator   Brachial artery   Flexor carpi radialis

CHAPTER 4

THE WRIST
William D. Middleton, M.D.

The human wrist is composed of a plethora of anatomic structures including bones, tendons, ligaments, muscles, and neurovascular structures. Because there are so many anatomic structures located in a relatively confined area, the anatomy of the wrist can be intimidating when seen in cross section. However, careful analysis of cross-sectional images and anatomic sections reveals a relatively detailed, yet understandable, portrayal of articular and periarticular structures.

The carpal bones are arranged in a proximal and distal row. The proximal row is composed of the scaphoid, lunate, triquetrum, and pisiform bone and the distal row is composed of the trapezium, trapezoid, capitate, and hamate. With the exception of the pisiform, the bones of the proximal carpal row articulate with the radius, the distal carpal row, and each other. The pisiform articulates only with the triquetrum. The bones of the distal carpal row articulate with the proximal carpal row, each other, and the metacarpals. Their complex interrelations are shown in Fig. 4–1.

The triangular fibrocartilage separates the scaphoid and lunate from the ulna and attaches the distal radius and ulna to each other. It is ligamentous peripherally and this ligamentous portion extends from the ulnar styloid to the dorsal and palmar aspect of the radius.

A number of ligaments support the carpus. The radiocarpal articulations are supported on their palmar and dorsal aspects by broad, thin ligaments extending from the distal radius and ulna to the scaphoid, lunate, and triquetrum. These are called the palmar and dorsal radial carpal ligaments. The radial and ulnar collateral ligaments extend from the radial styloid to the scaphoid and from the ulnar styloid to the triquetrum and pisiform, respectively.

In addition to these ligaments, a complex arrangement of ligaments connect the carpal bones to each other. Numerous palmar and dorsal ligaments connect the superficial surfaces of the carpal bones and multiple interosseous ligaments connect the deep surfaces of the carpal bones.

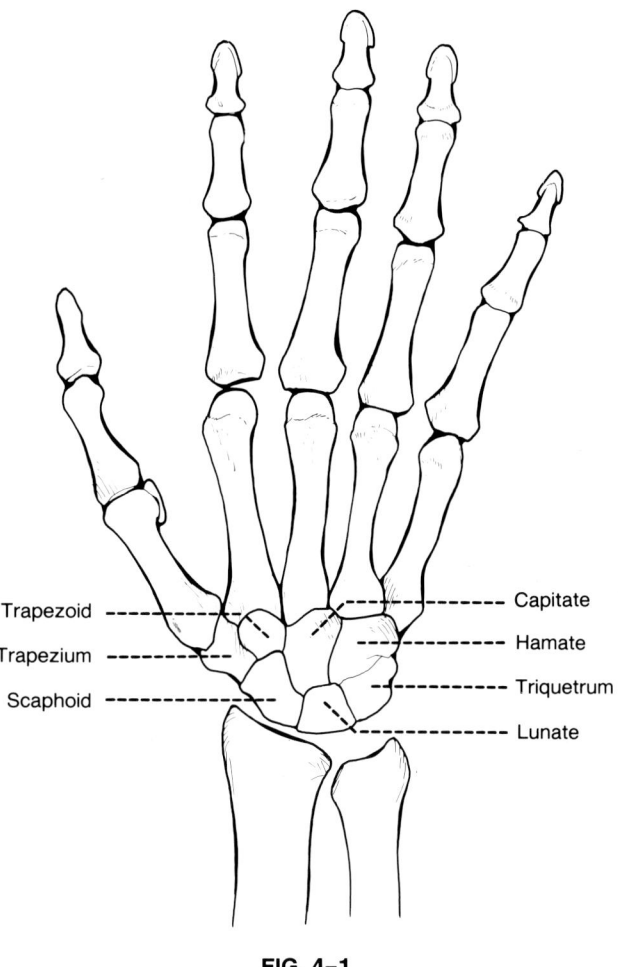

FIG. 4–1

The flexor retinaculum is a thick ligamentous band that attaches primarily to the hook of the hamate and the tubercle of the trapezium. It is thinner proximally where attenuated strands attach to the pisiform and the tubercle of the scaphoid. The flexor retinaculum forms the superficial border of the carpal tunnel, with the carpal bones forming the deep border.

The extensor retinaculum is much thinner than the flexor retinaculum. It forms multiple fibro-osseous tunnels along the dorsal aspect of the wrist, through which pass the extensor tendons.

The major muscles of the wrist are limited to those of the thenar and hypothenar eminence, shown in Fig. 4–2. The three thenar muscles all arise from the flexor retinaculum. The abductor pollicis brevis and flexor pollicis brevis are superficial and both insert at the base of the first phalanx. The opponens pollicis is deep and has a broad insertion on the shaft of the first metacarpal. The origins and insertions of the three hypothenar muscles are similar to those of the thenar muscles, except the insertions are onto the fifth digit.

The adductor pollicis is located deep to the thenar muscles. It arises from the capitate and the third metacarpal and inserts at the base of the first phalanx. It is divided into an oblique (proximal) and transverse (distal) portion by the radial artery. There is no adductor muscle to the fifth digit.

Other muscles which are not strictly part of the wrist but which are seen in images of the wrist are the pronator quadratus and the lumbrical muscles. The pronator quadratus arises from the palmar aspect of the distal ulna and inserts on the palmar aspect of the distal radius. It is the major pronator of the wrist. The four lumbricals arise from the tendons of the flexor digitorum profundus and insert on the radial aspect of the dorsal extensor tendon expansion.

Normally all of the muscles of the forearm become tendinous prior to the wrist. Because of their number, these tendons can become confusing when seen in cross section. However, their arrangement is relatively constant and they are actually fairly easy to identify and separate from each other. They are best understood by dividing them into dorsal and palmar groups.

The palmar group includes the flexors of the wrist and fingers. The superficial flexors of the forearm include the flexor carpi radialis, flexor carpi ulnaris, and palmaris longus. The tendon of the flexor carpi radialis travels su-

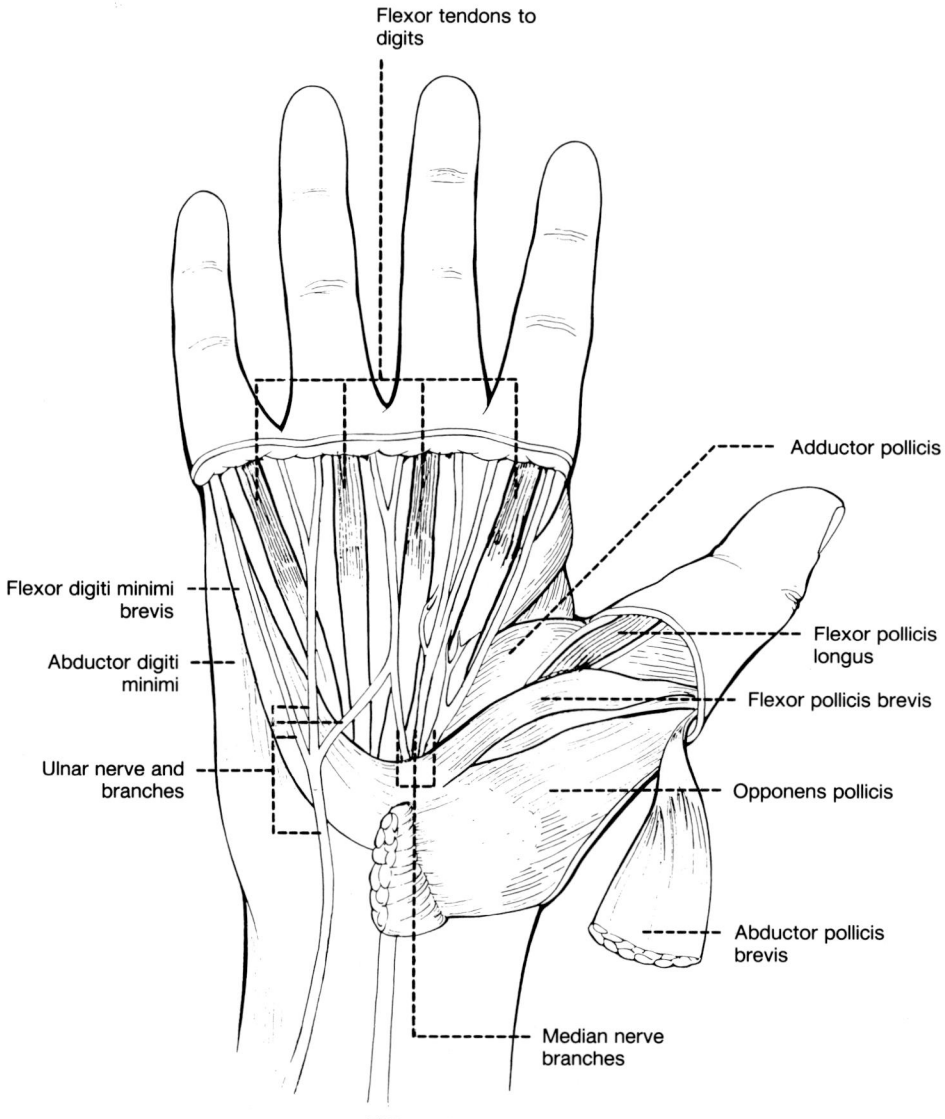

FIG. 4–2

perficial to the distal scaphoid and pierces the radial aspect of the flexor retinaculum. It then runs in its own fibro-osseous tunnel formed by two layers of the flexor retinaculum and the vertical groove of the trapezium. It inserts primarily on the base of the second metacarpal, although some fibers do extend to the base of the third metacarpal. The flexor carpi ulnaris tendon inserts onto the pisiform bone and continues beyond the pisiform to the hamate and fifth metacarpal as the pisohamate and pisometacarpal ligaments. The palmaris longus tendon is flattened and less bulky than the other flexor tendons. It runs superficial to the flexor retinaculum and eventually blends into the palmar aponeurosis.

The intermediate flexor of the forearm is the flexor digitorum superficialis. This muscle divides into four tendons prior to reaching the wrist. These four tendons pass just beneath the flexor retinaculum and eventually extend to the sides of the second phalanges. Within the carpal tunnel, the tendons of the third and fourth digits are relatively superficial, while those to the second and fifth digits are deeper. Because of this arrangement, the four tendons are situated in an arc just deep to the flexor retinaculum. This arrangement is shown in Fig. 4–3.

The deep flexors of the forearm are the flexor digitorum profundus and flexor pollicis longus. Similar to the flexor digitorum superficialis, the flexor digitorum profundus divides into four tendons prior to reaching the wrist. These tendons occupy the deepest portion of the carpal tunnel. As they extend distally to insert at the distal phalanges, they diverge from one another and pair up with the corresponding tendons of the flexor digitorum superficialis (Fig. 4–3).

The flexor pollicis longus tendon occupies the most radial aspect of the carpal tunnel (Fig. 4–3). Beyond the carpal tunnel it runs between the flexor pollicis brevis and the adductor pollicis brevis muscles. It inserts onto the base of the first distal phalanx.

The dorsal tendon group includes the extensors of the digits and wrist and the long abductor tendon of the thumb. All of the tendons pass beneath the extensor retinaculum and are divided into groups by six fibro-osseous tunnels formed by the retinaculum and grooves within the distal radius. The overall arrangement of the dorsal tendons is shown in Fig. 4–4.

The most lateral of these groups are the abductor pollicis longus and extensor pollicis brevis. The extensor pollicis brevis runs just dorsal to the abductor pollicis longus. The extensor pollicis brevis inserts on the base of the first proximal phalanx and the abductor pollicis longus inserts at the base of the first metacarpal.

Just medial to the extensor pollicis brevis and abductor pollicis longus are the extensor carpi radialis longus and brevis. These tendons run together along the radial border of the radius with the brevis position medially and dorsally. After they run beneath the thin extensor retinaculum, they separate from each other and proceed to their insertions on the base of the second (longus) and third (brevis) metacarpals.

The extensor pollicis longus originates medial to the extensor carpi radialis longus and brevis. After passing through its own tunnel in the extensor retinaculum, it passes over the extensor carpi radialis longus and brevis and eventually lies lateral to these tendons. The extensor pollicis longus inserts on the base of the first distal phalanx.

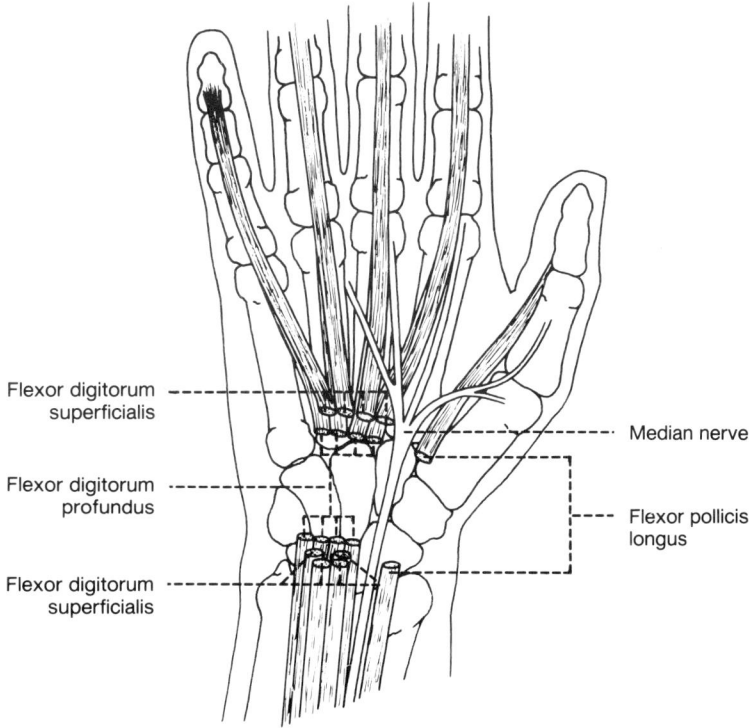

FIG. 4–3

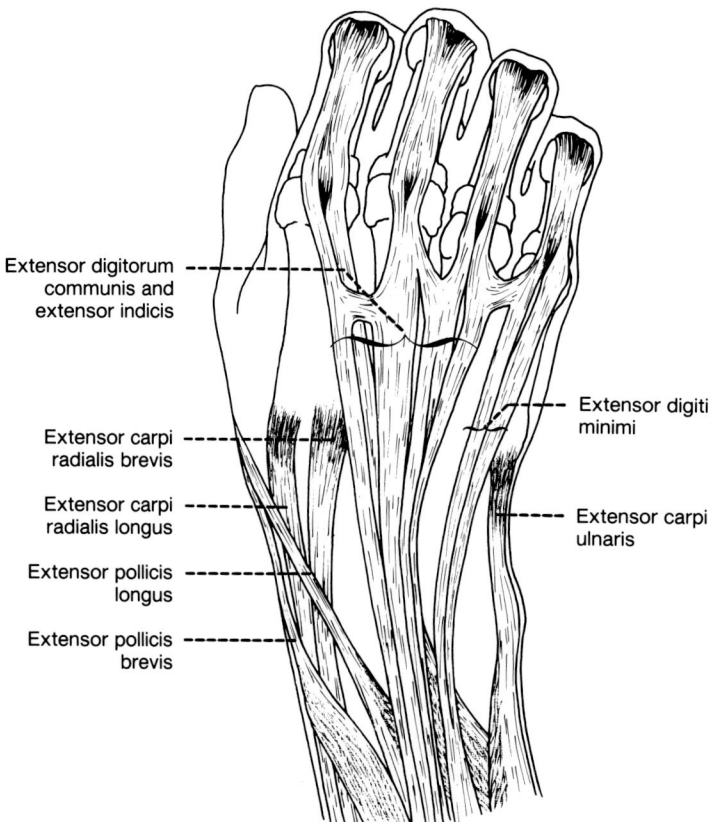

FIG. 4-4

The extensor digitorum communis lies medial to the extensor pollicis longus. Like the flexor tendons of the fingers, it divides into four tendons prior to reaching the wrist. These four tendons pass within their own compartment (along with the extensor indicis) through the extensor retinaculum. Distally the four tendons contribute to the dorsal extensor tendon expansion of the second through fifth digits. The separate tendons of the extensor digiti minimi and extensor indices accompany the tendon of the extensor digitorum communis to the index and small fingers. The extensor digiti minimi travels in its own fibro-osseous tunnel medial to that of the extensor digitorum communis and extensor indicis.

The most medial of the extensor tendons is the extensor carpi ulnaris. It runs in a separate compartment of the extensor retinaculum within a groove formed between the styloid process and head of the ulna. Distally it inserts at the base of the fifth metacarpal.

The blood supply to the hand and wrist comes from the radial and ulnar arteries. The radial artery travels along the radial aspect of the forearm to reach the wrist, where it is located lateral to the flexor carpi radialis tendon. At the wrist, the radial artery descends under the abductor pollicis longus and extensor pollicis brevis and longus into the "anatomical snuff box." As it reaches the interosseous space between the thumb and index finger, it perforates the first interosseous muscle to enter the palm of the hand deep to the adductor pollicis longus and lumbrical muscle. There it anastomoses with the deep palmar branch of the ulnar artery to form the deep palmar arch. At the level of the wrist the radial artery also gives off a small superficial branch which anastomoses with the ulnar artery to form the superficial palmar arch.

The ulnar artery travels in the forearm deep to the flexor carpi ulnaris muscle. At the wrist the ulnar artery remains superficial to the flexor retinaculum. It extends beyond the wrist to anastomose with the superficial branch of the radial artery to form the superficial palmar arch.

The ulnar nerve travels medial to the ulnar artery throughout most of its course. At the wrist it remains closely associated with the ulnar artery and travels superficially, sending branches to the fifth and fourth digits. It also has a deep branch that travels adjacent to the deep palmar branch of the ulnar artery.

Unlike the ulnar nerve, the median nerve is not associated with an artery in the wrist. In the forearm it travels deep to the muscle of the flexor digitorum superficialis. At the wrist it extends deep to the flexor retinaculum within the carpal tunnel (Fig. 4–3). As it exits the carpal tunnel, it divides into three branches that extend to the interosseous spaces between the first four digits.

THE WRIST

AXIAL
    Cryomicrotomes . . . . FIGS. 4–5 to 4–10
    MR Images . . . . FIGS. 4–11 to 4–16

SAGITTAL
    Cryomicrotomes . . . . FIGS. 4–17 to 4–22
    MR Images . . . . FIGS. 4–23 to 4–27

CORONAL
    Cryomicrotomes . . . . FIGS. 4–28 to 4–32
    MR Images . . . . FIGS. 4–33 to 4–37

Anatomy and MRI of the Joints

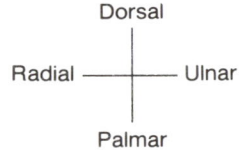

FIG. 4–5

AXIAL

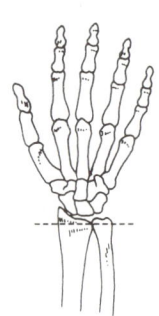

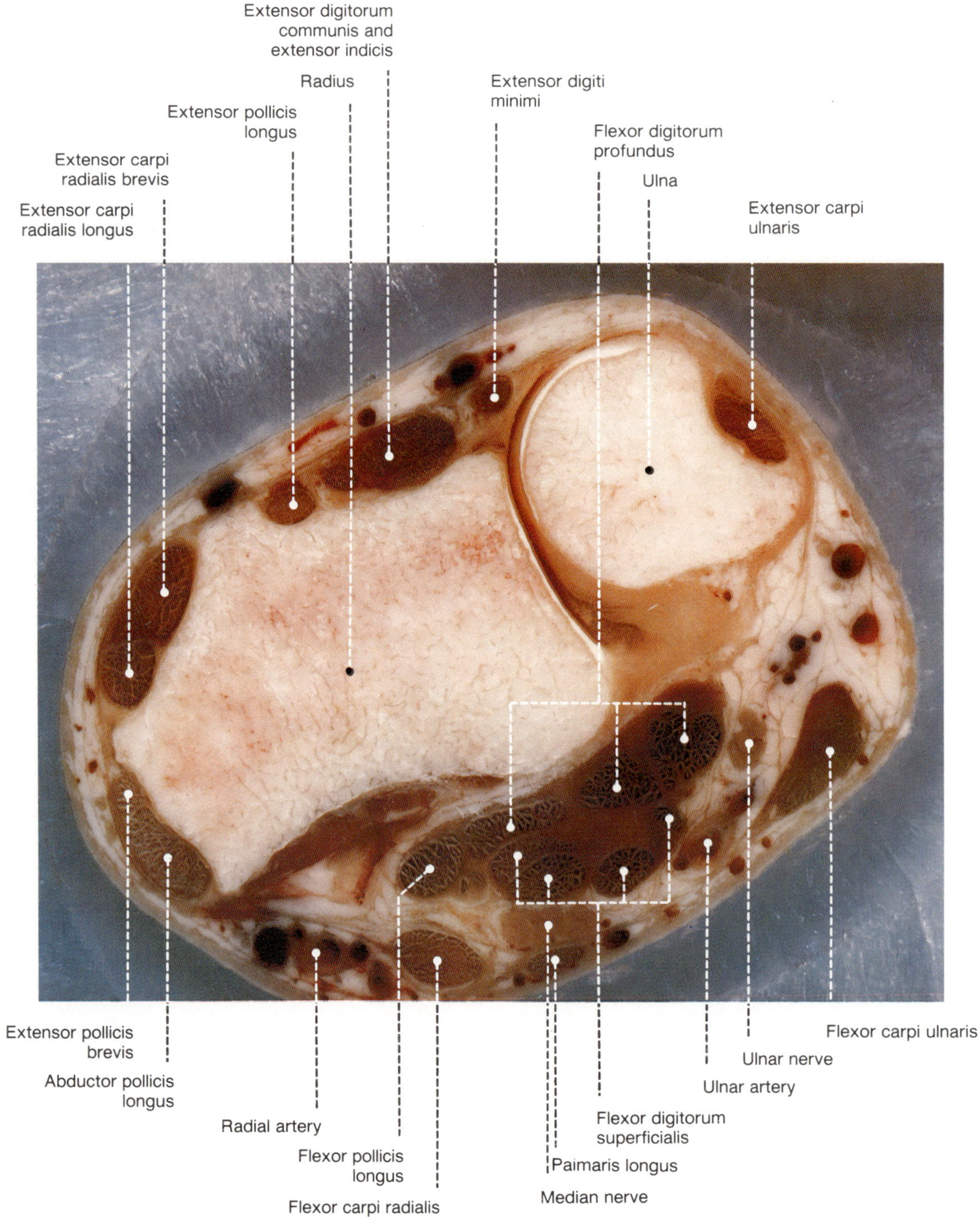

- Extensor carpi radialis longus
- Extensor carpi radialis brevis
- Extensor pollicis longus
- Radius
- Extensor digitorum communis and extensor indicis
- Extensor digiti minimi
- Flexor digitorum profundus
- Ulna
- Extensor carpi ulnaris

- Extensor pollicis brevis
- Abductor pollicis longus
- Radial artery
- Flexor pollicis longus
- Flexor carpi radialis
- Palmaris longus
- Median nerve
- Flexor digitorum superficialis
- Ulnar artery
- Ulnar nerve
- Flexor carpi ulnaris

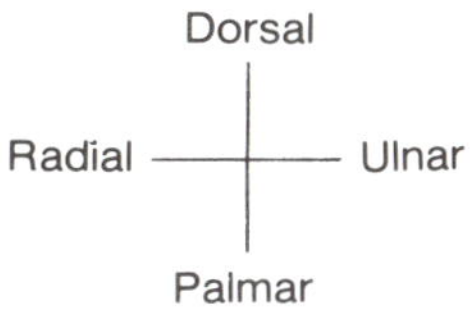

Dorsal
Radial
Ulnar
Palmar

FIG. 4–6

AXIAL

Extensor digitorum communis and extensor indicis
Scaphoid
Extensor pollicis longus
Extensor carpi radialis brevis
Extensor carpi radialis longus
Lunate
Extensor digiti minimi
Flexor digitorum profundus
Triquetrum
Extensor carpi ulnaris
Extensor pollicis brevis
Abductor pollicis longus
Radial styloid
Radial artery
Flexor carpi radialis
Flexor pollicis longus
Palmaris longus
Median nerve
Flexor digitorum superficialis
Ulnar artery
Ulnar nerve
Flexor carpi ulnaris

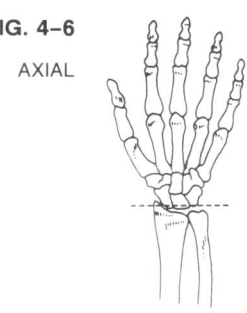

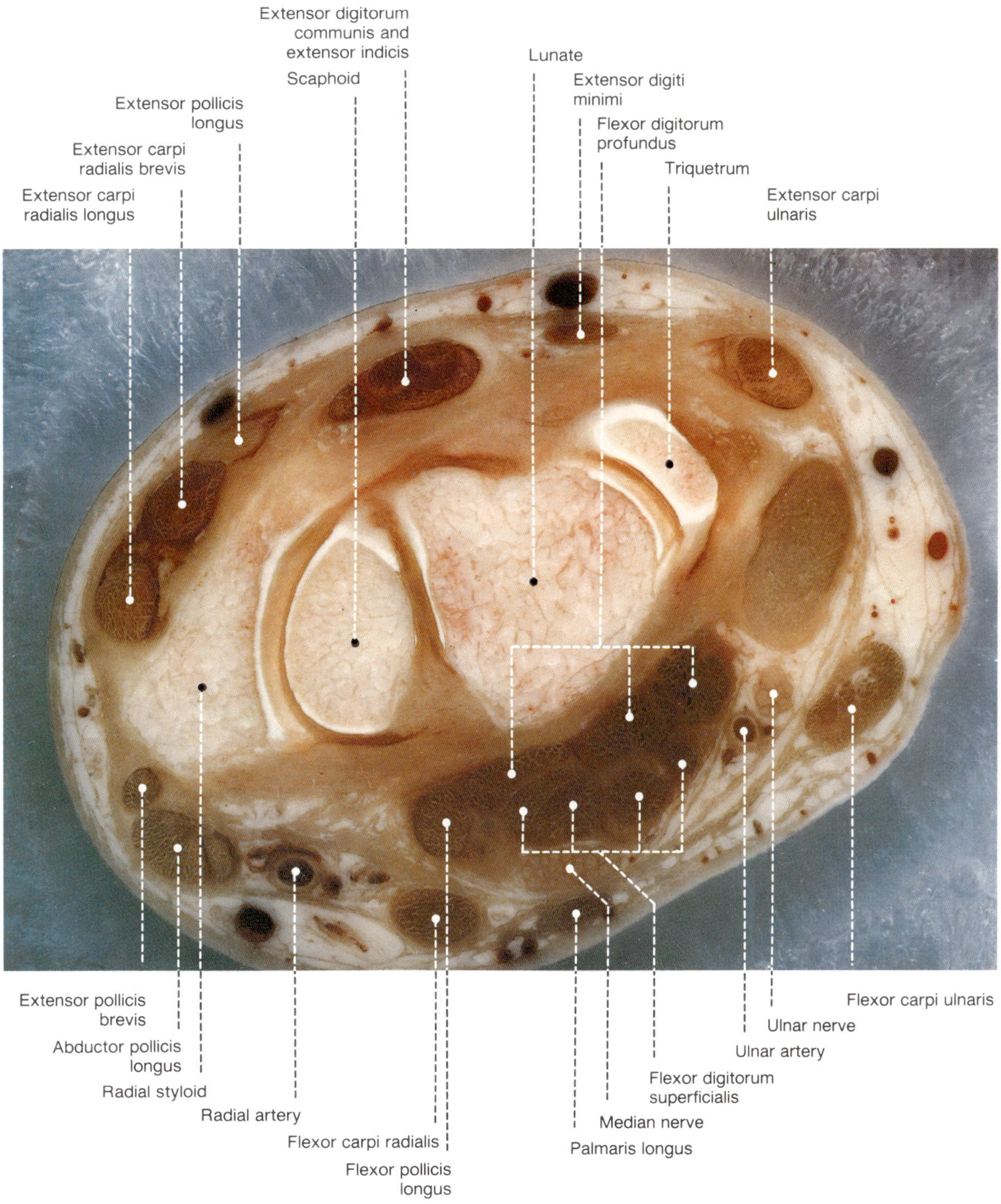

Anatomy and MRI of the Joints

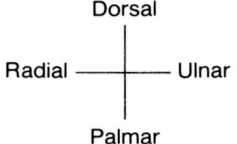

FIG. 4-7
AXIAL

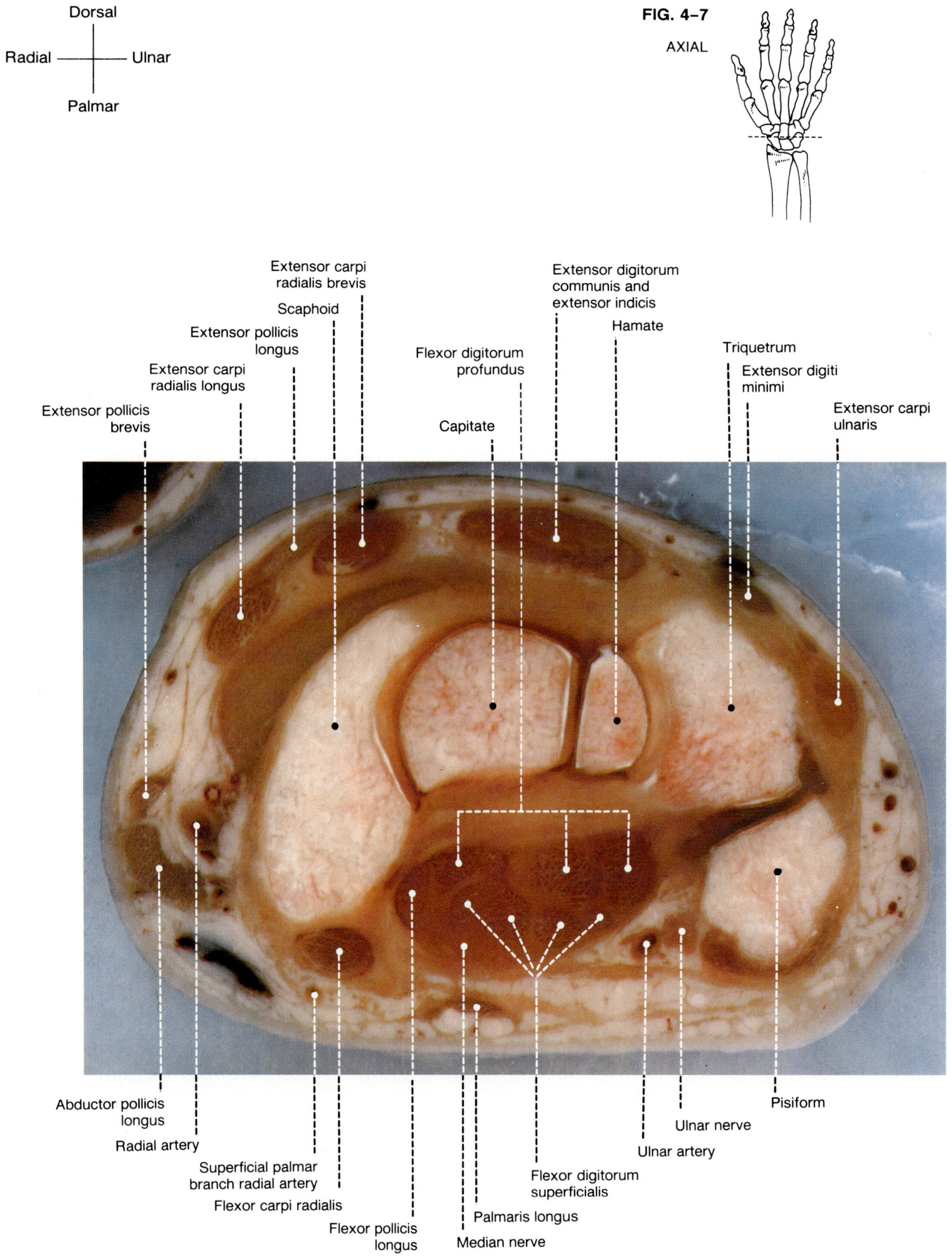

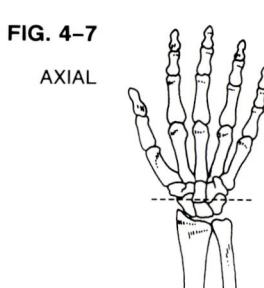

Labels (clockwise/around the axial section):
- Extensor pollicis brevis
- Extensor carpi radialis longus
- Extensor pollicis longus
- Extensor carpi radialis brevis
- Scaphoid
- Flexor digitorum profundus
- Capitate
- Extensor digitorum communis and extensor indicis
- Hamate
- Triquetrum
- Extensor digiti minimi
- Extensor carpi ulnaris
- Pisiform
- Ulnar nerve
- Ulnar artery
- Flexor digitorum superficialis
- Palmaris longus
- Median nerve
- Flexor pollicis longus
- Flexor carpi radialis
- Superficial palmar branch radial artery
- Radial artery
- Abductor pollicis longus

91 THE WRIST

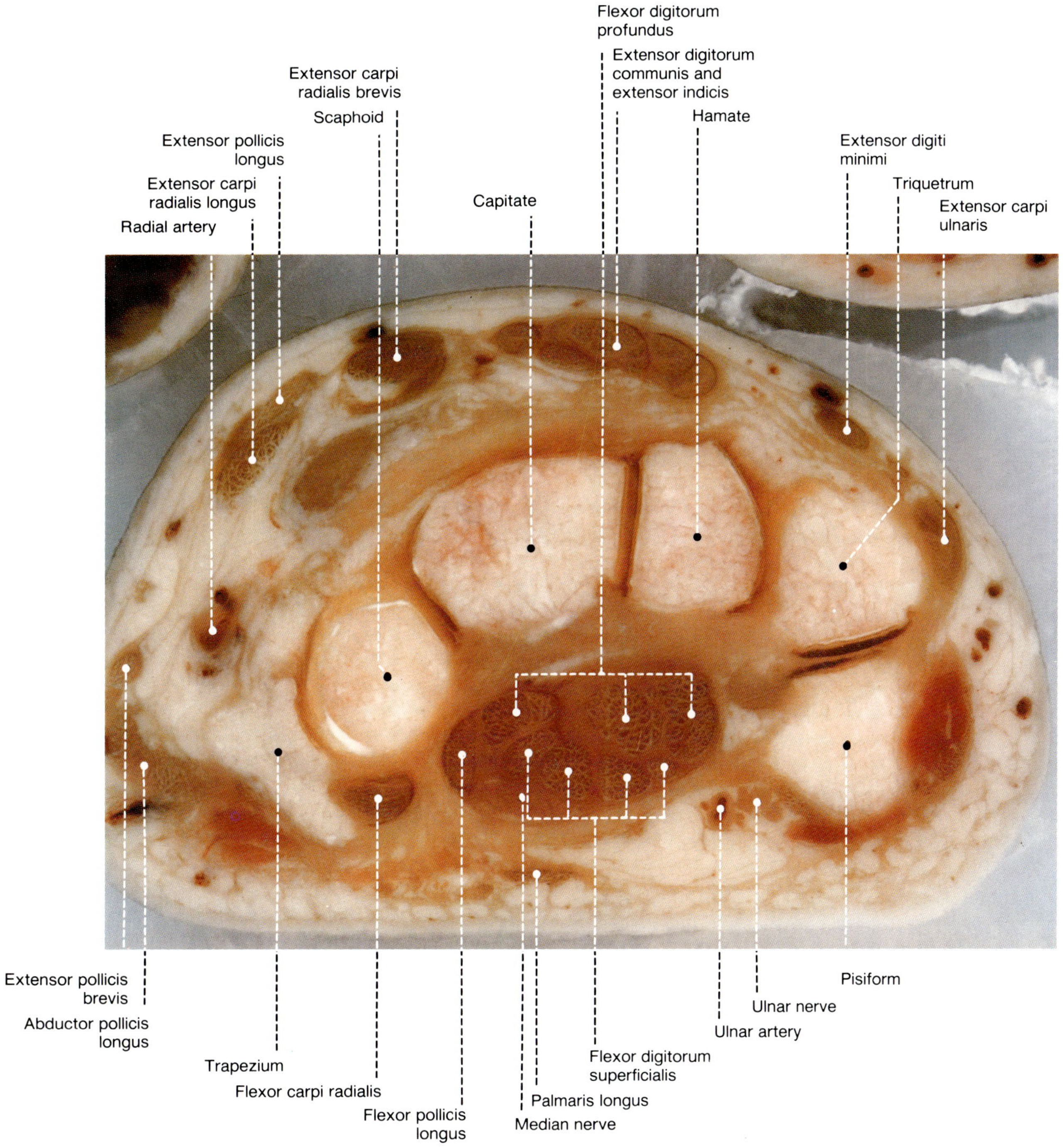

FIG. 4–8

AXIAL

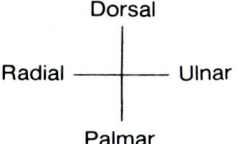
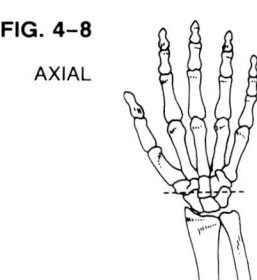

Anatomy and MRI of the Joints 92

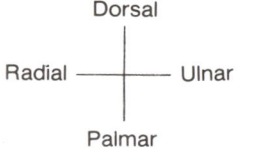

FIG. 4–9
AXIAL

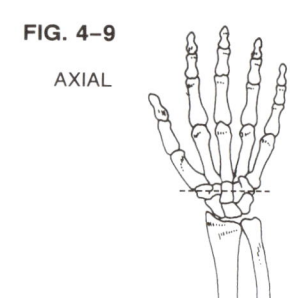

Figure labels (top, left to right): Extensor pollicis brevis; Radial artery; Extensor pollicis longus; Extensor carpi radialis longus; Trapezoid; Extensor carpi radialis brevis; Capitate; Flexor digitorum profundus; Extensor digitorum communis and extensor indicis; Hamate; Hook of hamate; Extensor digiti minimi; Extensor carpi ulnaris.

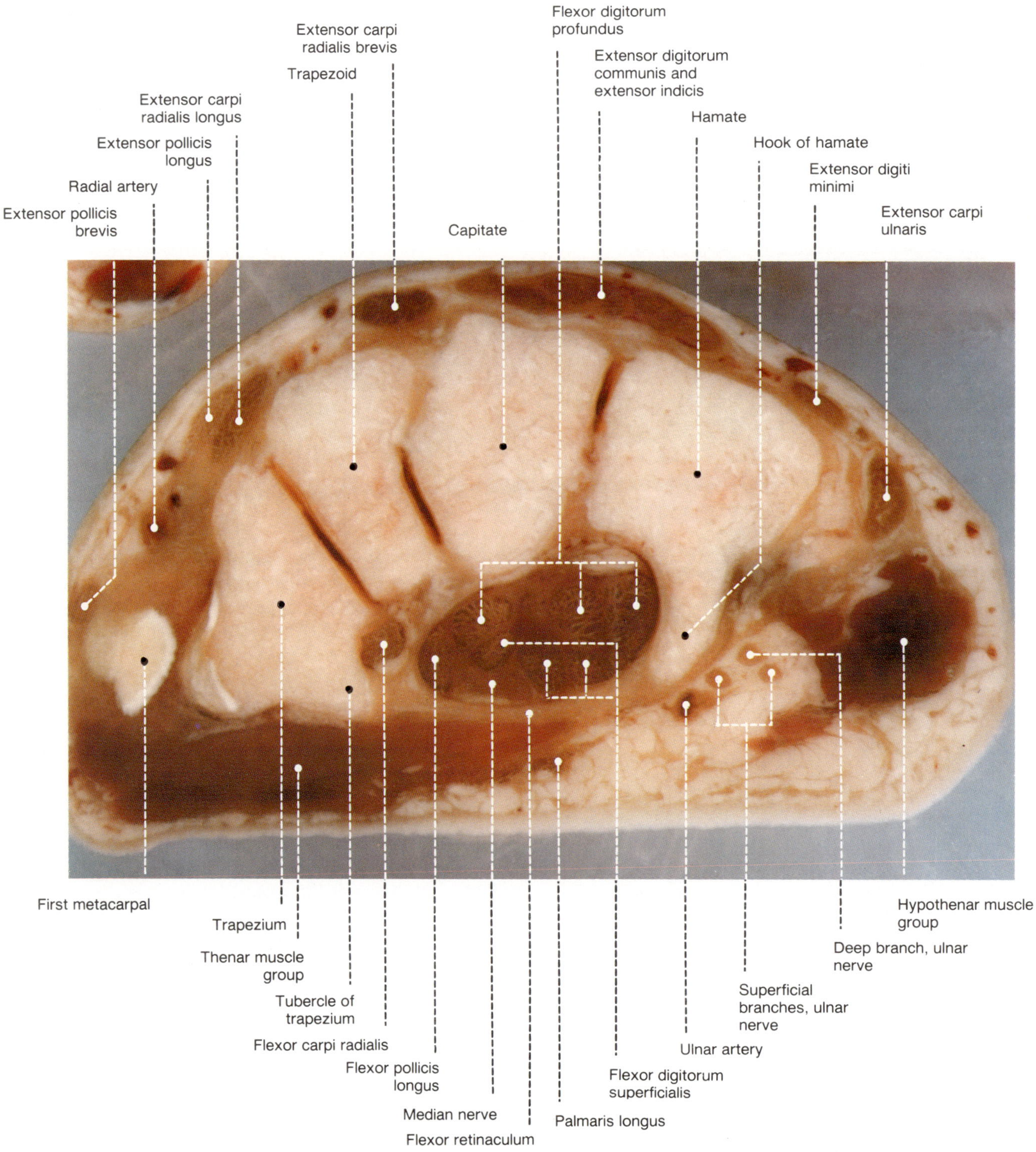

Figure labels (bottom, left to right): First metacarpal; Trapezium; Thenar muscle group; Tubercle of trapezium; Flexor carpi radialis; Flexor pollicis longus; Median nerve; Flexor retinaculum; Palmaris longus; Flexor digitorum superficialis; Ulnar artery; Superficial branches, ulnar nerve; Deep branch, ulnar nerve; Hypothenar muscle group.

Orientation: Dorsal / Palmar / Radial / Ulnar

93 THE WRIST

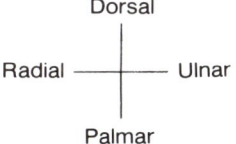

FIG. 4–10

AXIAL

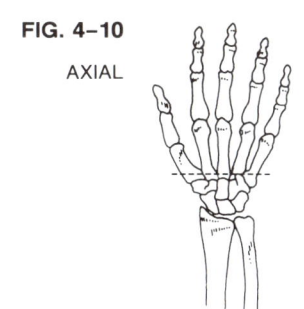

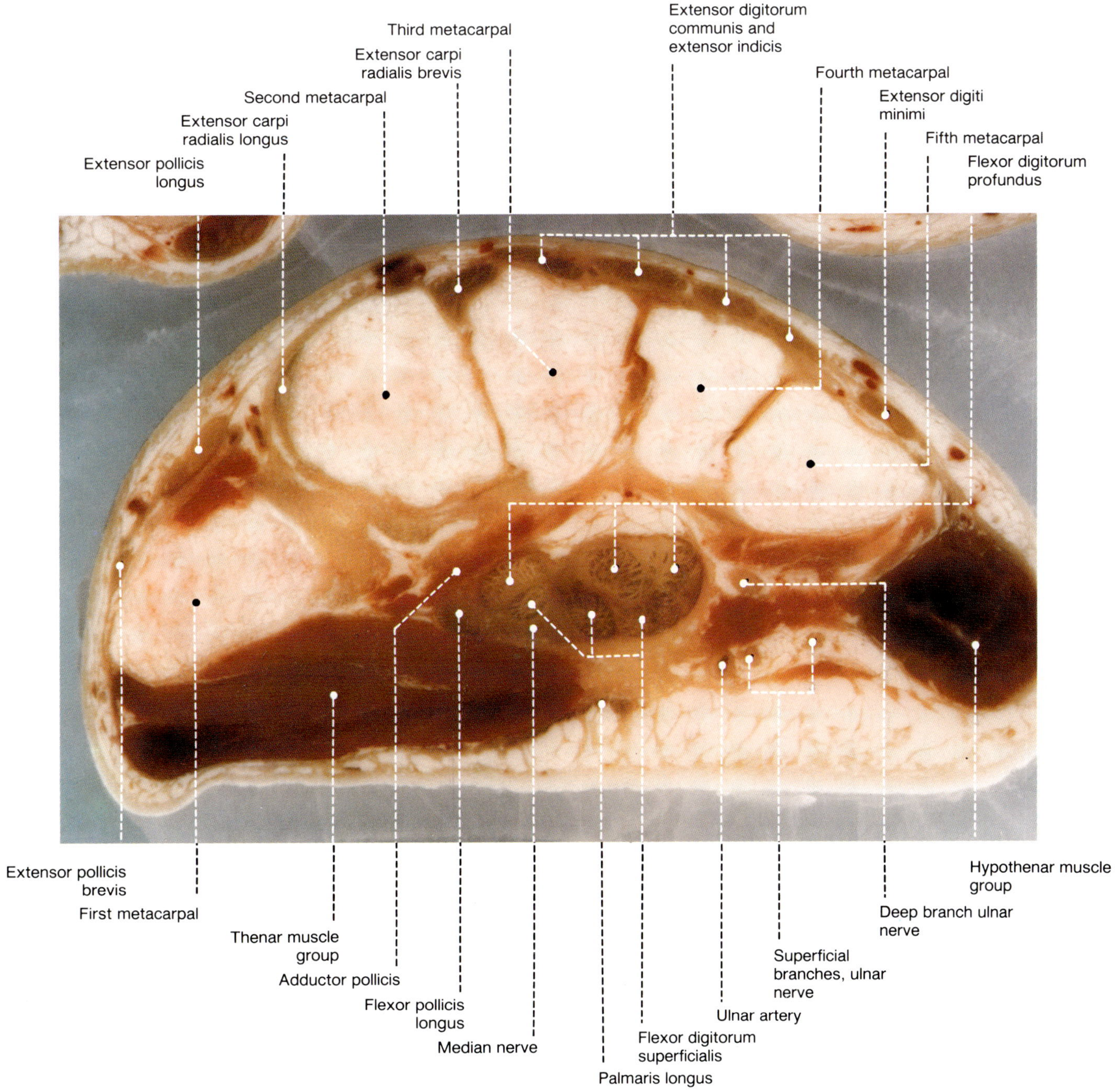

Labels (clockwise/around figure):
- Extensor pollicis longus
- Extensor carpi radialis longus
- Second metacarpal
- Extensor carpi radialis brevis
- Third metacarpal
- Extensor digitorum communis and extensor indicis
- Fourth metacarpal
- Extensor digiti minimi
- Fifth metacarpal
- Flexor digitorum profundus
- Hypothenar muscle group
- Deep branch ulnar nerve
- Superficial branches, ulnar nerve
- Ulnar artery
- Flexor digitorum superficialis
- Palmaris longus
- Median nerve
- Flexor pollicis longus
- Adductor pollicis
- Thenar muscle group
- First metacarpal
- Extensor pollicis brevis

Anatomy and MRI of the Joints 94

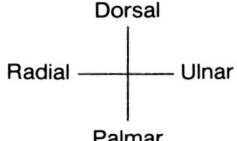

FIG. 4-11

AXIAL

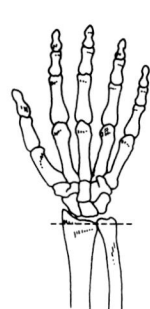

Extensor pollicis brevis
Extensor carpi radialis longus
Extensor carpi radialis brevis
Extensor pollicis longus
Radius
Flexor digitorum profundus
Extensor digitorum communis and extensor indicis
Extensor digiti minimi
Ulna
Extensor carpi ulnaris

Abductor pollicis longus
Radial artery
Flexor carpi radialis
Flexor pollicis longus
Median nerve
Palmaris longus
Flexor digitorum superficialis
Flexor carpi ulnaris
Ulnar nerve
Ulnar artery

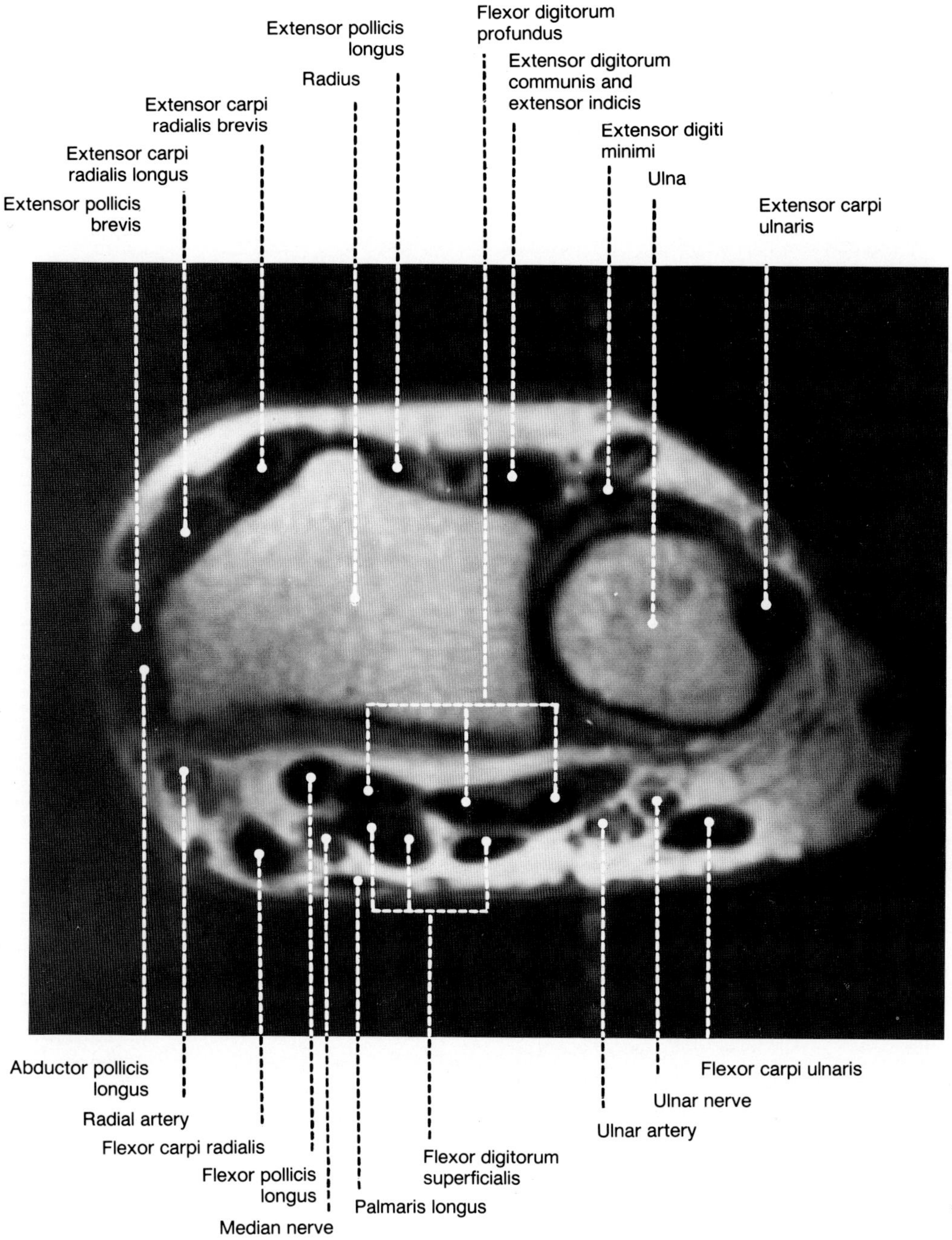

Dorsal
Radial Ulnar
Palmar

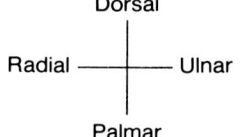

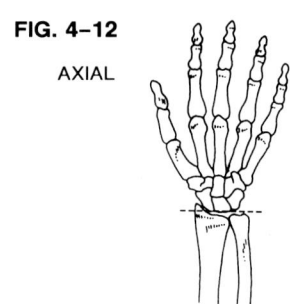

FIG. 4–12

AXIAL

Scaphoid
Extensor pollicis longus
Flexor digitorum profundus
Extensor carpi radialis brevis
Extensor digitorum communis and extensor indicis
Radial styloid
Lunate
Extensor carpi radialis longus
Extensor digiti minimi
Extensor pollicis brevis
Extensor carpi ulnaris
Abductor pollicis longus
Radial artery
Flexor carpi radialis
Flexor pollicis longus
Median nerve
Palmaris longus
Flexor digitorum superficialis
Ulnar artery
Ulnar nerve
Flexor carpi ulnaris

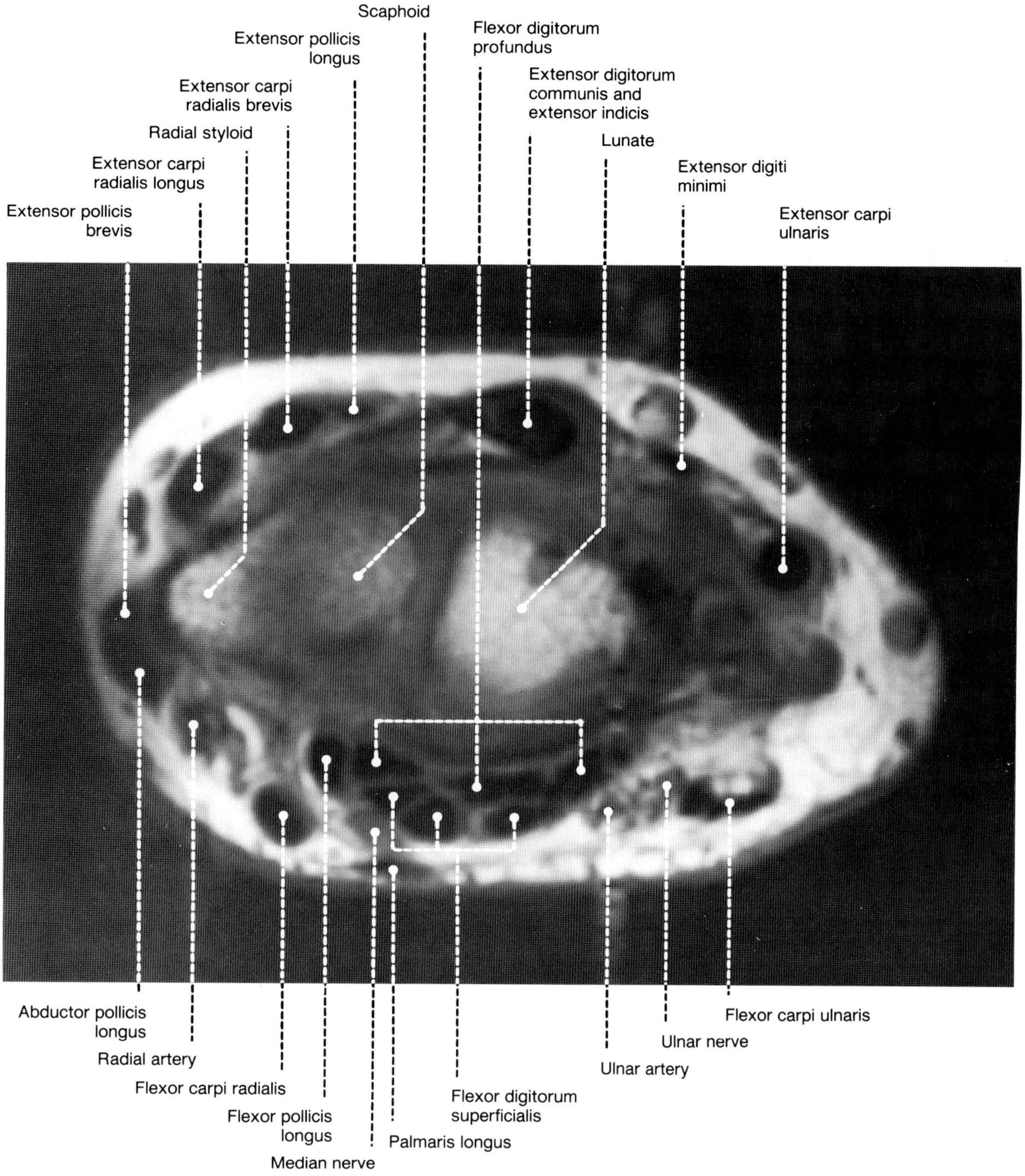

Anatomy and MRI of the Joints 96

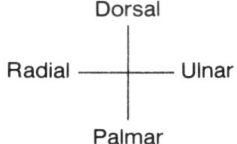

FIG. 4–13

AXIAL

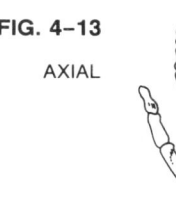

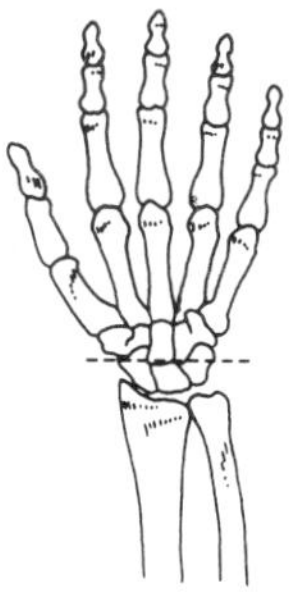

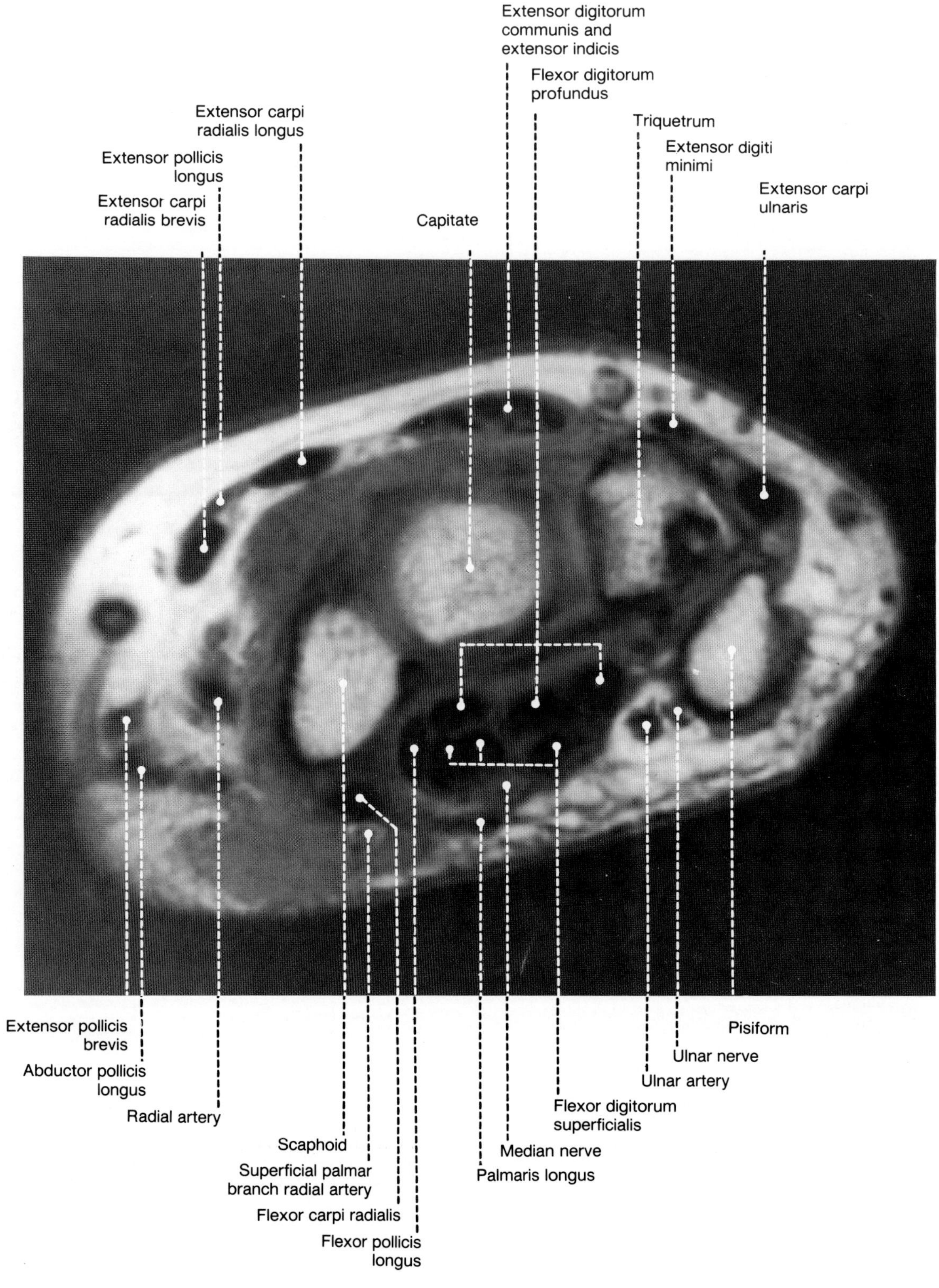

THE WRIST

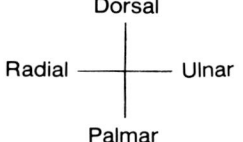

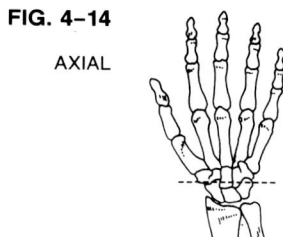

FIG. 4-14

AXIAL

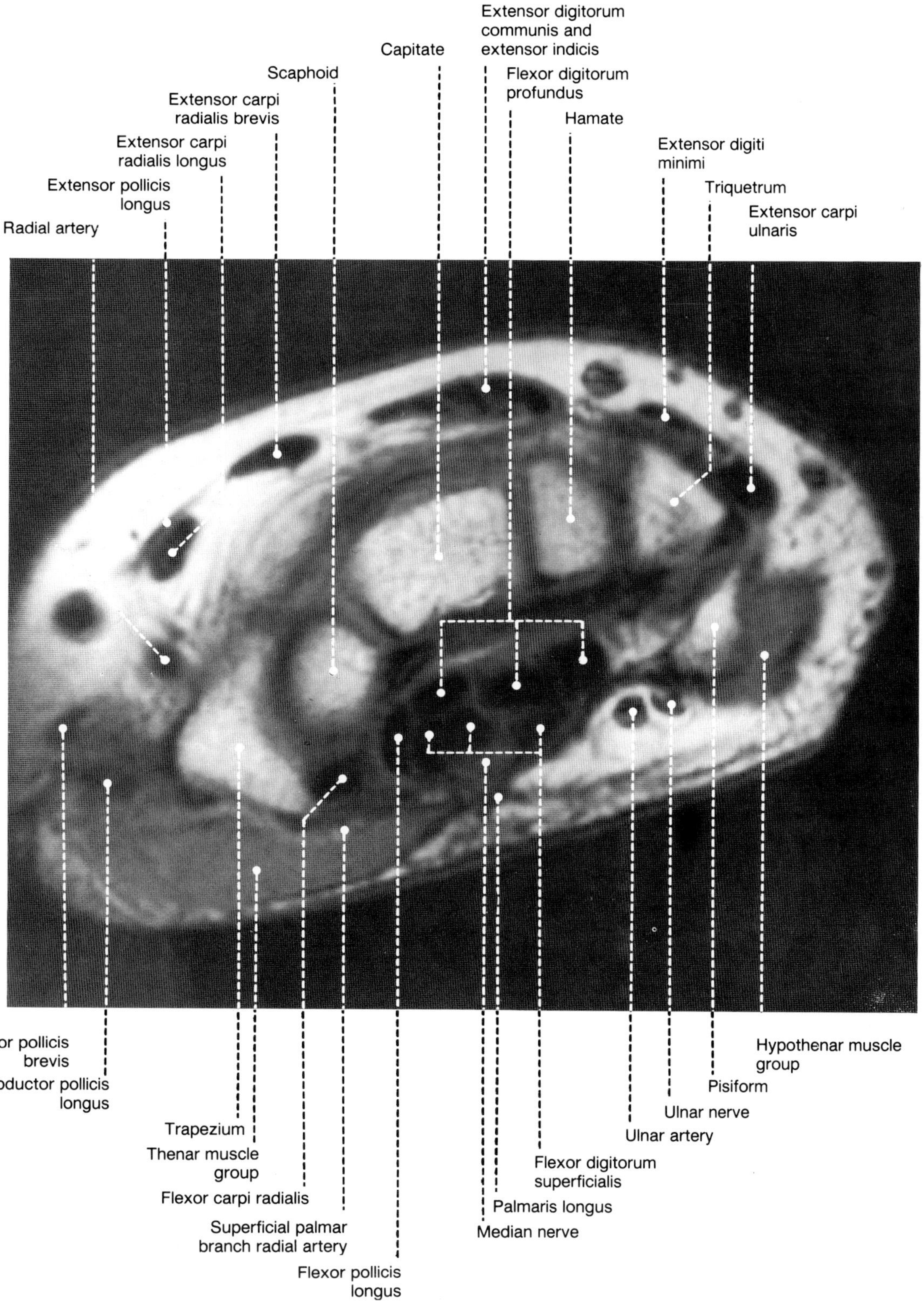

Anatomy and MRI of the Joints

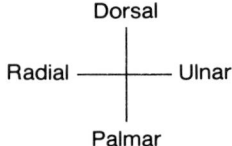

FIG. 4–15

AXIAL

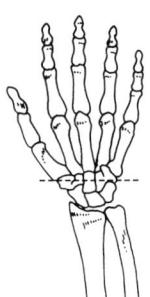

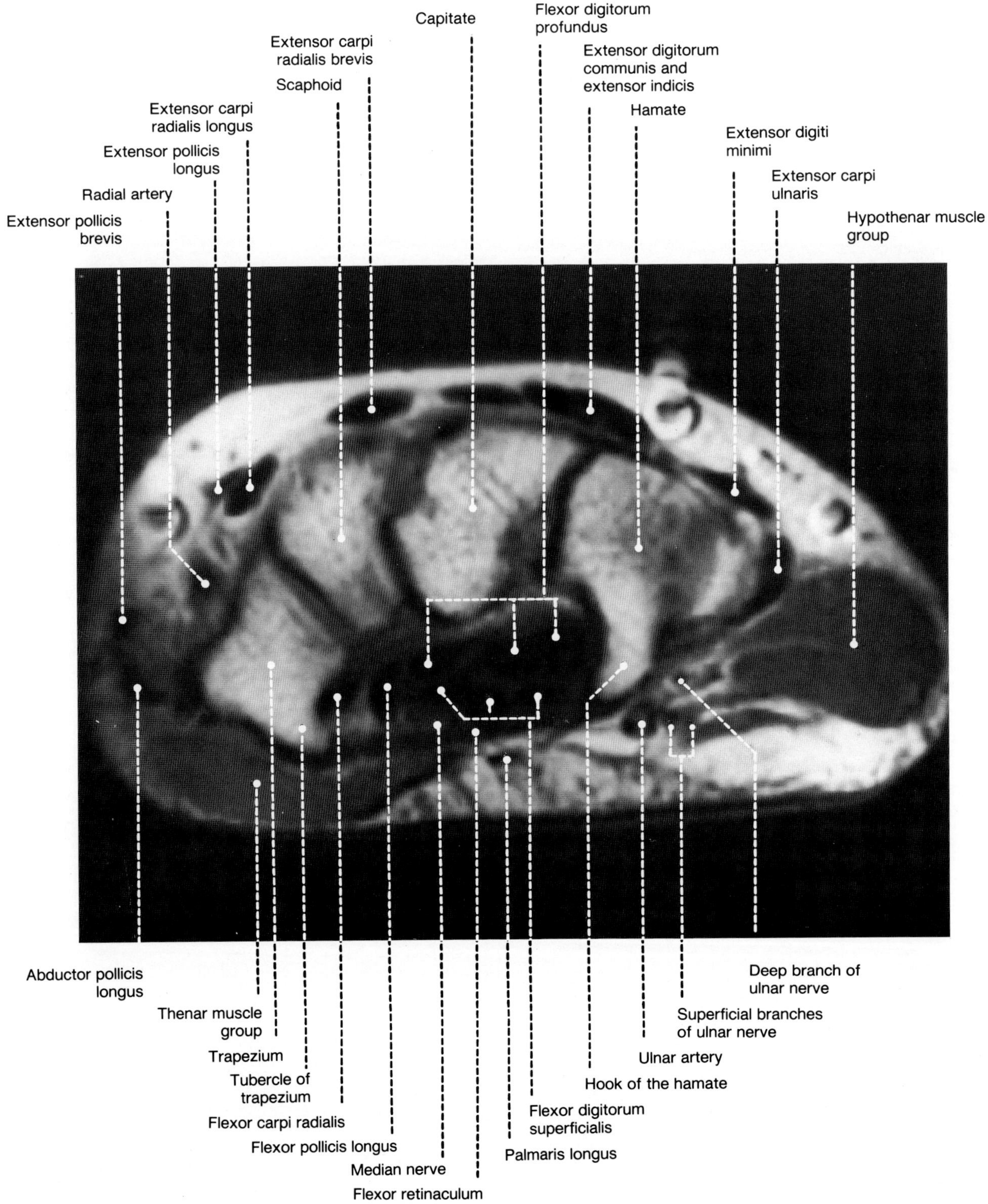

Labels (clockwise/around the axial MRI):
- Extensor pollicis brevis
- Radial artery
- Extensor pollicis longus
- Extensor carpi radialis longus
- Extensor carpi radialis brevis
- Scaphoid
- Capitate
- Flexor digitorum profundus
- Extensor digitorum communis and extensor indicis
- Hamate
- Extensor digiti minimi
- Extensor carpi ulnaris
- Hypothenar muscle group
- Abductor pollicis longus
- Thenar muscle group
- Trapezium
- Tubercle of trapezium
- Flexor carpi radialis
- Flexor pollicis longus
- Median nerve
- Flexor retinaculum
- Palmaris longus
- Flexor digitorum superficialis
- Hook of the hamate
- Ulnar artery
- Superficial branches of ulnar nerve
- Deep branch of ulnar nerve

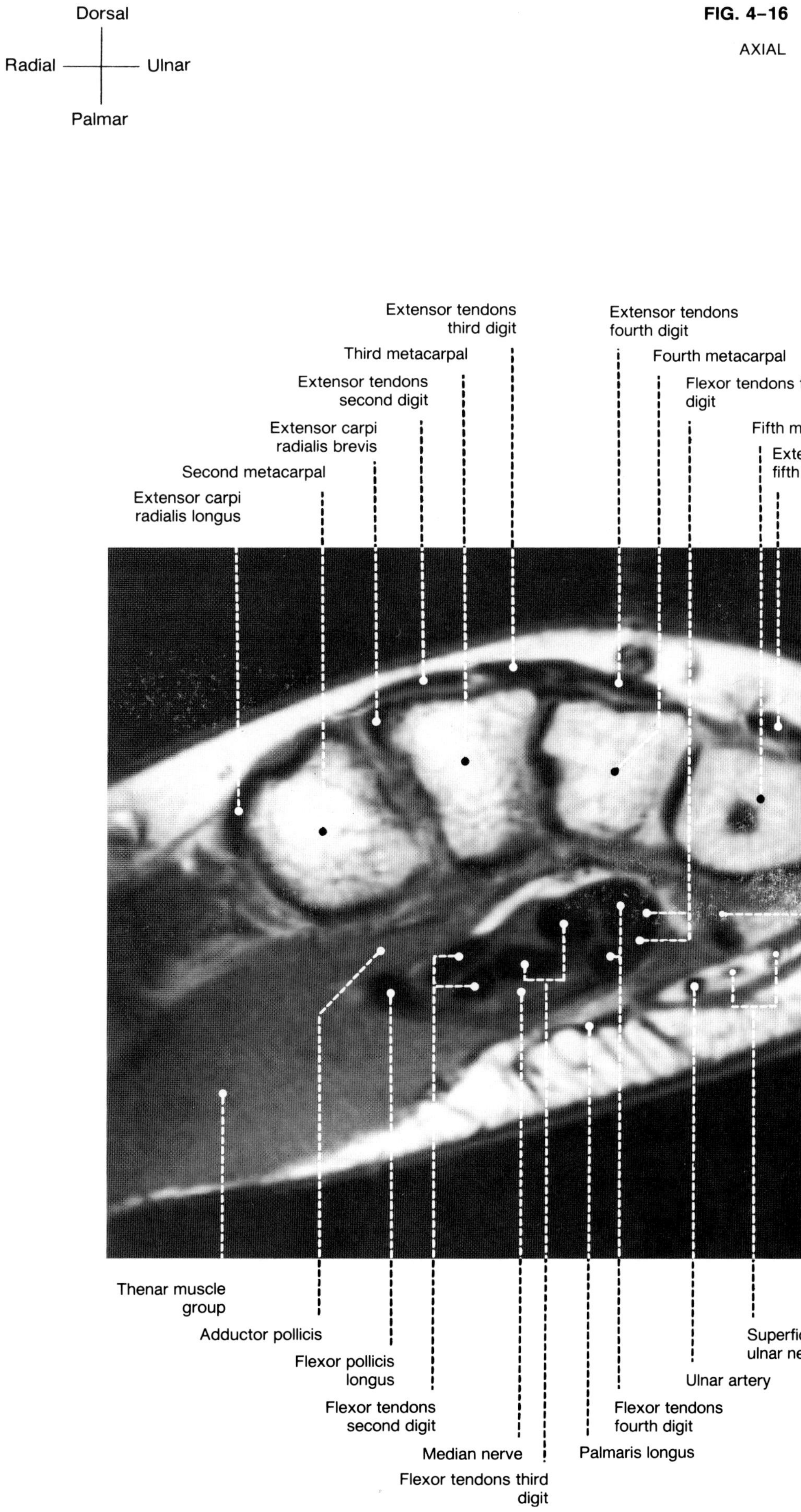

THE WRIST

FIG. 4-16

AXIAL

Dorsal / Radial — Ulnar / Palmar

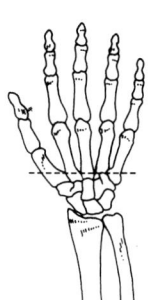

Labels (top, left to right):
- Extensor carpi radialis longus
- Second metacarpal
- Extensor carpi radialis brevis
- Extensor tendons second digit
- Third metacarpal
- Extensor tendons third digit
- Extensor tendons fourth digit
- Fourth metacarpal
- Flexor tendons fifth digit
- Fifth metacarpal
- Extensor tendons fifth digit
- Hypothenar muscle group

Labels (bottom, left to right):
- Thenar muscle group
- Adductor pollicis
- Flexor pollicis longus
- Flexor tendons second digit
- Median nerve
- Flexor tendons third digit
- Palmaris longus
- Flexor tendons fourth digit
- Ulnar artery
- Superficial branches ulnar nerve
- Deep branch ulnar nerve

Anatomy and MRI of the Joints

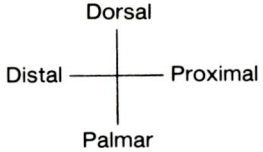

FIG. 4–17
SAGITTAL

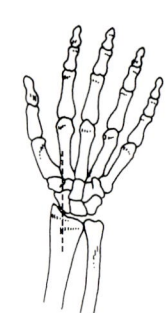

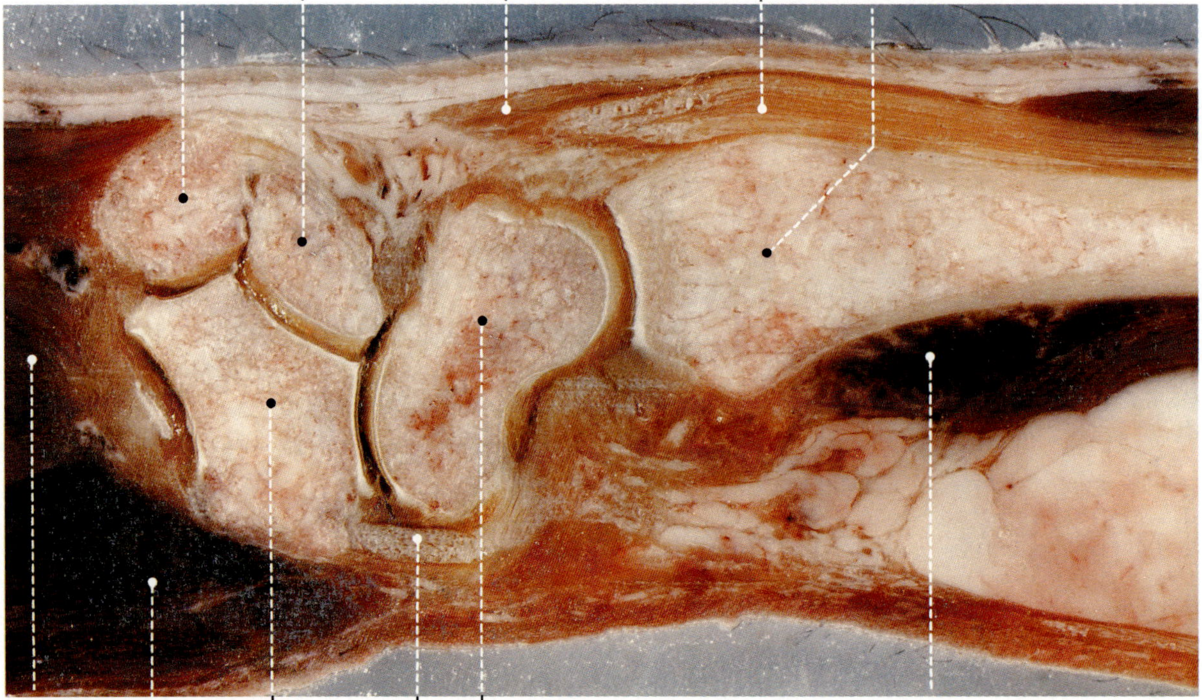

101 THE WRIST

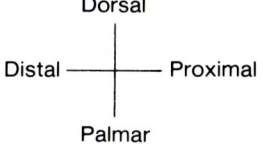

Dorsal
Distal — Proximal
Palmar

FIG. 4-18
SAGITTAL

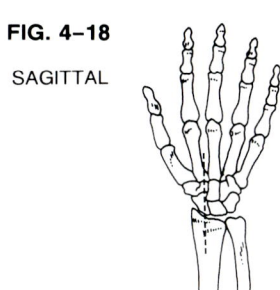

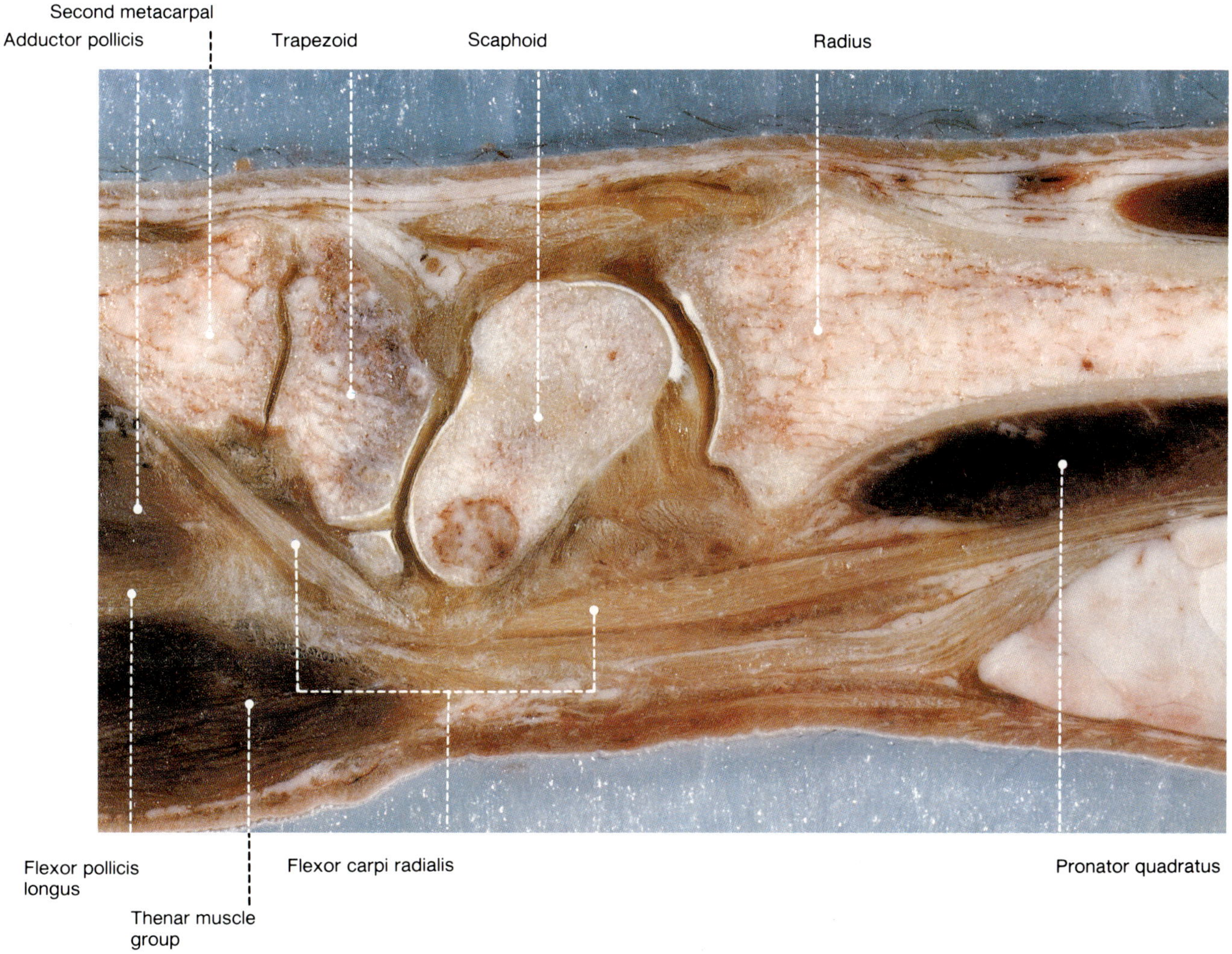

Second metacarpal · Adductor pollicis · Trapezoid · Scaphoid · Radius

Flexor pollicis longus · Thenar muscle group · Flexor carpi radialis · Pronator quadratus

Anatomy and MRI of the Joints   102

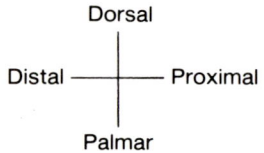
Dorsal
Distal —— Proximal
Palmar

FIG. 4–19
SAGITTAL
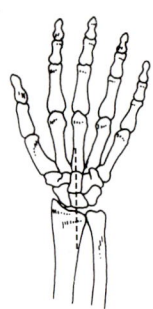

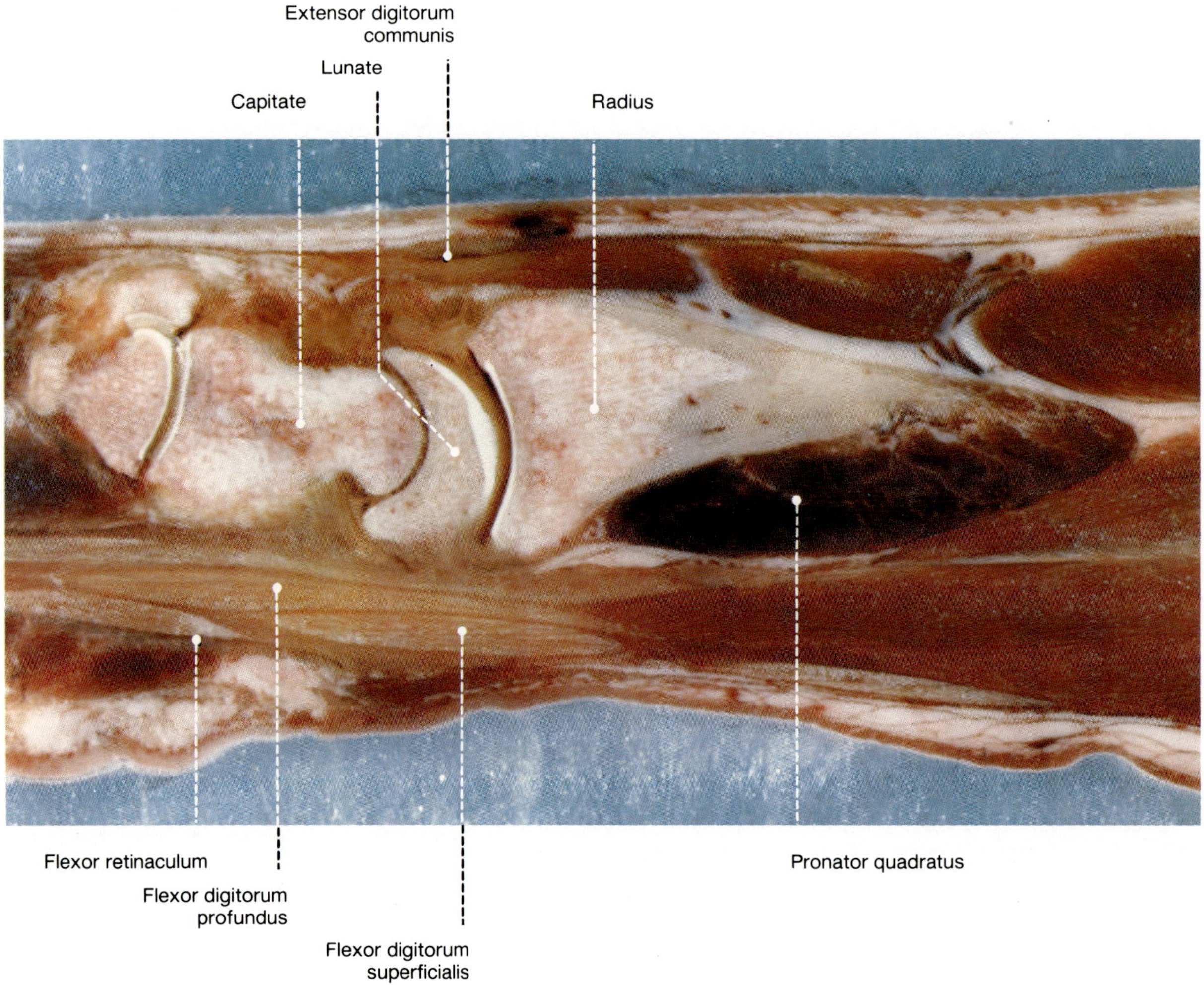

Capitate — Lunate — Extensor digitorum communis — Radius

Flexor retinaculum — Flexor digitorum profundus — Flexor digitorum superficialis — Pronator quadratus

Dorsal
Distal
Proximal
Palmar

FIG. 4–20

SAGITTAL

Hamate
Capitate
Lunate
Third metacarpal
Ulna
Flexor retinaculum
Flexor digitorum profundus
Flexor digitorum superficialis
Radius
Pronator quadratus

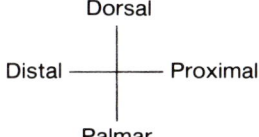

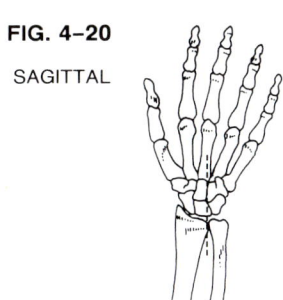

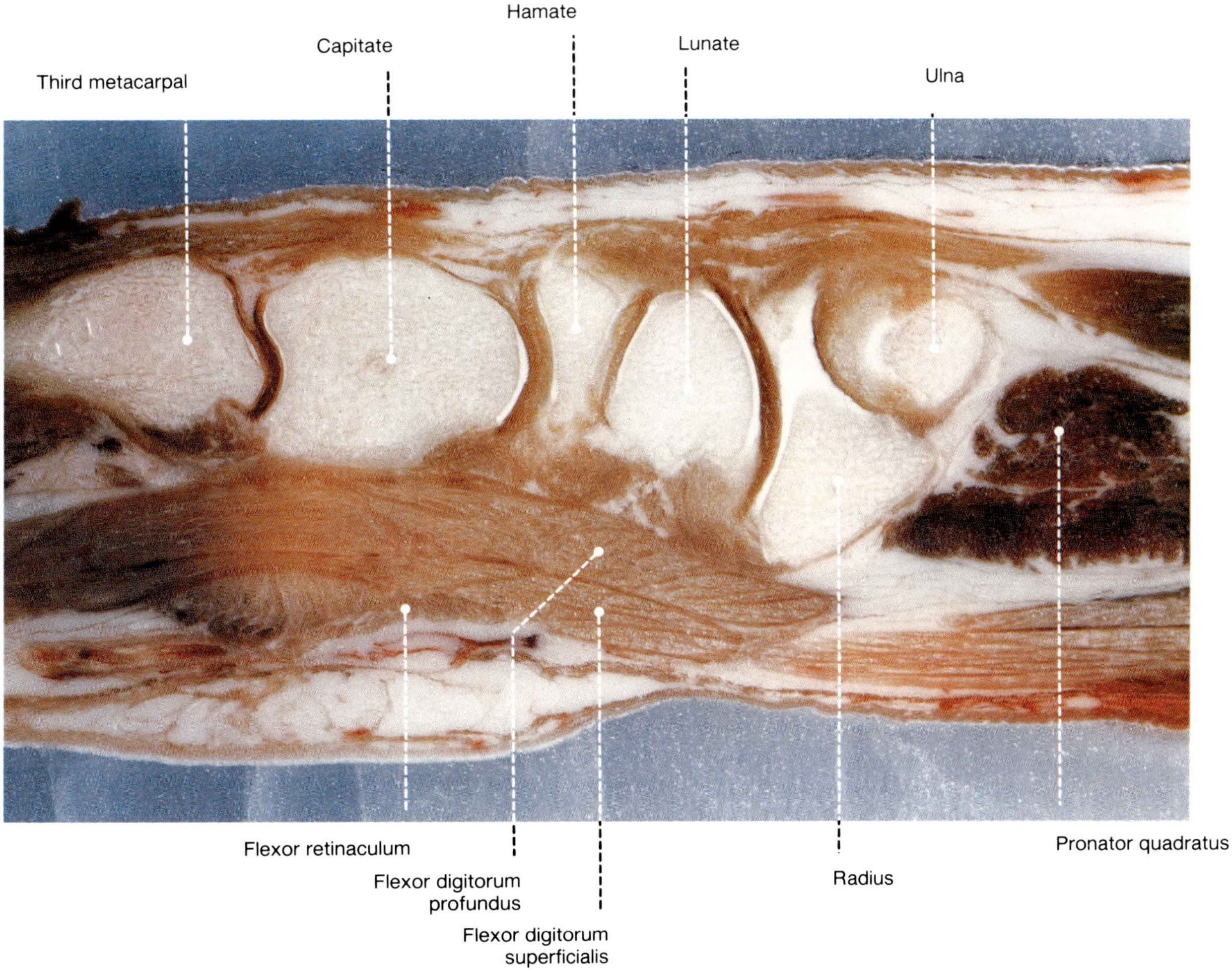

Anatomy and MRI of the Joints

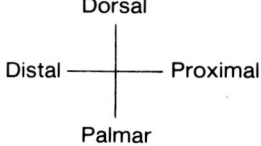

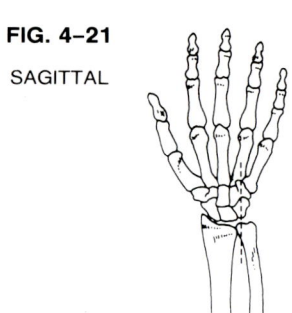

FIG. 4–21
SAGITTAL

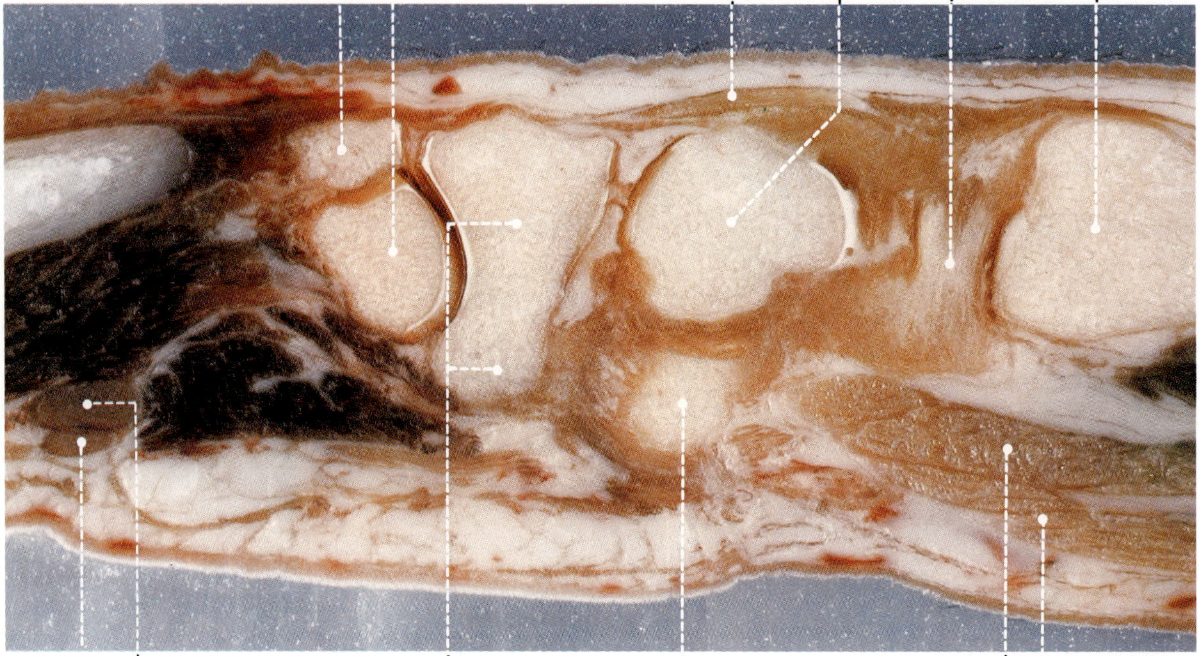

THE WRIST

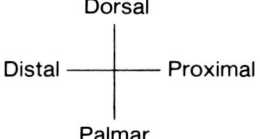

FIG. 4-22
SAGITTAL

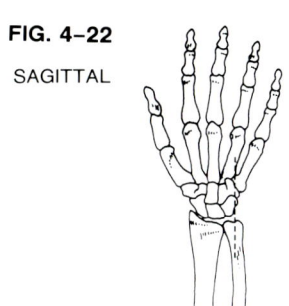

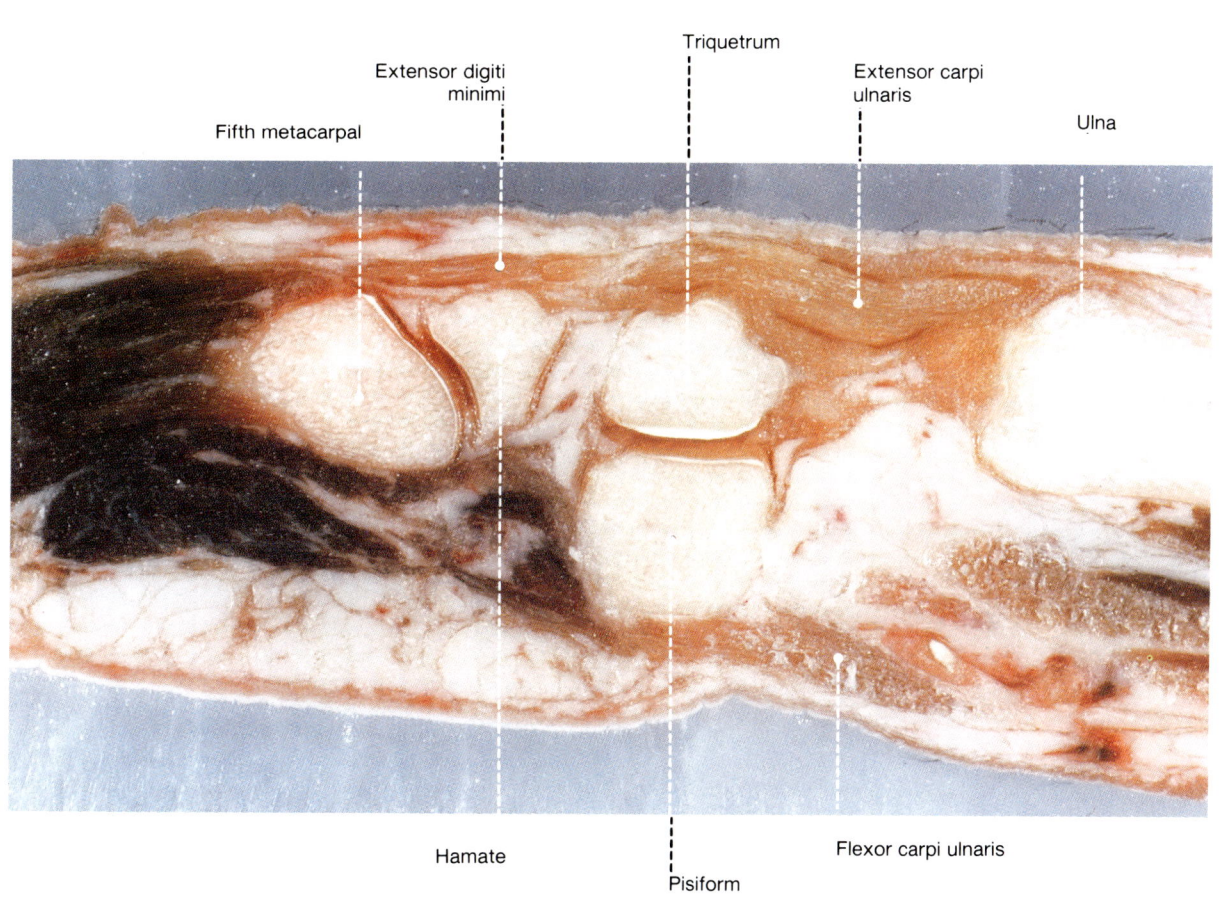

Anatomy and MRI of the Joints

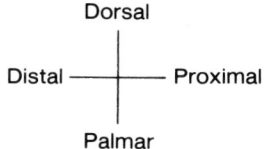

FIG. 4-23

SAGITTAL

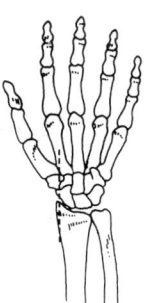

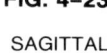

Adductor pollicis — Second metacarpal — Trapezoid — Extensor pollicis longus — Extensor carpi radialis longus

Flexor pollicis longus — Thenar muscle group — Trapezium — Scaphoid — Radius — Pronator quadratus

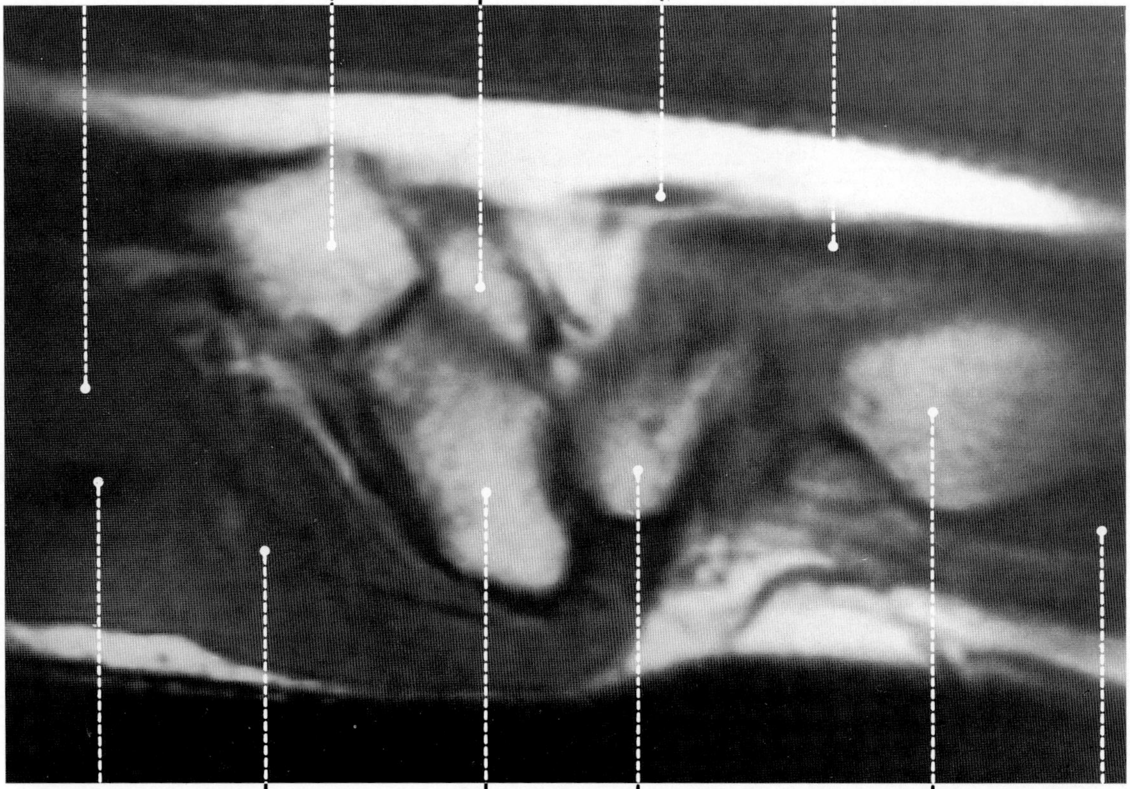

FIG. 4–24

SAGITTAL

Dorsal
Distal
Proximal
Palmar

Extensor pollicis longus
Extensor carpi radialis brevis
Trapezoid
Radius
Second metacarpal
Adductor pollicis
Flexor pollicis longus
Thenar muscle group
Flexor carpi radialis
Scaphoid
Pronator quadratus

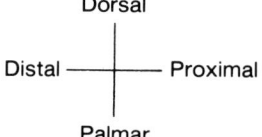

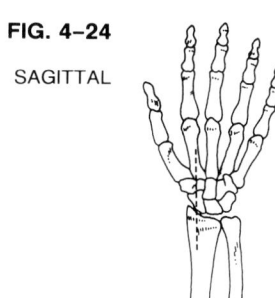

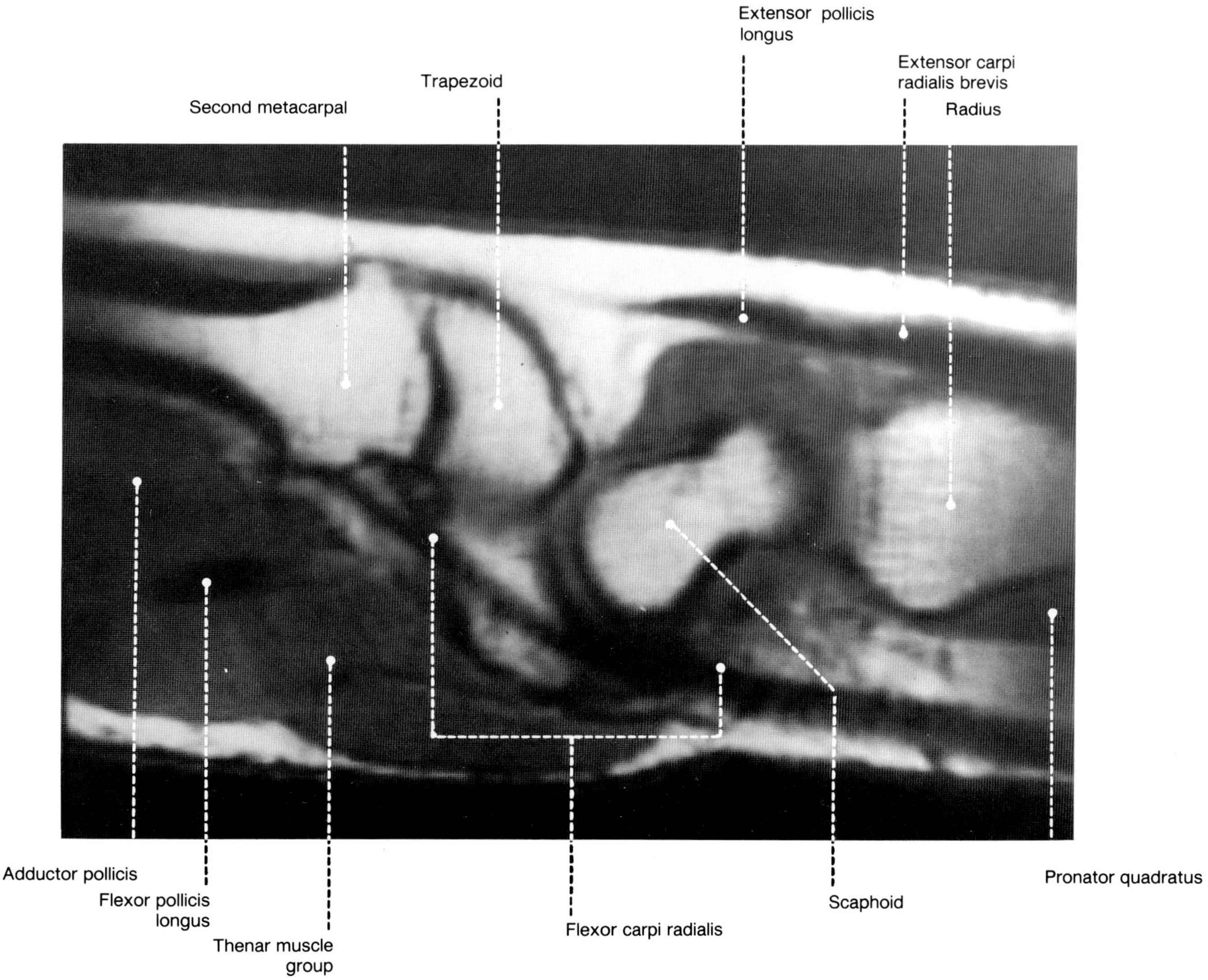

Anatomy and MRI of the Joints

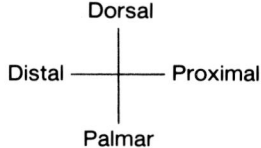

FIG. 4–25

SAGITTAL

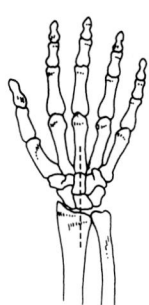

Third metacarpal | Capitate | Extensor digitorum communis and extensor indicis | Radius

Flexor retinaculum | Flexor digitorum superficialis | Flexor digitorum profundus | Lunate

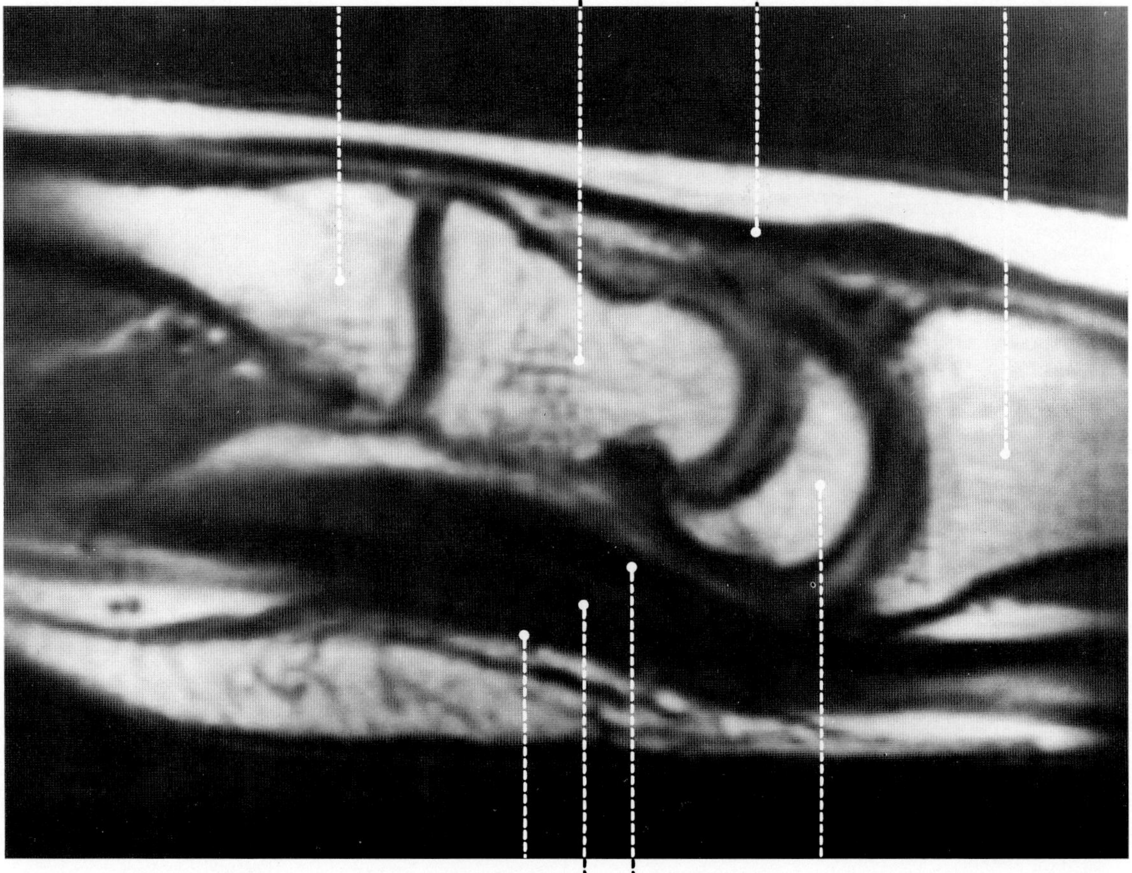

Dorsal
Distal
Proximal
Palmar

FIG. 4–26

SAGITTAL

Extensor digitorum communis and extensor indicis
Fourth metacarpal
Capitate
Flexor retinaculum
Flexor digitorum superficialis
Flexor digitorum profundus
Lunate
Radius

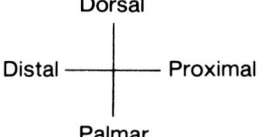

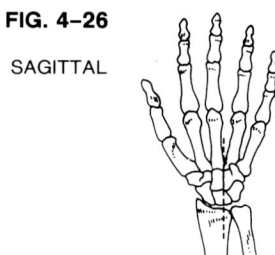

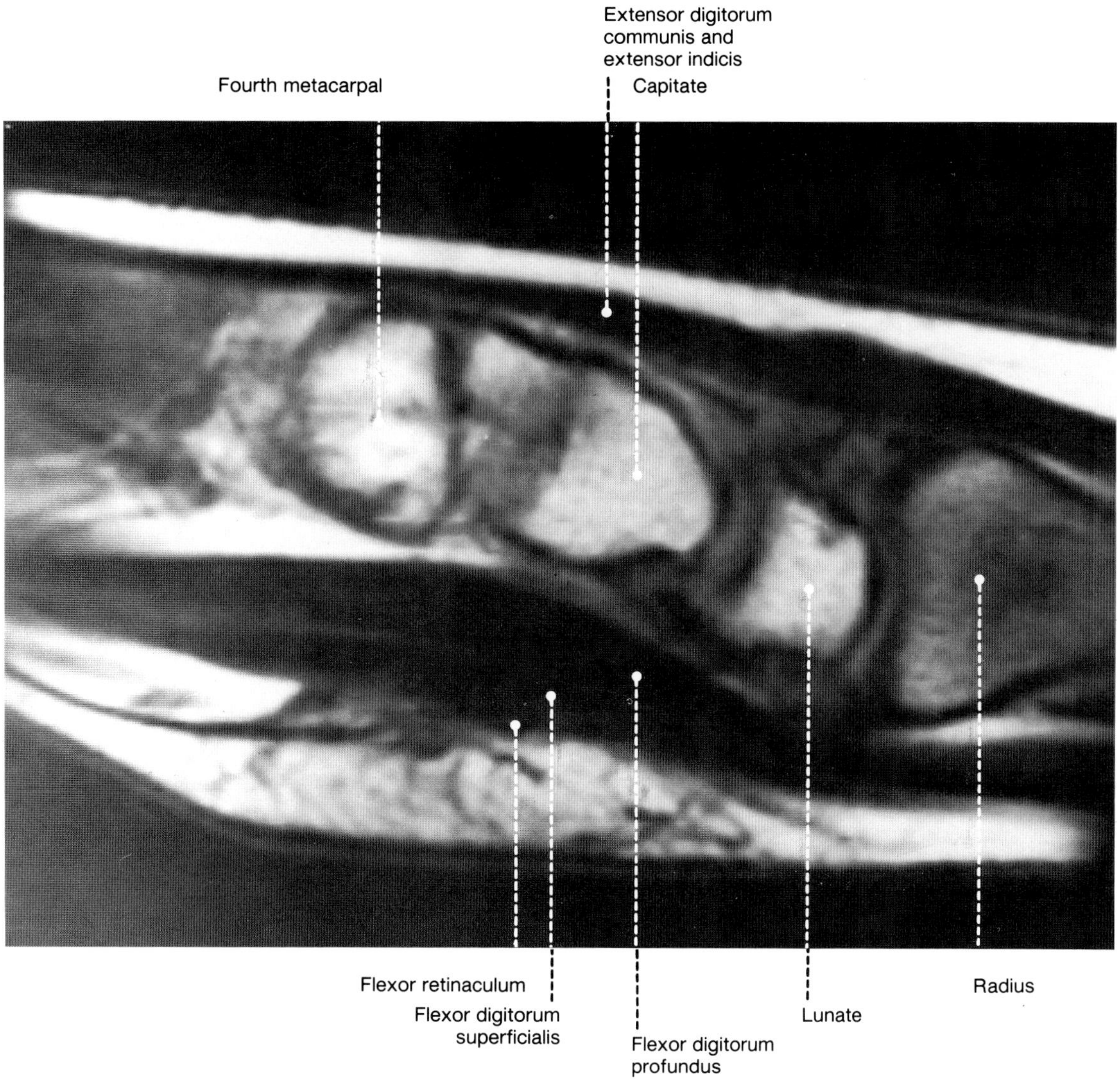

Anatomy and MRI of the Joints

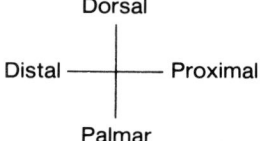

FIG. 4–27

SAGITTAL

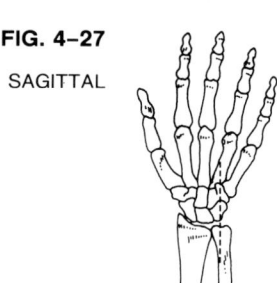

Flexor digitorum profundus — Fourth metacarpal — Extensor digitorum communis — Triquetrum — Extensor digiti minimi

Flexor digitorum superficialis — Hamate and hook of hamate — Ulnar artery — Pisohamate ligament — Triangular fibrocartilage — Ulna

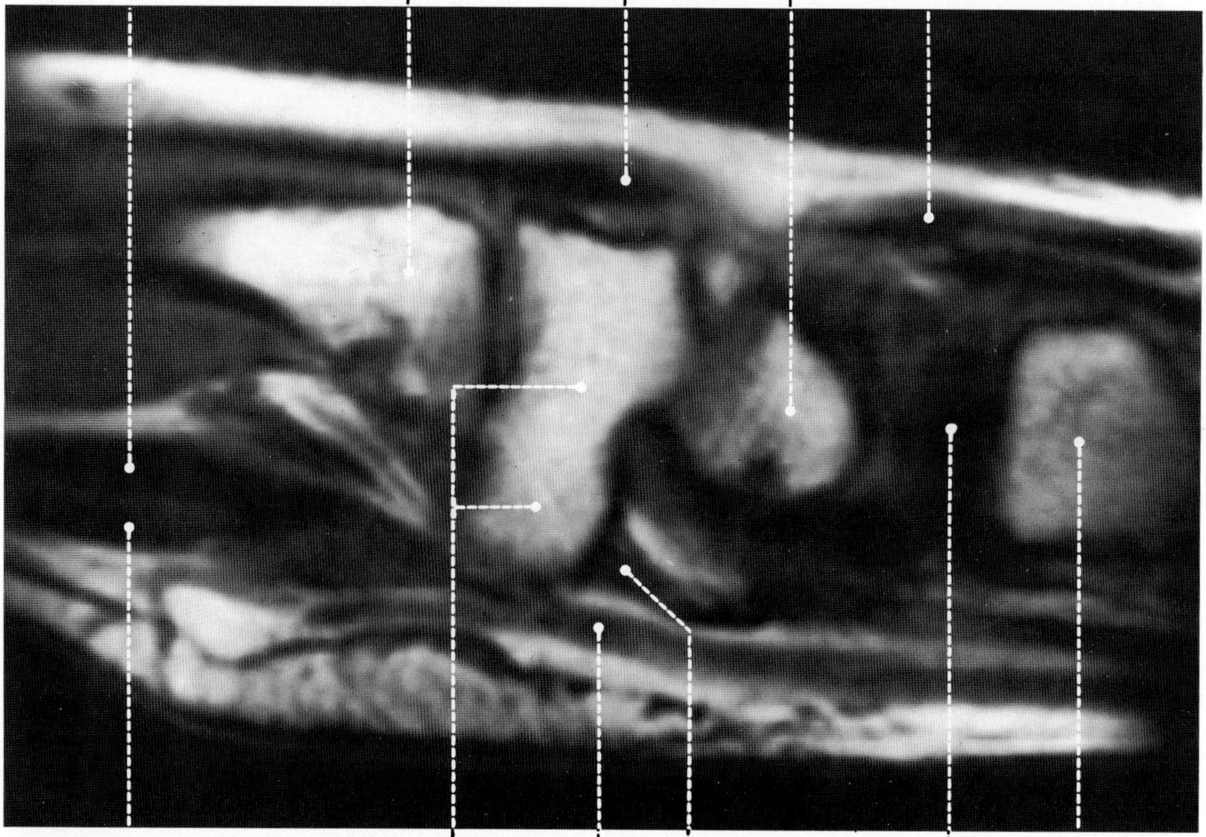

THE WRIST

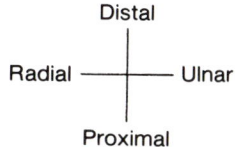
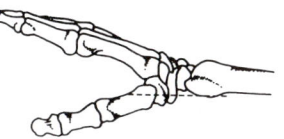

FIG. 4-28

CORONAL

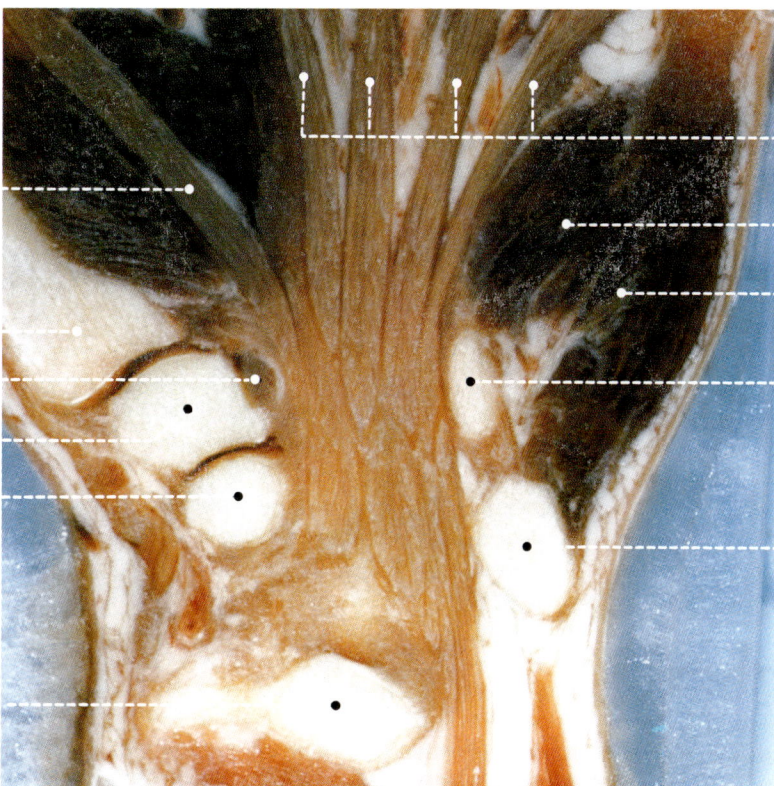

- Flexor pollicis longus
- First metacarpal
- Flexor carpi radialis
- Trapezium
- Distal scaphoid
- Distal radius
- Flexor digitorum superficialis tendons
- Opponens digiti minimi
- Abductor digiti minimi
- Hook of hamate
- Pisiform

Anatomy and MRI of the Joints

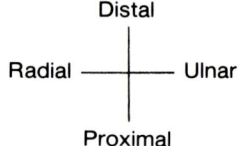

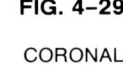
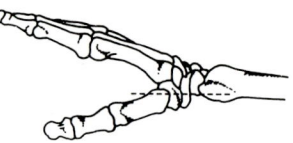

FIG. 4-29
CORONAL

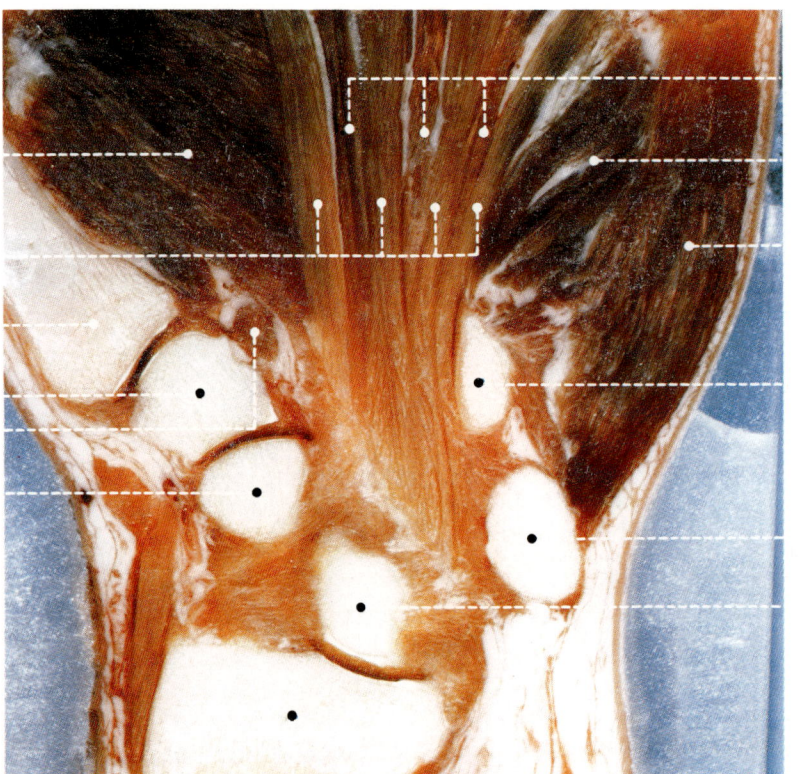

Adductor pollicis

Flexor digitorum profundus tendons

First metacarpal

Trapezium
Flexor carpi radialis

Distal scaphoid

Lumbricals

Opponens digiti minimi

Abductor digiti minimi

Hook of hamate

Pisiform

Lunate

Radius

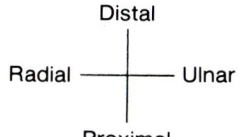
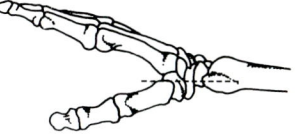

FIG. 4-30

CORONAL

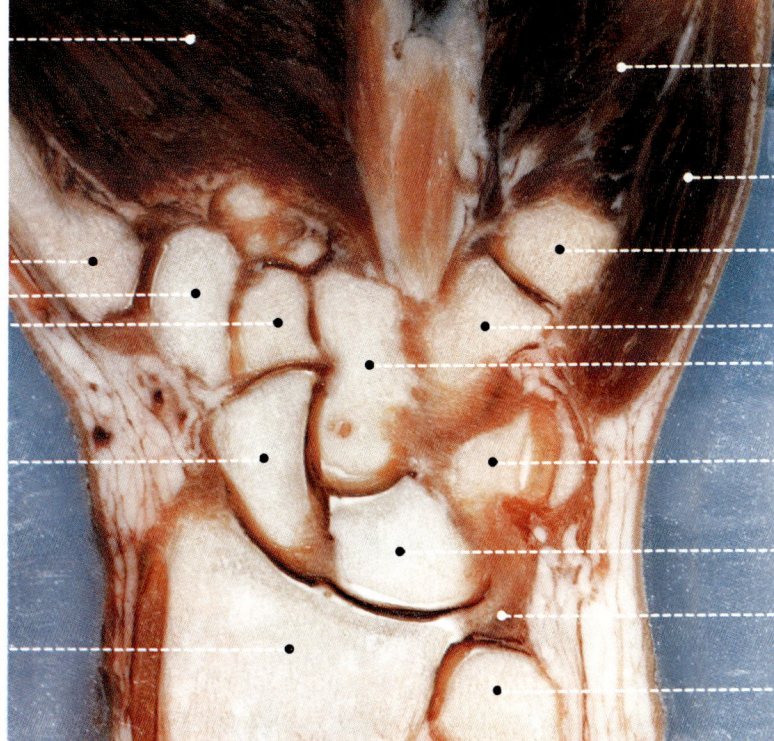

Anatomy and MRI of the Joints

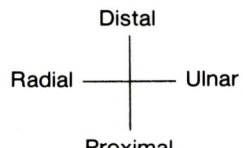

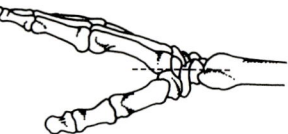

FIG. 4-31
CORONAL

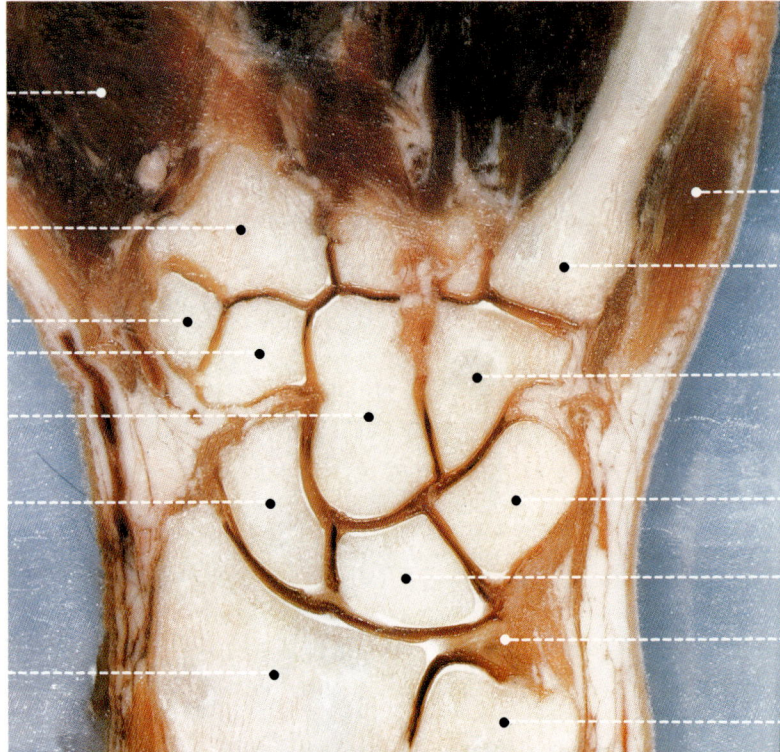

- Adductor pollicis
- Second metatarsal
- Trapezium
- Trapezoid
- Capitate
- Scaphoid
- Radius
- Abductor digiti minimi
- Fifth metatarsal
- Hamate
- Triquetrum
- Lunate
- Triangular fibrocartilage complex
- Ulna

THE WRIST

FIG. 4-32
CORONAL

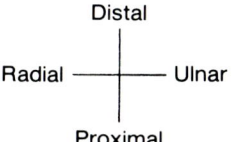
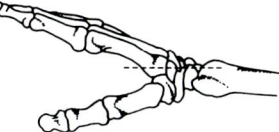
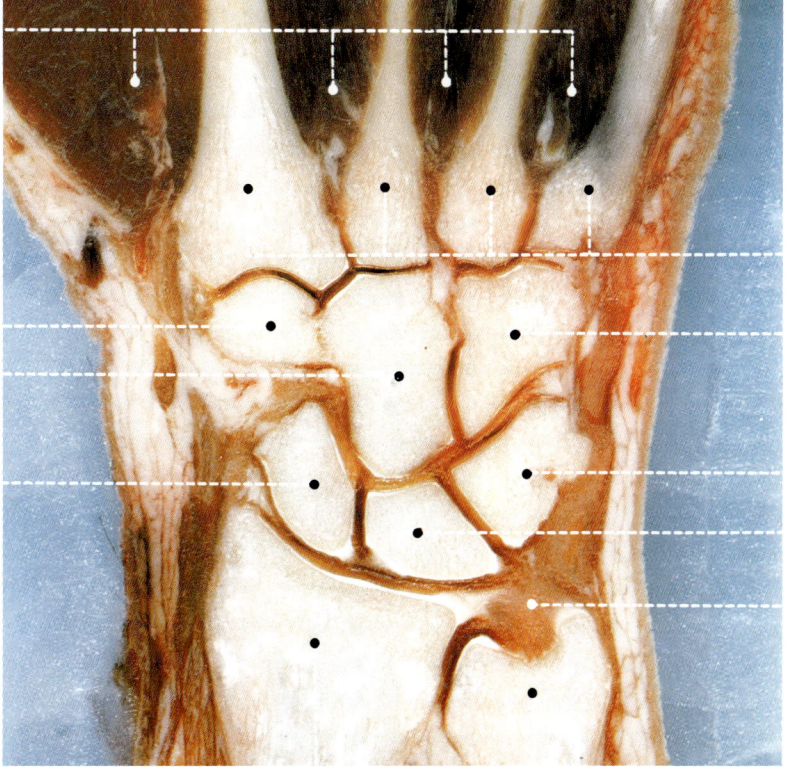

Anatomy and MRI of the Joints

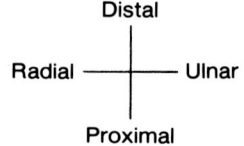

FIG. 4–33

CORONAL

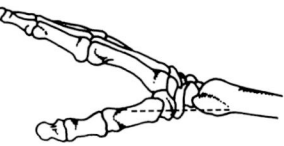

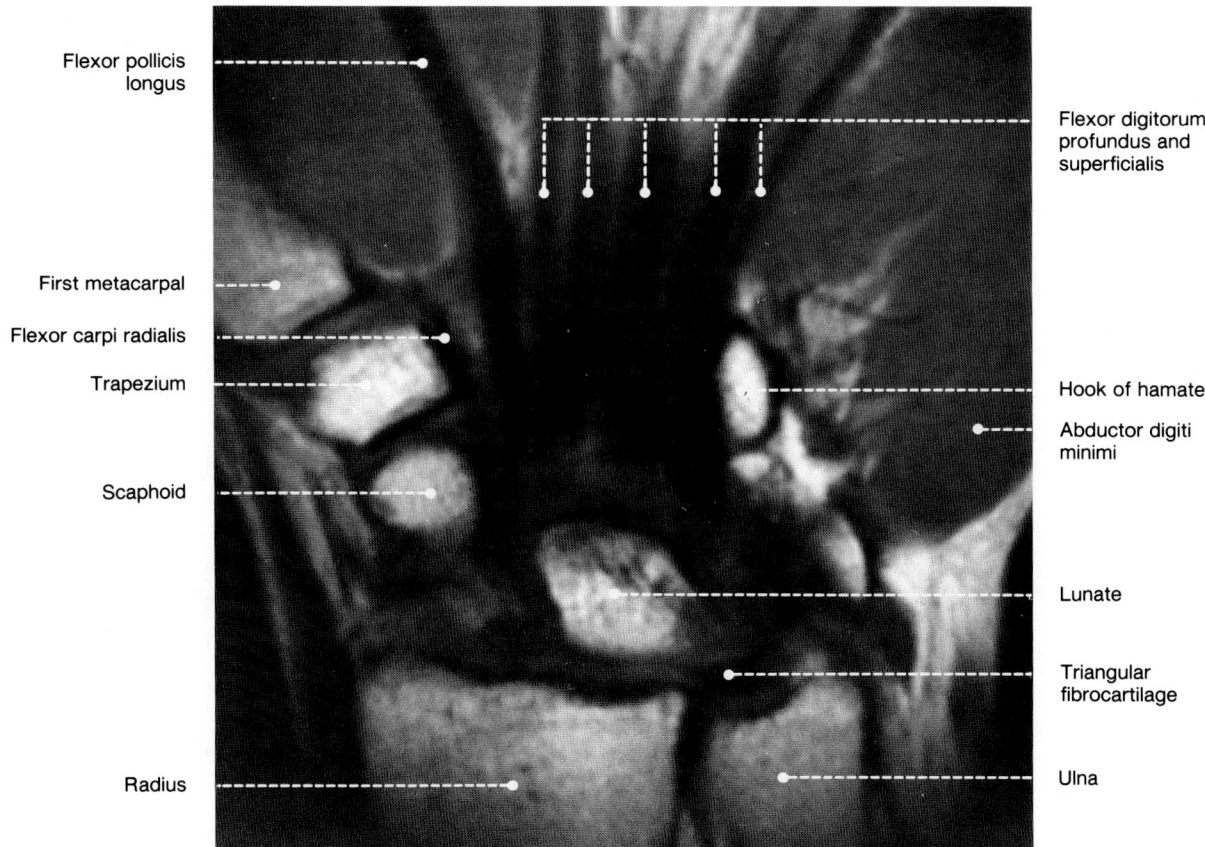

- Flexor pollicis longus
- Flexor digitorum profundus and superficialis
- First metacarpal
- Flexor carpi radialis
- Trapezium
- Hook of hamate
- Abductor digiti minimi
- Scaphoid
- Lunate
- Triangular fibrocartilage
- Radius
- Ulna

THE WRIST

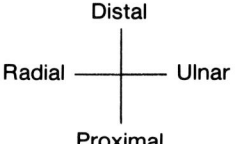

FIG. 4-34
CORONAL

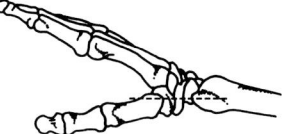

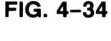

- Adductor pollicis
- Flexor carpi radialis
- First metacarpal
- Trapezium
- Trapezoid
- Scaphoid
- Radius
- Lumbricals
- Opponens digiti minimi
- Flexor digitorum profundus
- Abductor digiti minimi
- Fifth metacarpal
- Hamate
- Triquetrum
- Lunate
- Triangular fibrocartilage
- Ulna

Anatomy and MRI of the Joints

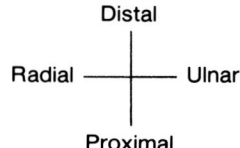

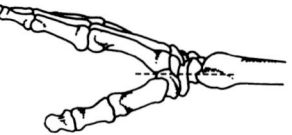

FIG. 4-35
CORONAL

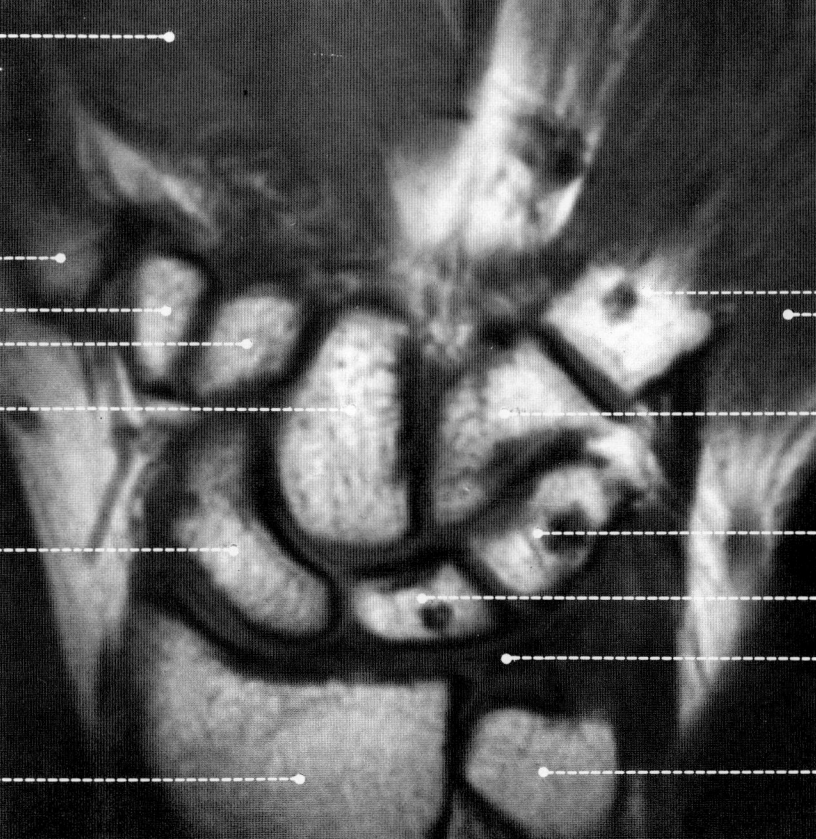

- Adductor pollicis
- First metacarpal
- Trapezium
- Trapezoid
- Capitate
- Scaphoid
- Radius
- Fifth metacarpal
- Abductor digiti minimi
- Hamate
- Triquetrum
- Lunate
- Triangular fibrocartilage
- Ulna

THE WRIST

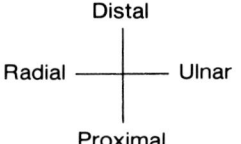

FIG. 4-36
CORONAL

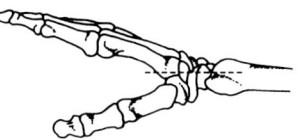

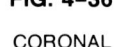

- Interossei
- Second metacarpal
- Third metacarpal
- Trapezoid
- Capitate
- Scaphoid
- Radius
- Fifth metacarpal
- Fourth metacarpal
- Hamate
- Triquetrum
- Lunate
- Triangular fibrocartilage
- Ulna

Anatomy and MRI of the Joints

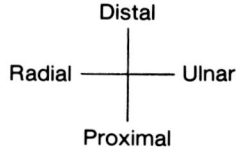

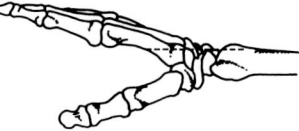

FIG. 4-37
CORONAL

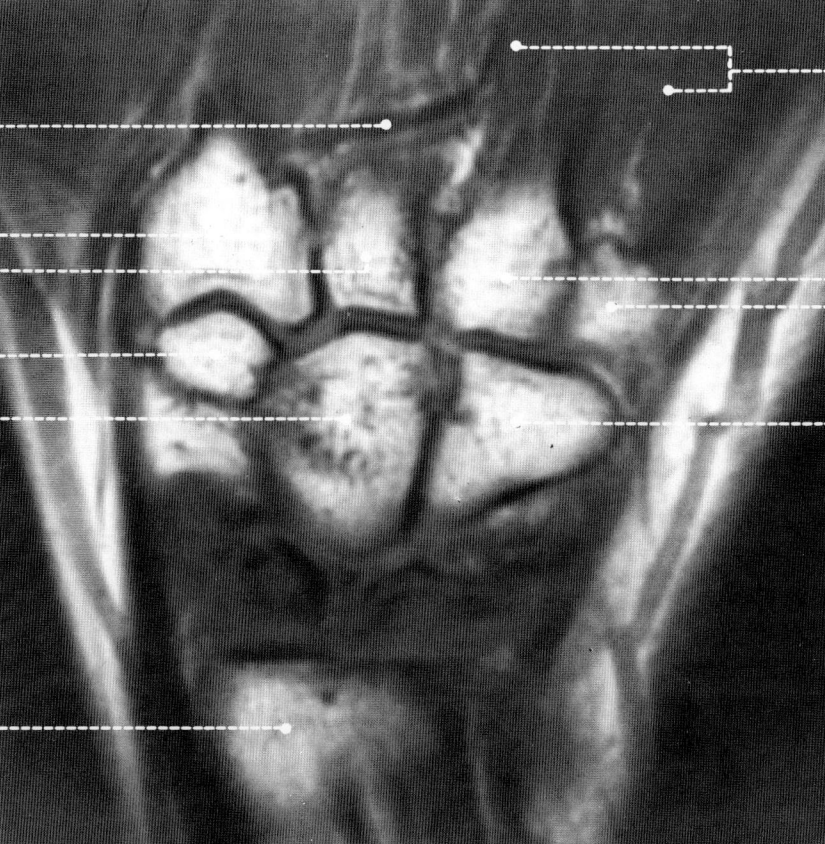

Chapter 5

THE FINGER
Scott Erickson, M.D.

The three articulations of the finger are the metacarpophalangeal joint, the proximal interphalangeal joint, and the distal interphalangeal joint. The metacarpophalangeal joint allows limited abduction and adduction as well as flexion and extension. The interphalangeal joints permit only flexion and extension.

A number of ligaments support the metacarpophalangeal joint. The palmar ligament, or volar plate, is a fibrocartilaginous plate extending from the base of the proximal phalanx to the head of the metacarpal. The transverse metacarpal ligament acts to unite the palmar ligaments. The collateral ligament is composed of two portions. The weaker, more proximal fanlike part acts to fix the palmar ligament to the metacarpal head. The stronger, cordlike part is the more distal component. The interphalangeal joints possess palmar and collateral ligaments having the same morphology as those of the metacarpophalangeal joint (Fig. 5-1).

The flexor digitorum tendons pass along the palmar surface of the digits. The flexor digitorum superficialis tendon is superficial to the flexor digitorum profundus tendon at the level of the metacarpophalangeal joint (Fig. 5-1). The superficialis tendon subsequently splits to lie first on either side of the profundus tendon at the level of the mid-proximal phalanx, then deep to the profundus at the level of the proximal interphalangeal joint, and finally deep and lateral to the profundus as it inserts onto the mid-portion of the middle phalanx. The flexor digitorum profundus tendon inserts onto the base of the distal phalanx (Fig. 5-1). The superficialis and profundus tendons each have their own synovial sheaths and also are surrounded by a common synovial sheath. This common sheath is then housed in a fibrous digital sheath, or fibrosseous tunnel.

The extensor expansion arises from the distal portion of the extensor digitorum tendon (Fig. 5-1). The central portion inserts onto the base of the middle phalanx along its dorsal aspect. The medial and lateral portions insert onto the base of the distal phalanx. The four lumbrical muscles arise from the flexor digitorum profundus tendons and insert onto the extensor expansion (Fig. 5-1). The dorsal and palmar interosseous muscles insert onto the expansion and also onto the bases of the proximal phalanges (Fig. 5-1).

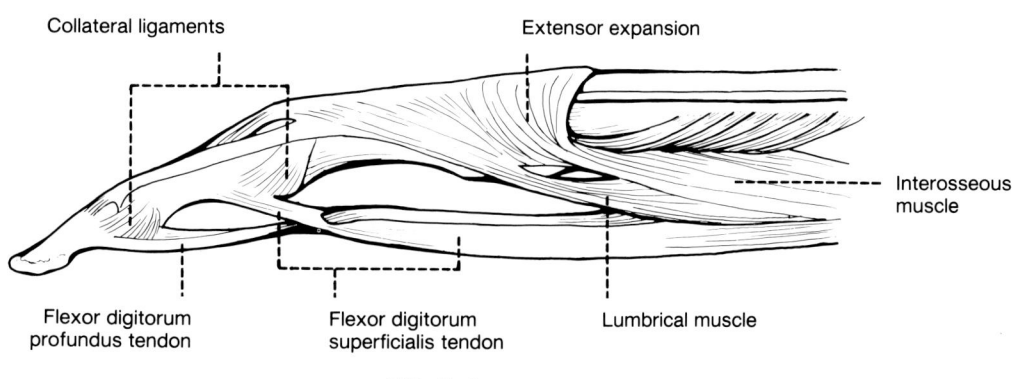

FIG. 5-1

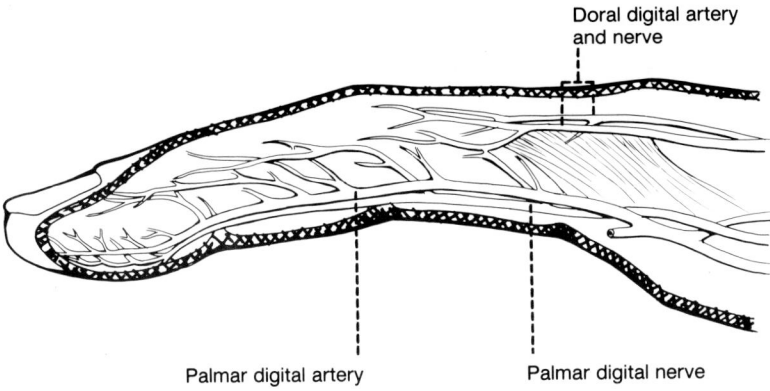

FIG. 5-2

The neurovascular supply to the finger consists of both palmar and dorsal digital branches of nerves, veins, and arteries (Fig. 5-2). The palmar digital arteries and nerves are larger than the dorsal arteries and nerves and are more easily seen on distal axial sections. The converse is true of the digital veins.

THE FINGER

AXIAL
    Cryomicrotomes..........................FIGS. 5–3 to 5–6
    MR Images..............................FIGS. 5–7 to 5–10

SAGITTAL
    Cryomicrotomes.........................FIGS. 5–11 to 5–12
    MR Images.............................FIGS. 5–13 to 5–14

CORONAL
    Cryomicrotome..........................FIG. 5–15
    MR Image..............................FIG. 5–16

Anatomy and MRI of the Joints   124   **FIG. 5–3**

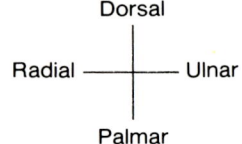

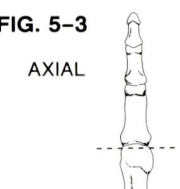

AXIAL

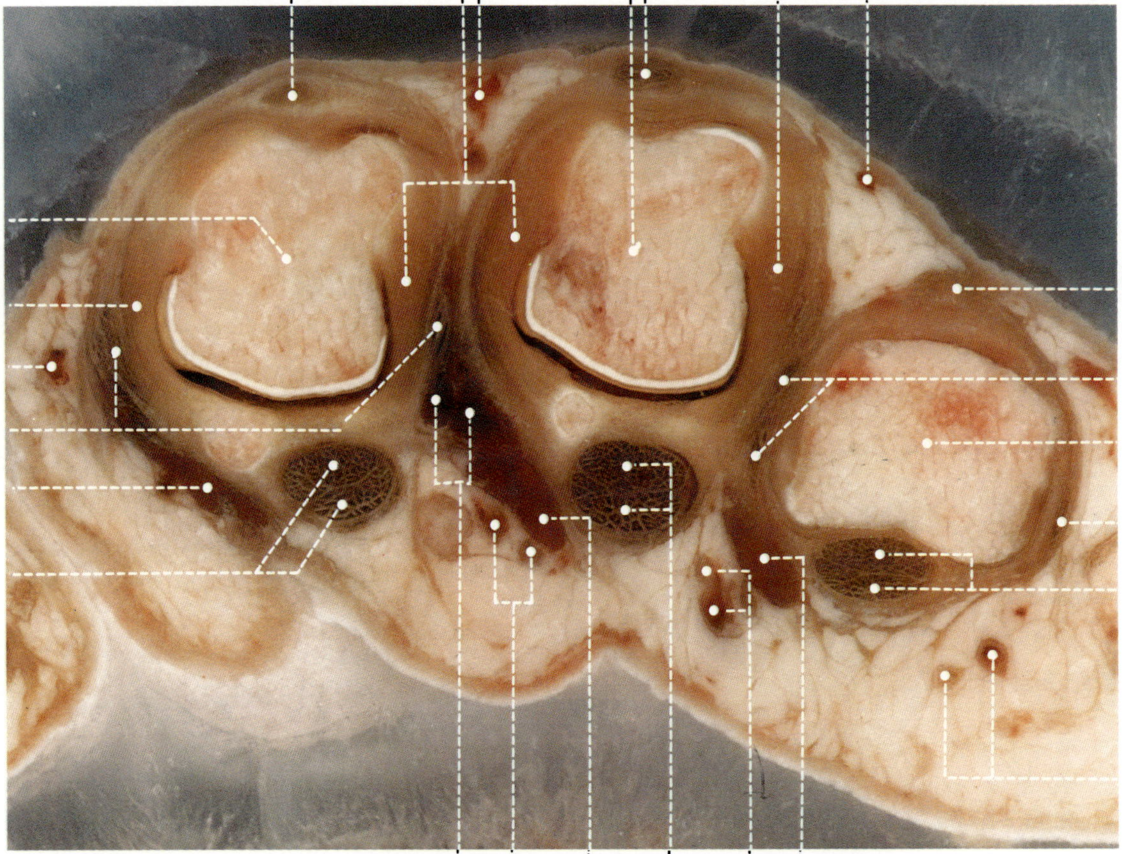

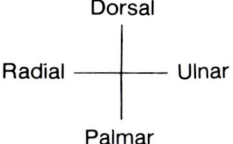

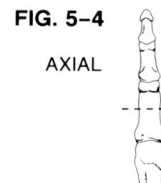

FIG. 5-4
AXIAL

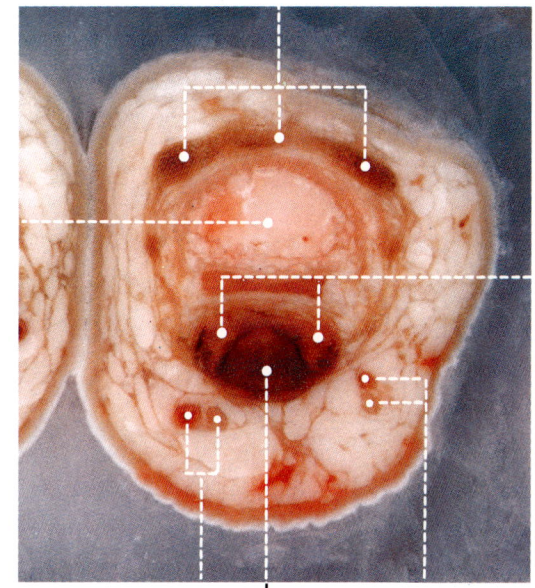

Extensor expansion

Proximal phalanx

Flexor digitorum superficialis tendon

Palmar digital artery and nerve

Flexor digitorum profundus tendon

Palmar digital artery and nerve

Anatomy and MRI of the Joints   126

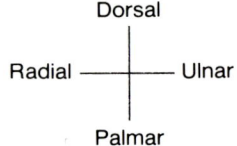

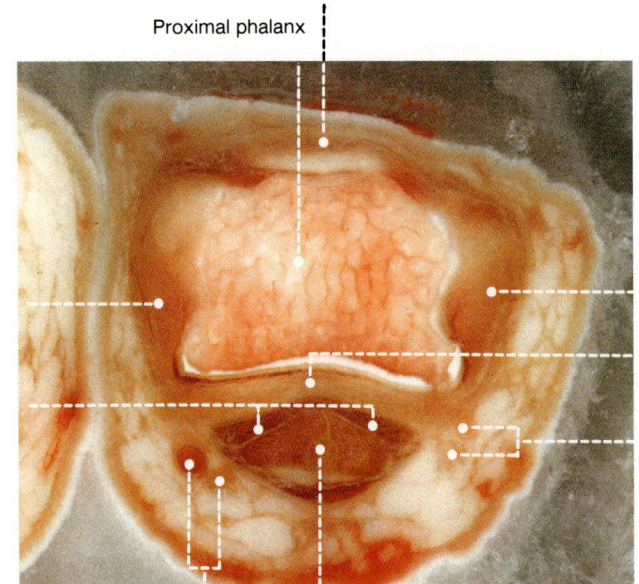

FIG. 5–5
AXIAL

127 THE FINGER

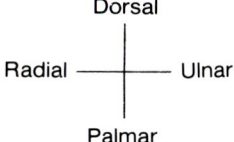

FIG. 5-6

AXIAL

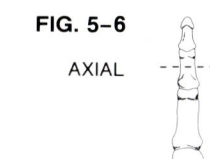

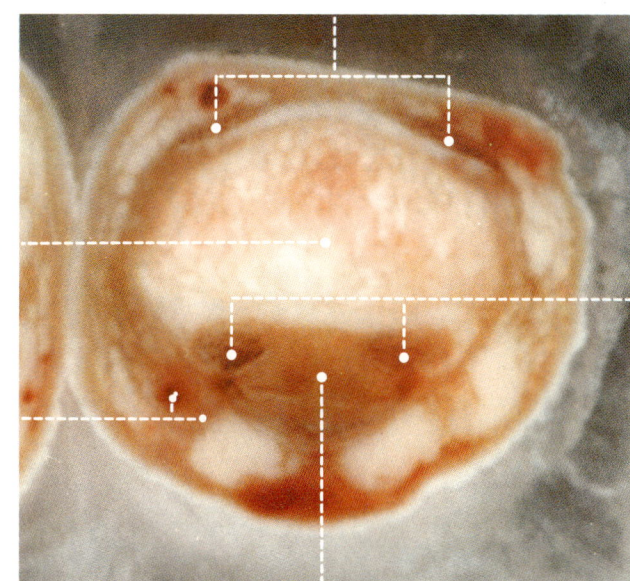

Extensor expansion

Middle phalanx

Flexor digitorum superficialis tendon

Palmar digital artery and nerve

Flexor digitorum profundus tendon

Anatomy and MRI of the Joints

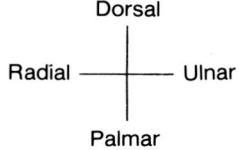

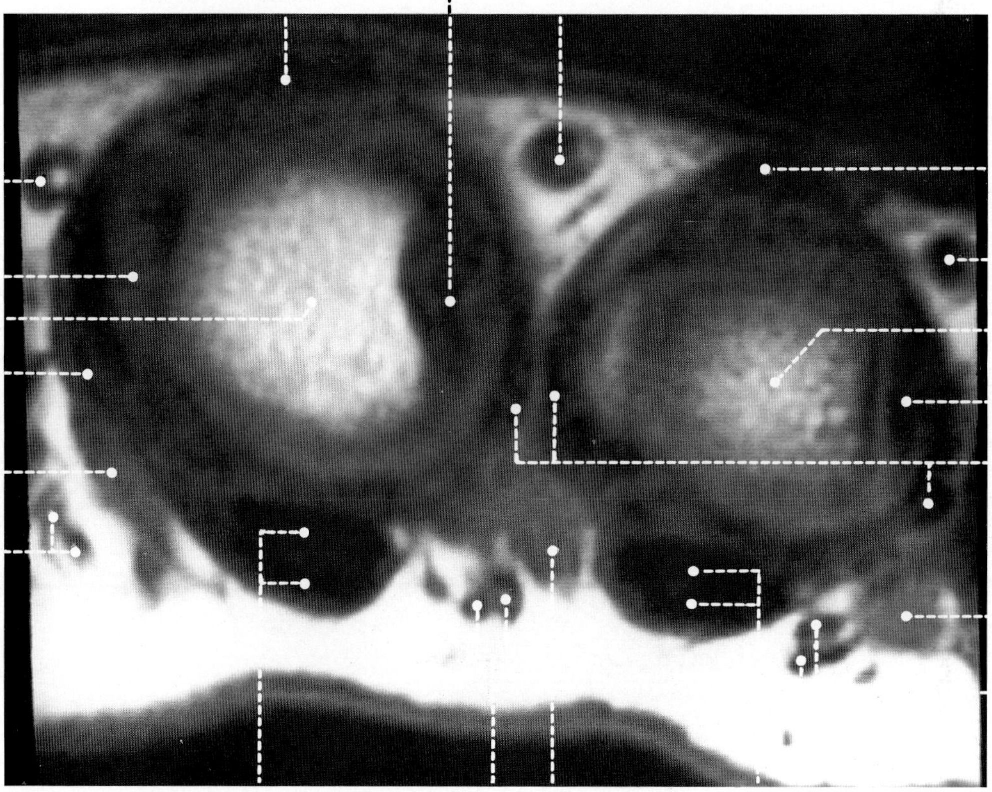

FIG. 5-7

AXIAL

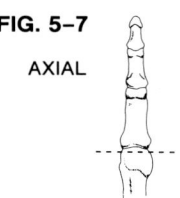

THE FINGER

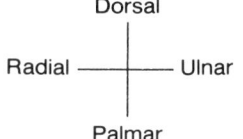

FIG. 5-8
AXIAL

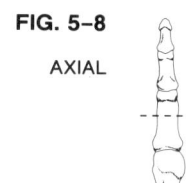

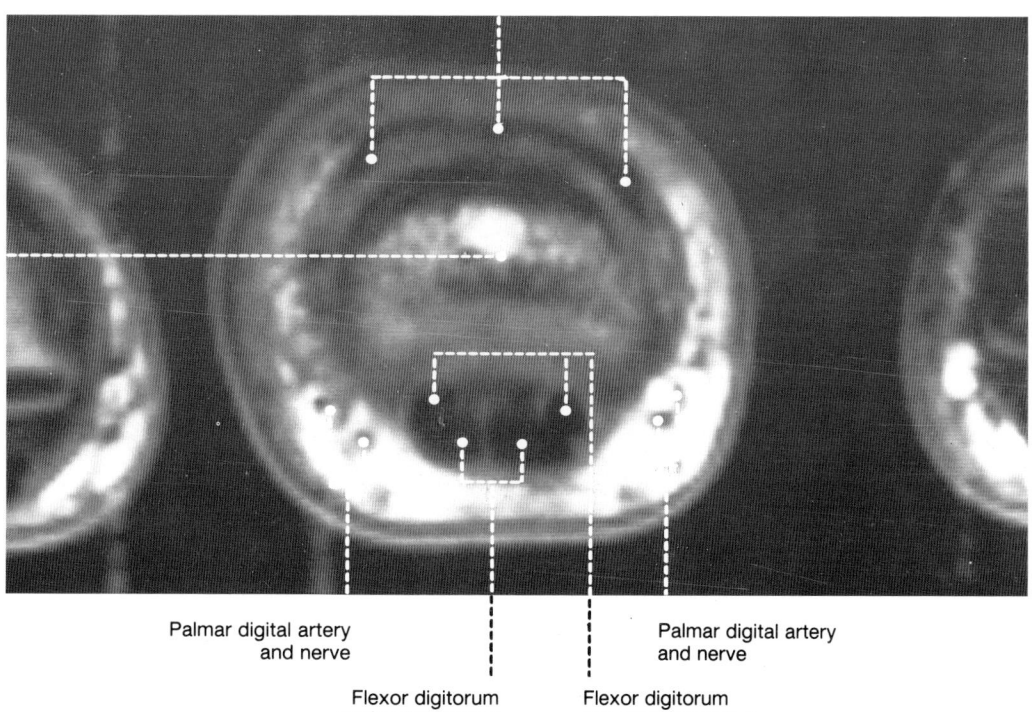

- Extensor expansion
- Proximal phalanx
- Palmar digital artery and nerve
- Flexor digitorum profundus tendon
- Flexor digitorum superficialis tendon
- Palmar digital artery and nerve

Anatomy and MRI of the Joints

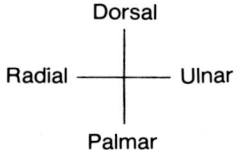

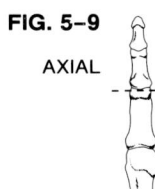

FIG. 5-9
AXIAL

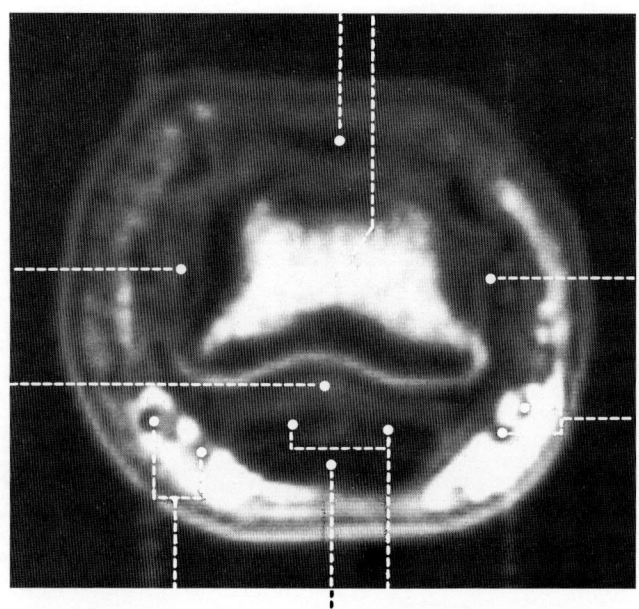

THE FINGER

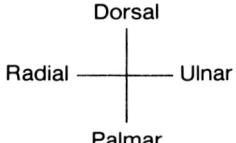

FIG. 5-10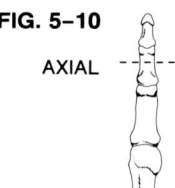
AXIAL

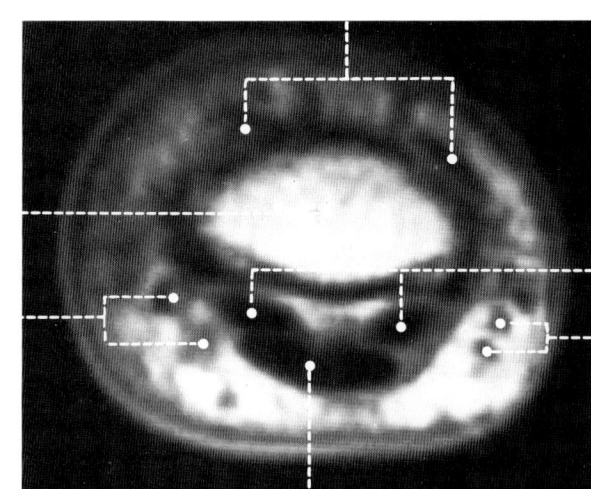

Extensor expansion

Middle phalanx

Palmar digital artery and nerve

Flexor digitorum superficialis tendon

Palmar digital artery and nerve

Flexor digitorum profundus tendon

Anatomy and MRI of the Joints   132

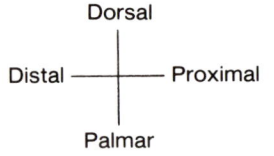

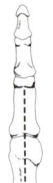

FIG. 5–11

SAGITTAL

Proximal phalanx — Extensor digitorum tendon — Metacarpal head — Interosseous muscle

Volar plate — Flexor digitorum profundus tendon — Flexor digitorum superficialis tendon — Lumbrical muscle

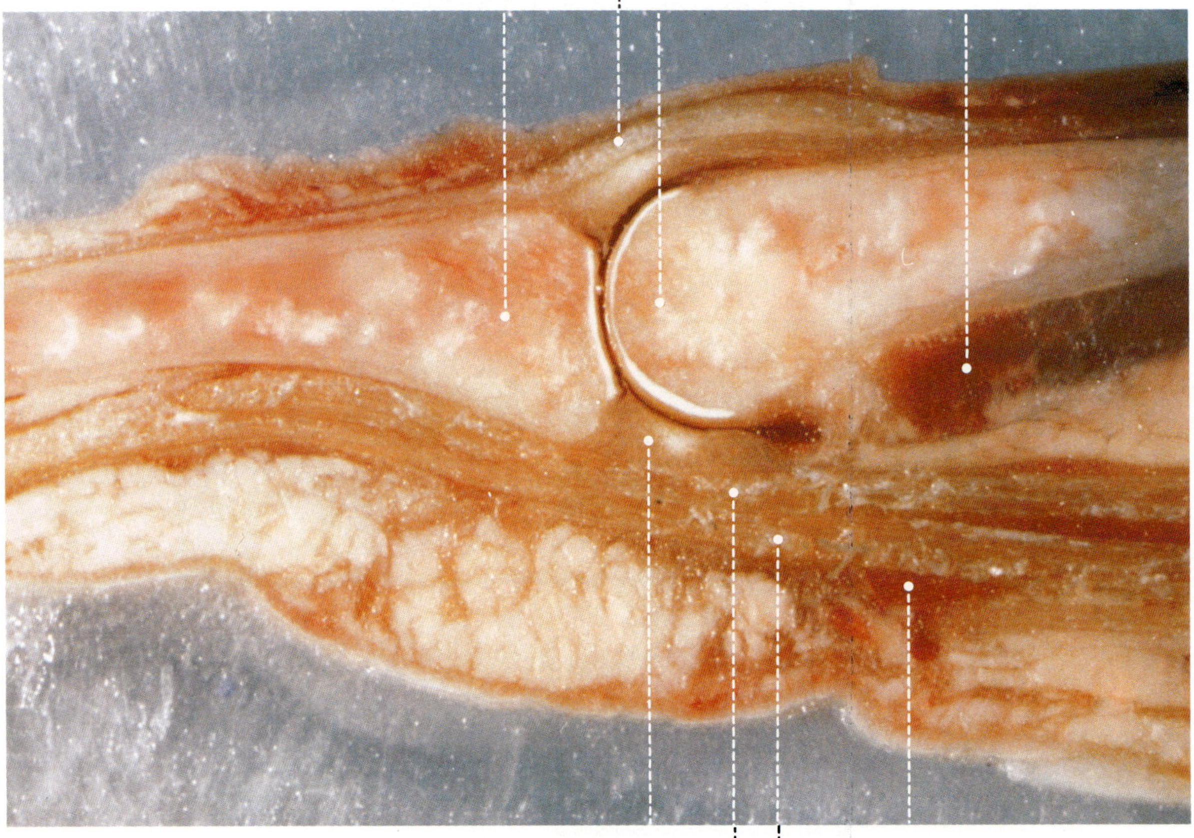

THE FINGER

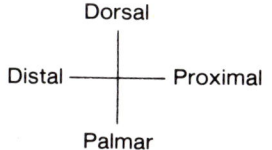

FIG. 5-12

SAGITTAL

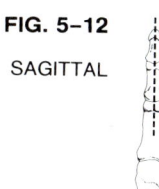

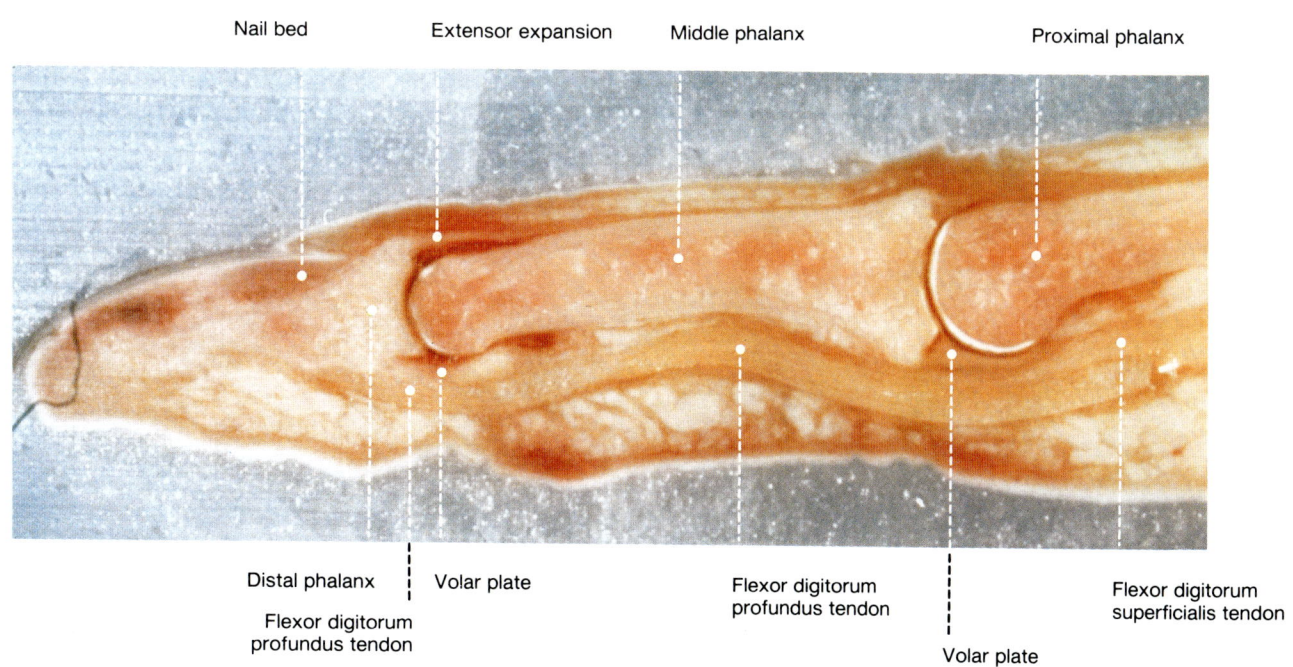

Nail bed — Extensor expansion — Middle phalanx — Proximal phalanx

Distal phalanx | Volar plate | Flexor digitorum profundus tendon | Flexor digitorum superficialis tendon
Flexor digitorum profundus tendon | | | Volar plate

Anatomy and MRI of the Joints

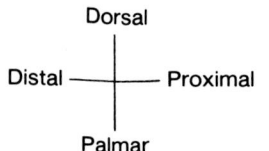

FIG. 5-13

SAGITTAL

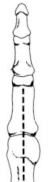

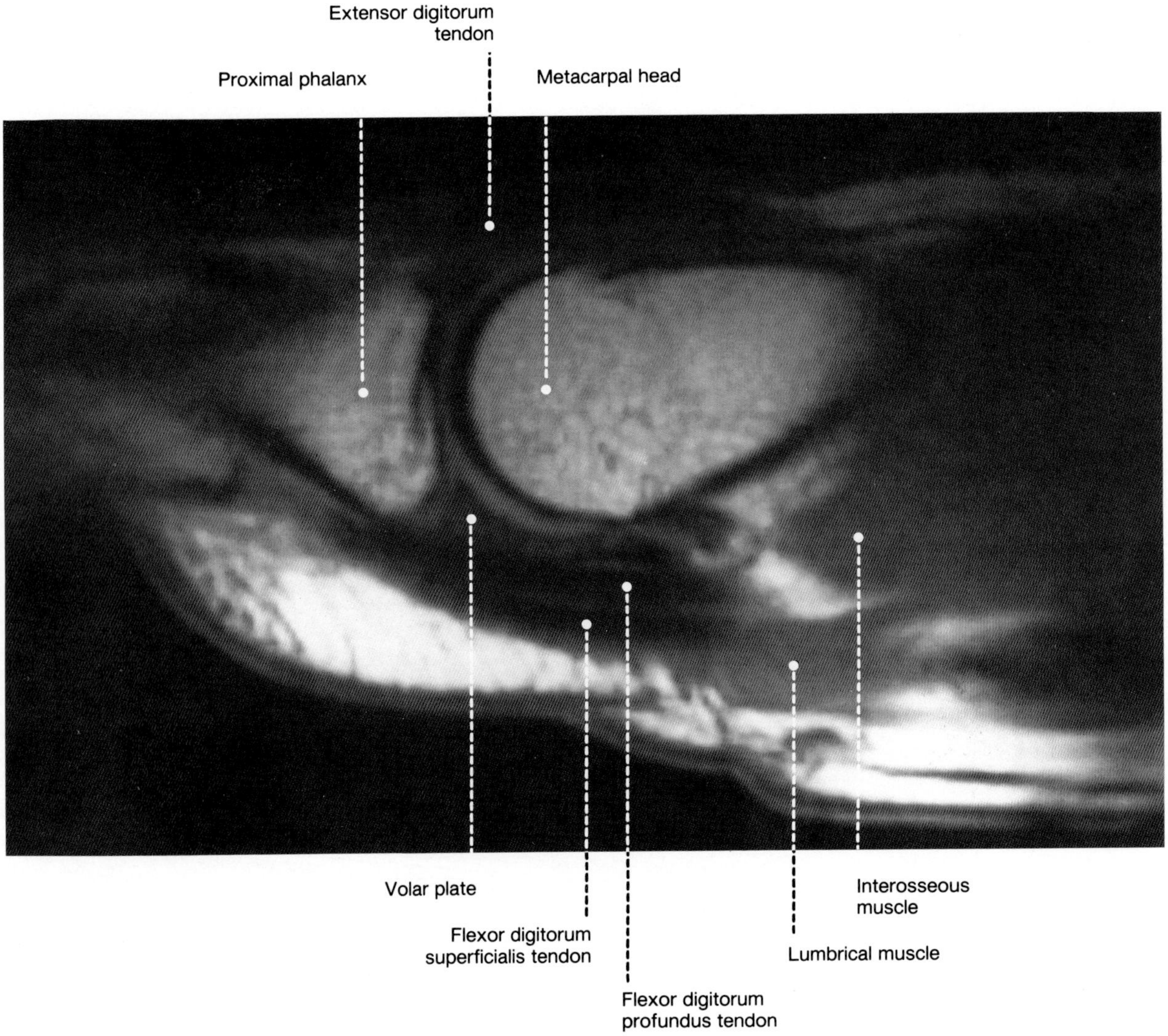

- Proximal phalanx
- Extensor digitorum tendon
- Metacarpal head
- Volar plate
- Flexor digitorum superficialis tendon
- Flexor digitorum profundus tendon
- Lumbrical muscle
- Interosseous muscle

THE FINGER

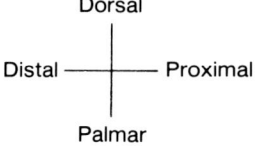

FIG. 5-14
SAGITTAL

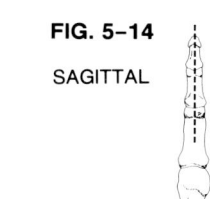

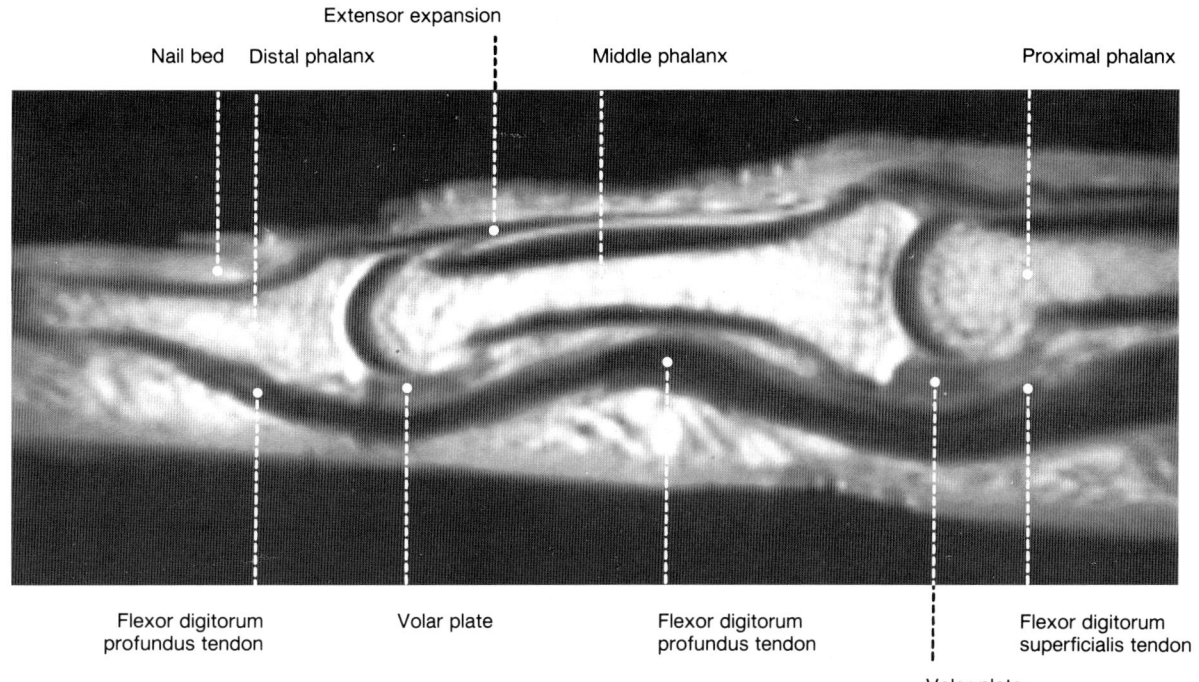

FIG. 5-15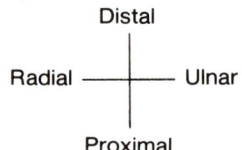
CORONAL

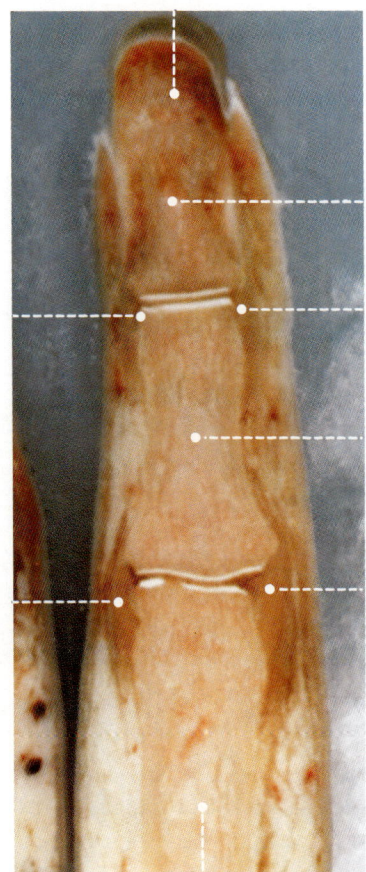

THE FINGER

FIG. 5-16

CORONAL

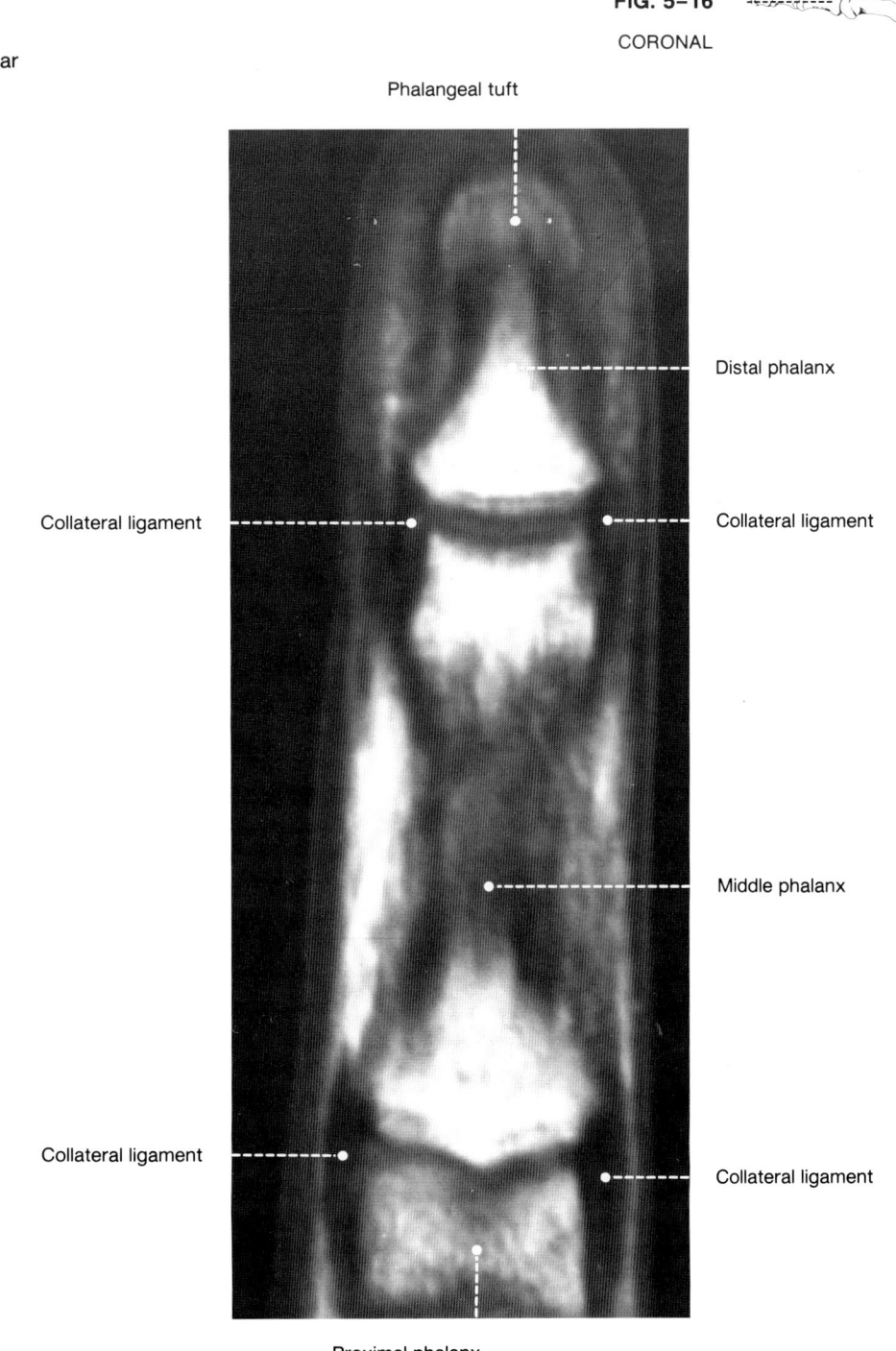

Chapter 6

THE VERTEBRAL COLUMN

Lowell Sether, Ph.D.

The vertebral column, in forming a flexible pillar of support for the trunk of the body and a protective skeleton for the spinal cord and nerve roots, consists of a series of bones (the vertebrae), ligaments, and the articulations between the movable vertebrae. While special joints make up the atlanto-occipital and atlanto-axial articulations, the intervertebral articulations from the second cervical vertebra to the sacrum are organized in a common pattern and include three types of joints: the fibrocartilaginous symphyses (intervertebral discs) between the vertebral bodies, the synovial zygapophyseal (facet) joints between the adjacent superior and inferior articular processes, and the fibrous joints of the vertebral arches between the adjacent laminae, transverse processes, and spinous processes. While the pattern of organization of the intervertebral joints is common at each segmental level of the vertebral column (Fig. 6–1), there are regional differences in the cervical, thoracic, and lumbar regions.

The vertebral bodies are firmly united by the intervertebral discs and by the anterior and posterior longitudinal ligaments. The intervertebral discs are a series of symphyses between the vertebral bodies while the longitudinal ligaments are fibrous structures that extend along the entire length of the vertebral column.

The intervertebral discs are composite plates of fibrocartilage interposed between the bodies of adjacent vertebrae from the axis to the sacrum and constitute the main bonds between the vertebral bodies. They are adherent to

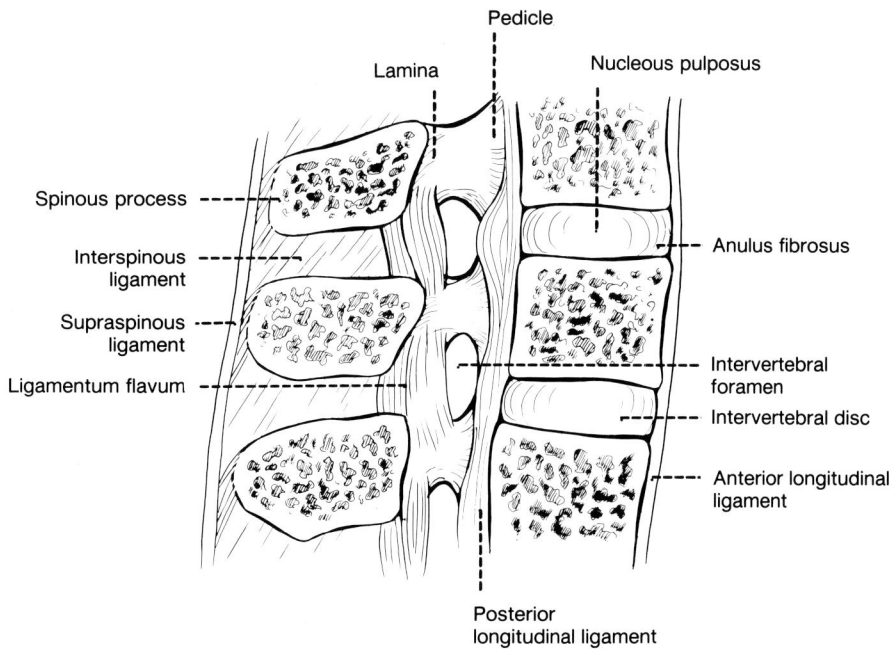

FIG. 6–1

the cartilage plates that cover the central parts of the ends of the bodies of the vertebrae and to the bony margins (ring apophyses) of the vertebral bodies. The discs make up nearly one-fourth of the total length of the vertebral column above the sacrum, varying in thickness in different regions. They are thickest in the lumbar region and narrowest in the thoracic region. The cervical and lumbar discs are wedge-shaped, being thicker anteriorly than posteriorly, while the thoracic discs are relatively uniform in thickness.

Each intervertebral disc consists of two parts: a firm outer fibrous ring, the anulus fibrosus, and a softer internal portion, the nucleus pulposus.

In the adult the anulus fibrosus is composed of concentric fibrocartilaginous lamellae in which the fibers extend obliquely from one vertebral body to the next. Its peripheral lamellae are composed mainly of densely arranged collagenous fibers which strongly unite the adjacent vertebral bodies by attaching to the ring apophyses as Sharpey's fibers. The lamellae of the inner portion of the anulus become progressively more fibrocartilaginous as they approach the nucleus pulposus and are attached to the edges of the cartilage plates on the ends of the vertebral bodies. The peripheral lamellae are convex, causing a slight bulging of the disc, while the innermost lamellae curve inward and blend with the nucleus in a fibrocartilaginous zone.

The internal part of the intervertebral disc, the nucleus pulposus, is usually described as a glistening white or yellowish gelatinous fibrocartilage. However, the structure, composition, and appearance of the nucleus pulposus undergo continuous changes throughout life. In the newborn and infant the nucleus is a centrally located and relatively large translucent structure composed of a soft semigelatinous matrix containing remnants of the notochord, fine collagenous fibers, and scattered connective tissue cells. Its periphery consists of fibrocartilage which blends with that of the inner portion of the anulus fibrosus and fuses with the cartilage plates of the adjacent vertebral bodies. During the first decade of life the nucleus becomes more fibrocartilaginous. More rapid growth of the anulus fibrosus leads to progressive displacement or replacement of the gelatinous matrix of the nucleus, resulting in a bilobed or multilocular-shaped nucleus. The nucleus pulposus also becomes eccentrically located within the disc, especially in the cervical and lumbar regions, usually being located more posteriorly than anteriorly. With increasing age the fibrocartilaginous tissues of the anulus fibrosus and nucleus pulposus blend with each other so that there is no distinct line of demarcation between them.

The anterior longitudinal ligament is a broad fibrous band located on the anterior and anterolateral surfaces of the vertebral bodies and intervertebral discs. It originates from a narrow attachment at the base of the occipital bone anterior to the foramen magnum and extends to the anterior surface of the upper sacrum where it blends with the periosteum. This ligament is firmly attached to, and strengthens, the anterior part of the anulus fibrosus of each intervertebral disc.

The posterior longitudinal ligament is located inside the vertebral canal on the posterior surfaces of the vertebral bodies and intervertebral discs. It extends from the intracranial base of the occipital bone down to a narrow attachment on the coccyx. This ligament is of nearly uniform width in the cervical region, covering the entire posterior surfaces of the vertebral bodies and intervertebral discs. In the thoracic and lumbar regions the ligament is narrowed as it crosses the vertebral bodies but broader over the intervertebral discs where thin dentate expansions cover the discs. The ligament consists of connective tissue fibers that are firmly attached to the anulus fibrosus of each intervertebral disc and the adjacent margins of the vertebral bodies. It is not attached to the midportions of the vertebral bodies where it is separated from the vertebrae by small spaces containing the emerging basivertebral veins and veins draining into the internal vertebral plexus.

The vertebral arches are united bilaterally by synovial joints between the superior and inferior articular processes (zygapophyses) of the adjacent vertebrae. Because these processes have articular facets on them they are commonly referred to as the facet joints. The articular surfaces of these joints are oriented differently in the different regions of the vertebral column. On the cervical vertebrae the orientation is in an oblique transverse plane, the superior articular surface facing posterosuperiorly and the inferior facing anteroinferiorly. In the thoracic region the plane of articulation is nearly in the coronal plane, with the superior articular surface facing posteriorly and the inferior facing anteriorly. In the lumbar region the plane of articulation is nearly sagittal, as the superior articular surface faces medially and slightly posteriorly and the inferior faces laterally and slightly anteriorly. The articulating surfaces (facets) are covered by articular cartilage, and are generally ovoid in shape. Small menisci are found in the periphery of some of these joints in the cervical and lumbar regions to accommodate the concavities and convexities of the articular facets and to aid in even distribution of pressure. Each joint is enclosed by a thin articular capsule which is attached to the margins of the articular processes and lined by a synovial membrane.

Fibrous joints unite the laminae, transverse processes, and spinous processes of the vertebral arches. These structures act as accessory ligaments of the synovial joints of the vertebral arches. The laminae of adjacent vertebrae from the axis to the sacrum are connected segmentally by the ligamenta flava (yellow ligaments) which are thick, flat membranes consisting of dense, elastic connective tissue fibers. These are the strongest and most important of the posterior ligaments of the vertebral arches. Each ligamentum flavum extends from the posterior edge of the intervertebral foramen on one side to a corresponding site on the opposite side. Because of their elastic nature, the ligamenta flava easily accommodate flexion and extension of the vertebral column. The interspinous ligaments are thin membranes that connect adjoining spinous processes. Their fibers extend obliquely from the base of the spinous process of one vertebra to the apex of the next spinous process. Anteriorly they blend with the ligamenta flava and posteriorly with the supraspinous ligament. The supraspinous ligament is a strong band that connects the tips of the spinous processes from the lower lumbar level to the spine of the seventh cervical vertebra where it becomes continuous with the ligamentum nuchae, which is a thick fibroelastic intermuscular septum attached to the spinous processes of the cervical vertebrae and the external occipital protuberance.

The intrinsic (true) muscles of the back comprise several columns of muscle tissue located in the deep grooves at the sides of the vertebral arches deep to the thoracolumbar fascia. The largest and most superficial of these muscles are the erector spinae (sacrospinalis) muscles. These muscles extend from the posterior aspect of the sacrum and iliac crests to the skull and consist of a lateral portion (the iliocostalis), an intermediate column of muscle (the longissimus), and a small medial muscle (the spinalis). In the cervical region the splenius muscles are included with this group. A group of muscles lying deep to the erector spinae muscles are collectively called the transversospinal muscles because they consist of a series of muscles that extend from the transverse processes to the spinous processes of most of the vertebrae. This group of muscles includes the semispinalis, multifidus, and rotatores muscles.

The spinal cord, located in the vertebral canal formed by the articulated vertebrae, begins as a nearly cylindrical continuation of the medulla at the foramen magnum and terminates at or near the level of the intervertebral disc between the first and second lumbar vertebrae. It is surrounded and protected by the meninges, the cerebrospinal fluid, and the vertebrae and their ligaments. Two rows of nerve roots, dorsal and ventral, arise on either side of the cord and pass laterally to emerge through the intervertebral foramina. The dorsal roots have spinal (or dorsal root) ganglia which are located in the intervertebral foramina. Just distal to the ganglia and outside the intervertebral foramina the dorsal and ventral roots of each segment unite to form spinal nerves which almost immediately divide into anterior primary divisions (ventral rami) and posterior primary divisions (dorsal rami). Because the spinal cord does not extend the entire length of the vertebral canal, most spinal cord segments are located at higher levels than the corresponding vertebral levels, resulting in elongation of the dorsal and ventral roots from their origins on the spinal cord to their entrance into the proper intervertebral foramina. Below the level of the first lumbar vertebra the large collections of these roots form the cauda equina, which is enclosed in a dural sac, from which the spinal nerves are distributed at corresponding vertebral levels.

The vasculature of the spinal cord and vertebrae is complex. Superiorly, the spinal cord receives a blood supply from three descending arteries, the anterior spinal artery and the paired posterior spinal arteries which originate from the vertebral arteries at the level of the hindbrain. Additional blood supply is derived segmentally from spinal radicular arteries which are branches of the vertebral, deep cervical, posterior intercostal, lumbar, and lateral sacral arteries. The spinal arteries enter the vertebral canal through the intervertebral foramina, divide into anterior and posterior radicular branches, supply the vertebrae and meninges, and follow the dorsal and ventral roots to supply the spinal cord by anastomoses with the anterior and posterior spinal arteries.

The venous drainage of the spinal cord follows a pattern similar to the distribution of the spinal arteries but is much more plexiform as the veins interconnect freely. Venous blood from the vertebrae drains into an external vertebral plexus by numerous small veins and into a rich internal vertebral plexus of valveless veins located inside the vertebral canal in an extradural position by means of the basivertebral vein. The veins of the vertebral plexuses communicate via longitudinal veins or sinuses with the dural venous sinuses. Most of the venous drainage of the spinal cord and vertebral plexuses is by way of radicular and intervertebral veins that pass through the intervertebral foramina into the vertebral veins, ascending lumbar veins, and azygos venous system.

THE VERTEBRAL COLUMN

AXIAL
    Cryomicrotome........................... FIG. 6–2
    MR Image................................. FIG. 6–3

SAGITTAL
    Cryomicrotomes........................ FIGS. 6–4 to 6–6
    MR Images............................. FIGS. 6–7 to 6–9

Anatomy and MRI of the Joints

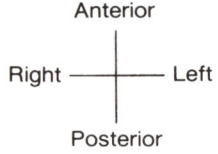

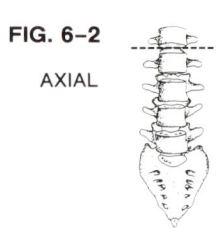

FIG. 6-2
AXIAL

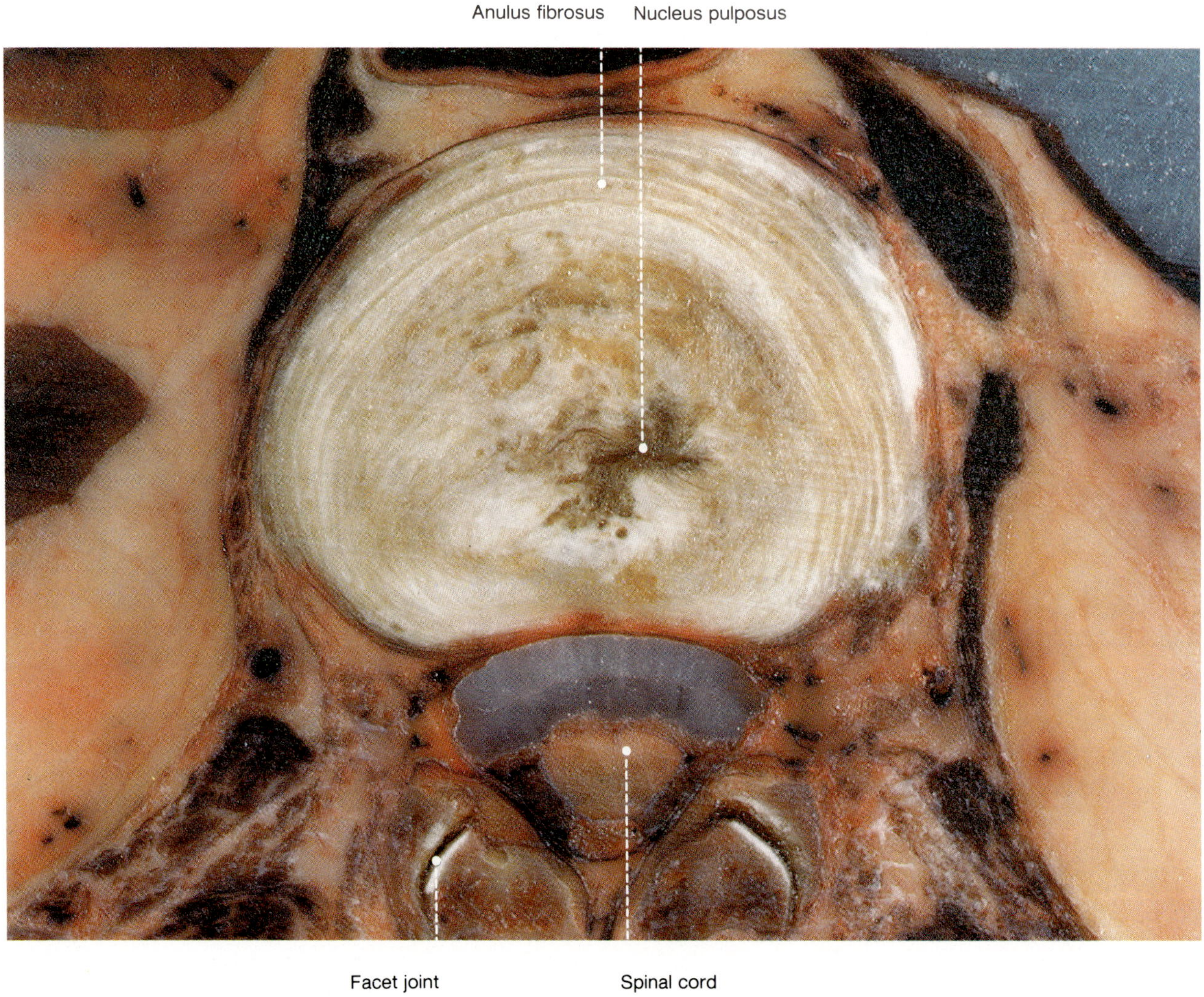

Anulus fibrosus   Nucleus pulposus

Facet joint   Spinal cord

THE VERTEBRAL COLUMN

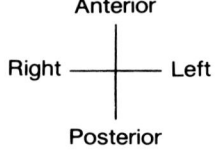

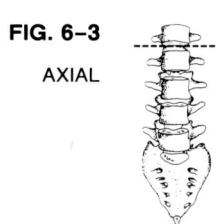

FIG. 6-3
AXIAL

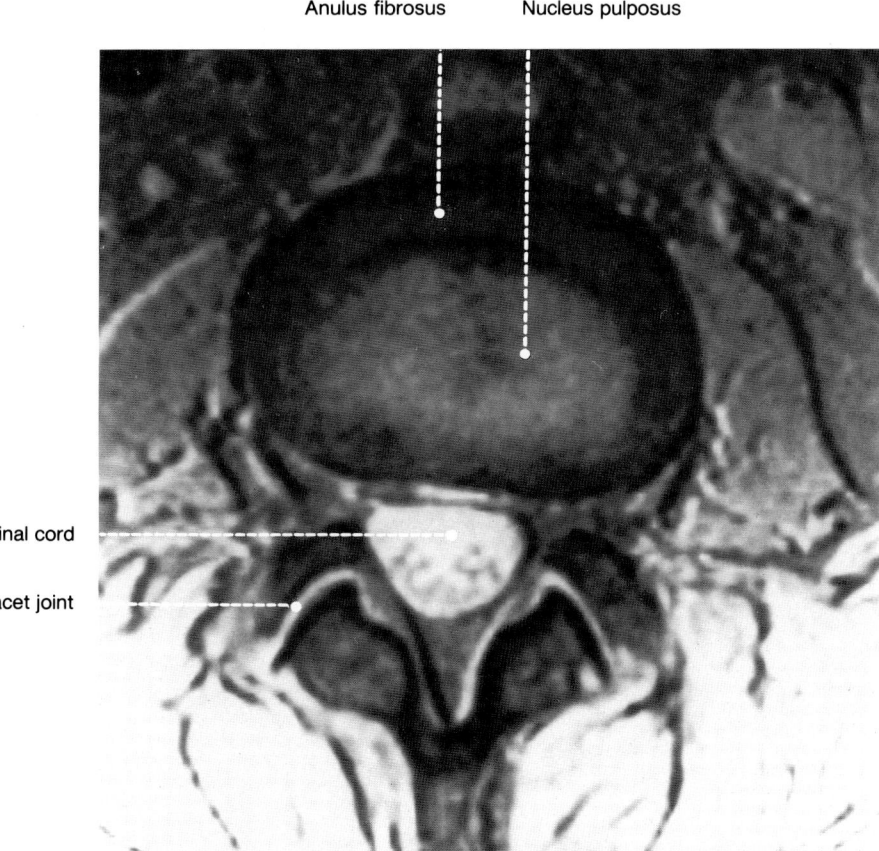

Anatomy and MRI of the Joints 146

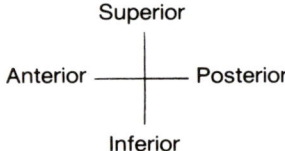

FIG. 6-4
SAGITTAL

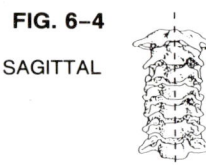

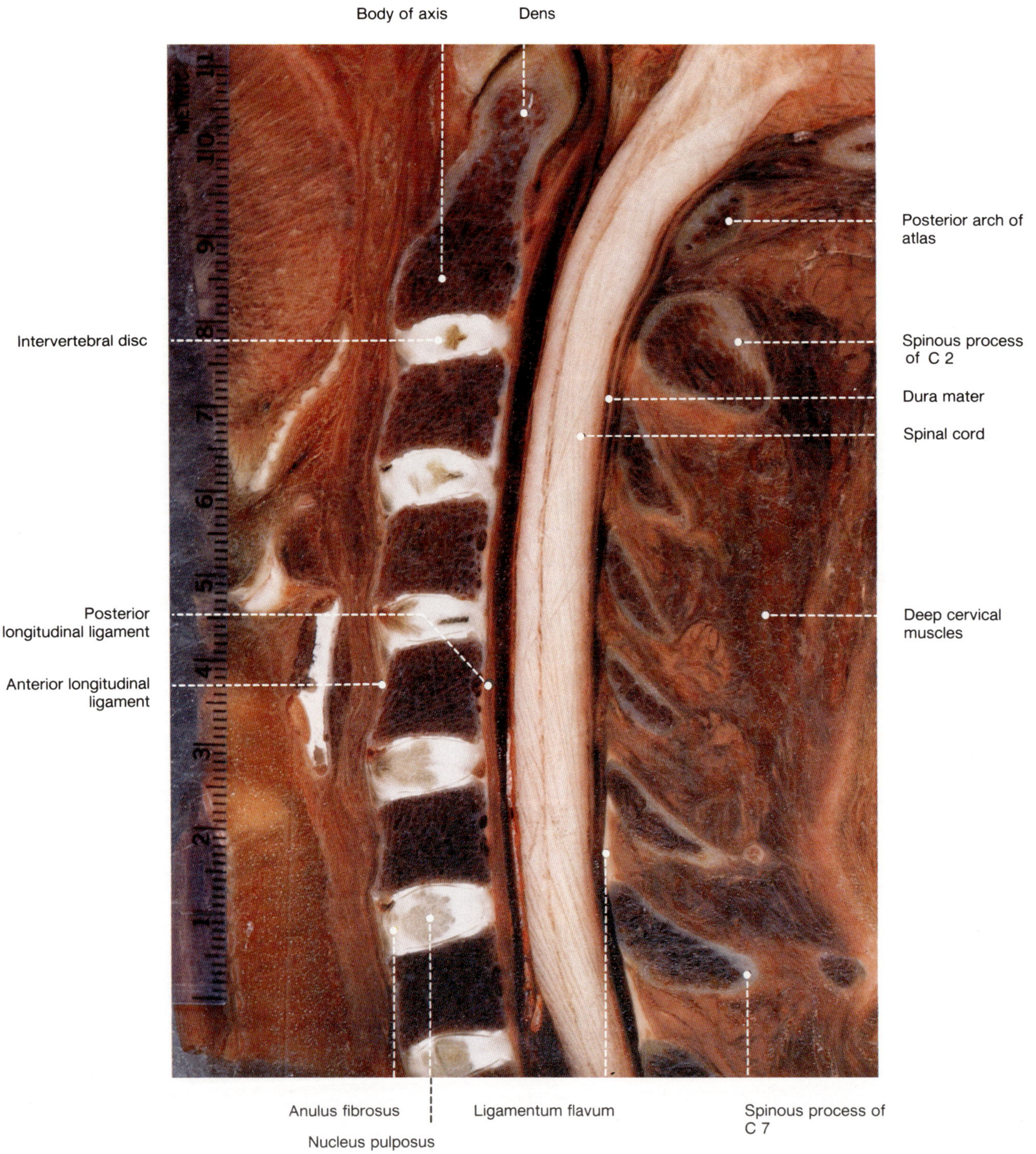

Superior
Anterior — Posterior
Inferior

FIG. 6–5

SAGITTAL

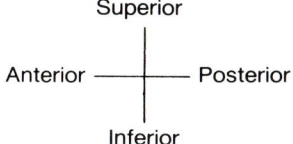

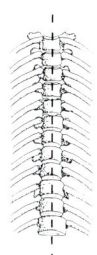

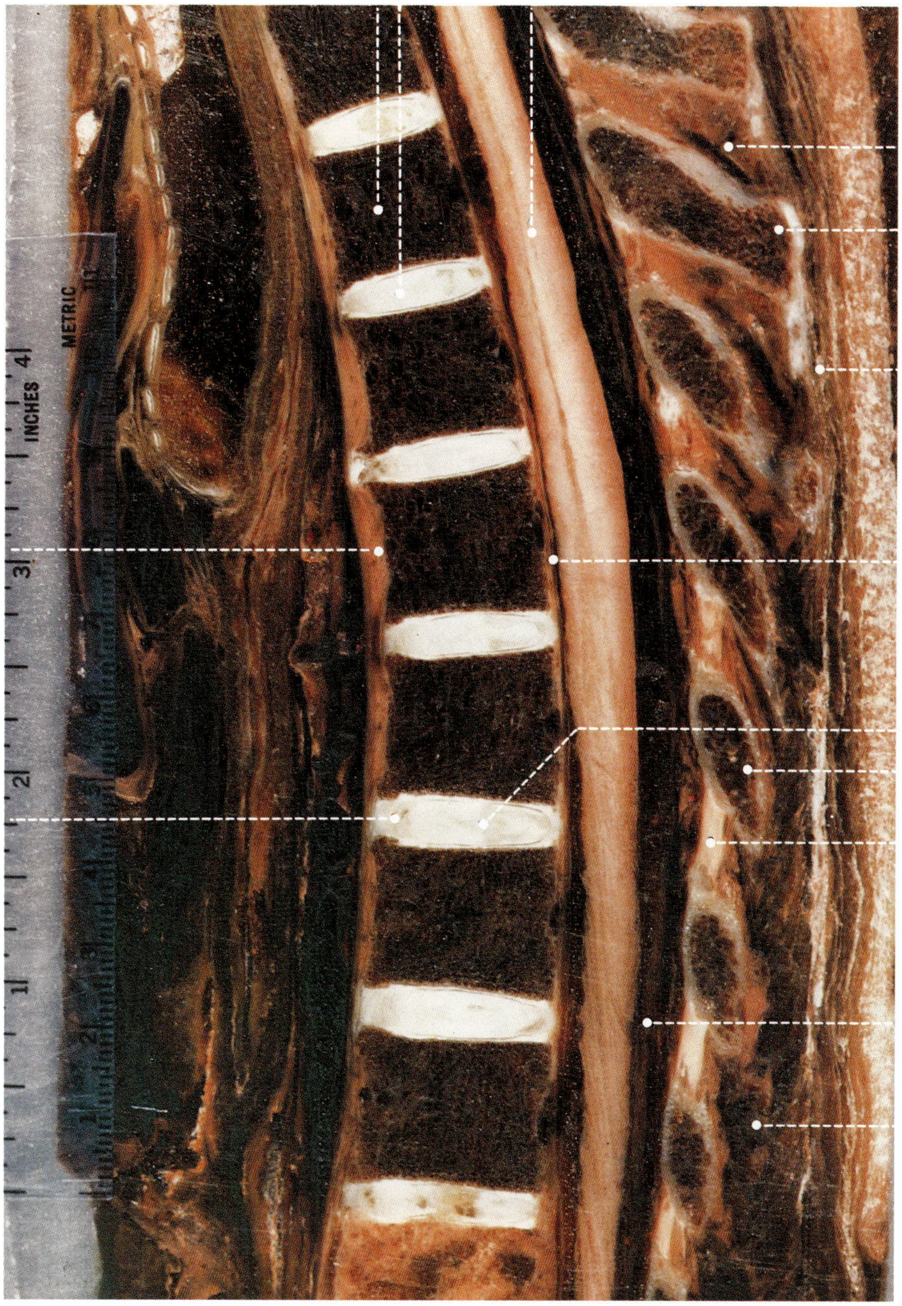

Anatomy and MRI of the Joints 148

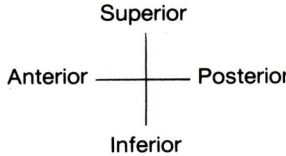

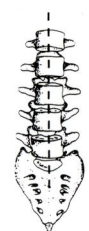

FIG. 6-6
SAGITTAL

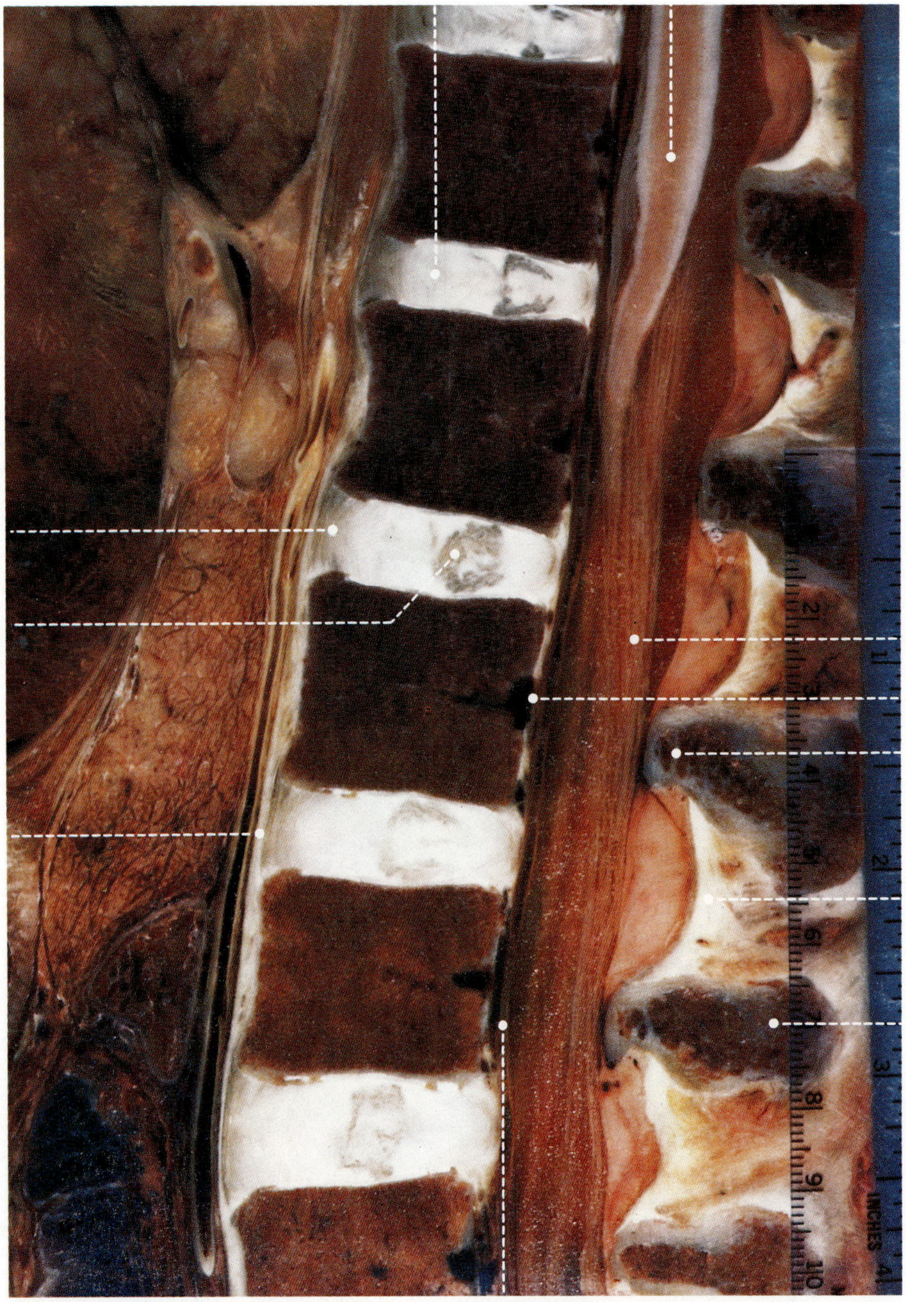

THE VERTEBRAL COLUMN

FIG. 6-7

SAGITTAL

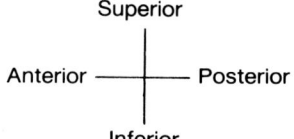
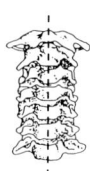

- Superior
- Anterior — Posterior
- Inferior

Labels:
- Medulla
- Cerebellum
- Dens
- Body of axis
- Intervertebral disc
- Spinal cord
- Anterior longitudinal ligament
- Posterior longitudinal ligament
- Nucleus pulposus
- Anulus fibrosus
- Posterior arch of atlas
- Spinous process of C 2

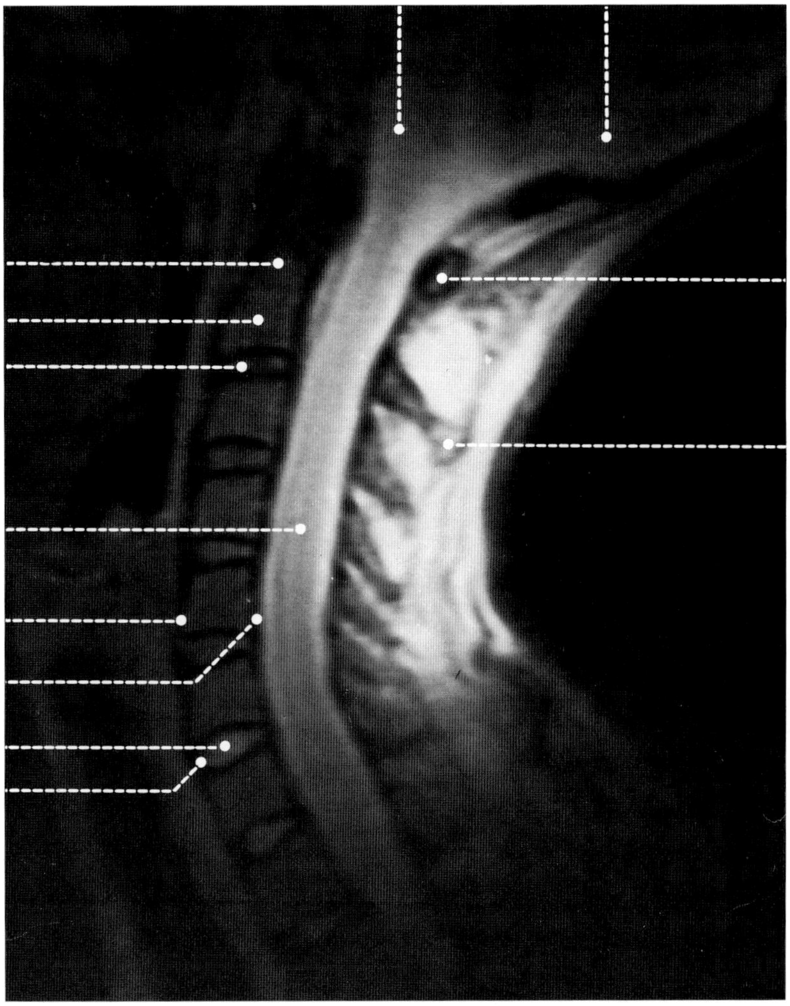

Anatomy and MRI of the Joints 150

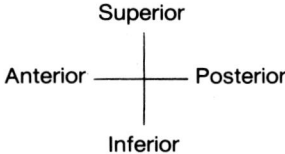

FIG. 6–8

SAGITTAL

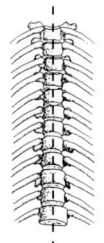

- Vertebral body
- Intervertebral disc
- Anterior longitudinal ligament
- Anulus fibrosus
- Nucleus pulposus
- Posterior longitudinal ligament
- Spinal cord
- Cerebrospinal fluid
- Lamina
- Ligamentum flavum

FIG. 6-9

SAGITTAL

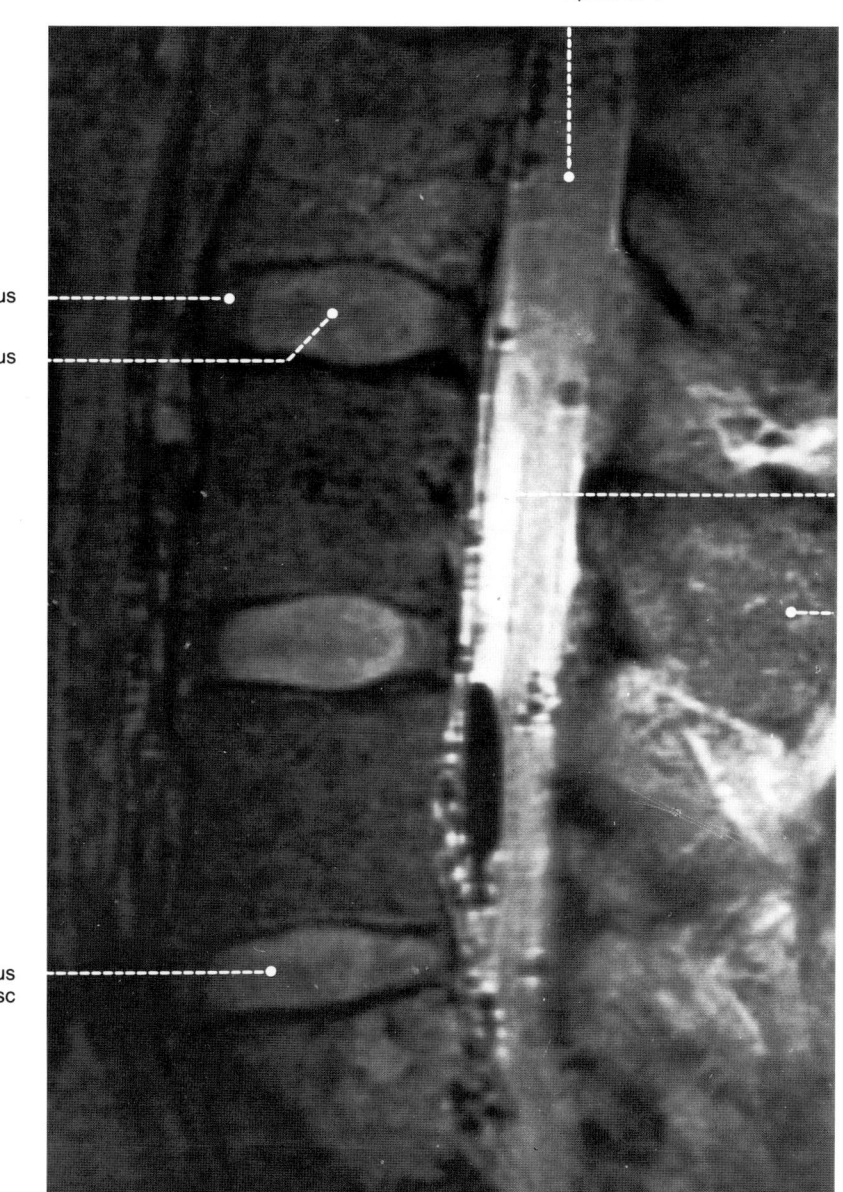

CHAPTER 7

THE HIP

Thomas L. Lawson, M.D. and William D. Middleton, M.D.

The function of the bony pelvis is to aid in the distribution and transmission of body weight to the limbs and to help absorb the stress of the muscular activity in the erect posture. The articulations of the bony pelvis include the hip joint, sacroiliac joint, and the pubic symphysis. In these latter two joints, free motion has been sacrificed in favor of stability and strength of union. The hip joint is the major joint of motion associated with the pelvis. It must be a strong joint and able to withstand great stresses and weight and also provide flexibility for motion of the lower extremity. The hip is structurally complex and reinforced by ligaments and bony struts to aid in this function. The hip joint allows for extensive motion: flexion, extension, adduction, abduction, circumduction, and rotation. The hip joint is well designed to allow not only for this wide range of motion, but also to provide the stability and strength to carry the weight of the body in an erect posture.

The hip is a ball and socket or an enarthrodial joint (Fig. 7–1). It is formed by the spherical-shaped head of the femur and the cup-shaped cavity of the acetabulum. The wall of the acetabulum is thick and heavily reinforced to support the weight of the body. The semilunar articular portion is open below and has a deep central nonarticular portion. The acetabulum is contributed to and is formed by the three component bones of the pelvis. One-fifth of the smooth lunate surface of the articular portion of the acetabulum is formed from the body of the pubis, two-fifths from the ilium, and two-fifths from the body of the ischium. The prominent osseous rim of the acetabulum forms the attachment of the labrum or cotyloid ligament of the hip joint. The uneven internal edge provides an attachment for the synovial membrane of the joint.

The articulating surfaces of the hip are covered with cartilage and lubricated by synovial fluid. The cartilage on the head of the femur covers the entire surface of the femoral head with the exception of a depression just below its center for the attachment of the ligamentum teres.

Conversely, the cartilage of the acetabulum is an incomplete cartilage ring of a horseshoe shape, with the opening of the horseshoe directed caudally.

The central acetabular fossa is a deep, irregular nonarticular portion of the joint. It is formed mainly from the ischium. In the fossa a small mass of fat can be found as well as the attachment of the ligamentum teres, one of the principle ligaments of the joint.

The acetabular fossa is open inferiorly as the acetabular notch. This notch is bridged by the transverse ligament. Just caudal to the acetabular notch is the obturator foramen, a large apperture surrounded by the bodies and rami of the ischium and the pubis.

The second component of the hip joint is the femoral head. The head of the femur is smooth and forms an approximate two-thirds of a sphere. The articular surface of the head of the femur is largest in its craniad and anterior portion, where the greatest weight is directed. Along its medial surface there is a small irregular depression, the fovea capitis or centralis, which forms the site of attachment of the ligamentum teres.

The head of the femur is attached to the body of the bone via the neck. This is a strong buttress of bone of about 5 cm in length. Its function is to displace the femoral shaft away from the pelvis to allow freedom of motion and to minimize contact of the leg with the pelvis. The neck forms an angle with the shaft of the femur which varies from approximately 115° to 140°. The head also points somewhat forward or anterior and as a result an anterior angle between the neck and shaft of the femur is formed that averages about 8°.

The greater trochanter is a large bony prominence along the lateral and craniad aspect of the base of the femoral neck. Along the medial and caudal aspect of the femoral neck is a smaller prominence called the lesser trochanter. Between the two bony masses there is an irregular ridge along the anterior aspect of the femur called the intertrochanteric line. Posteriorly, the two trochanters are joined

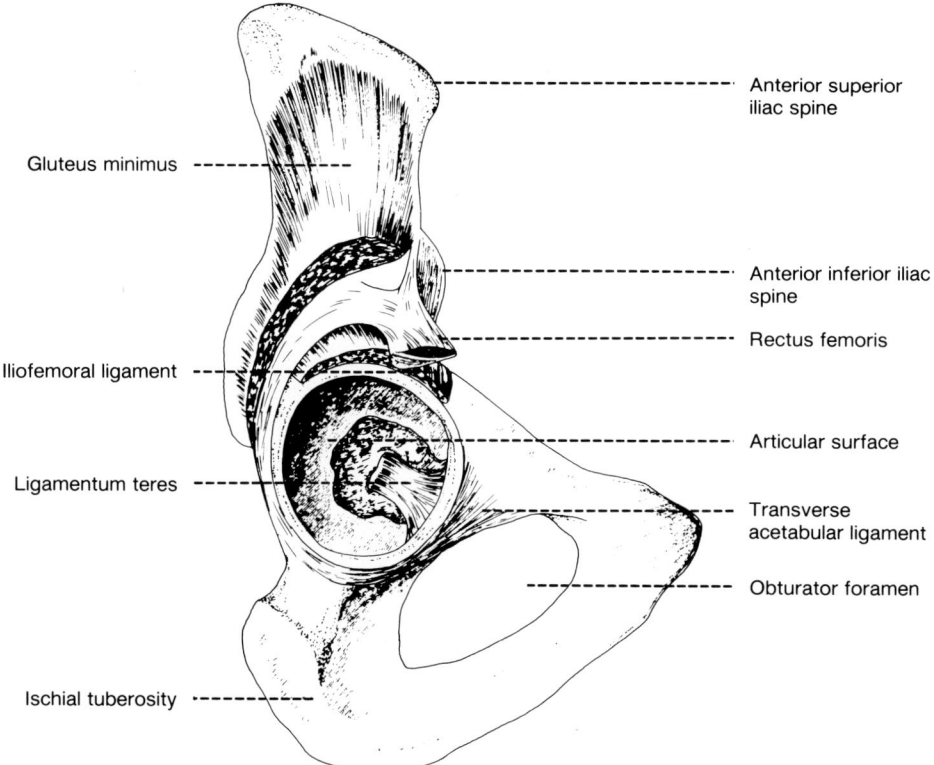

FIG. 7-1

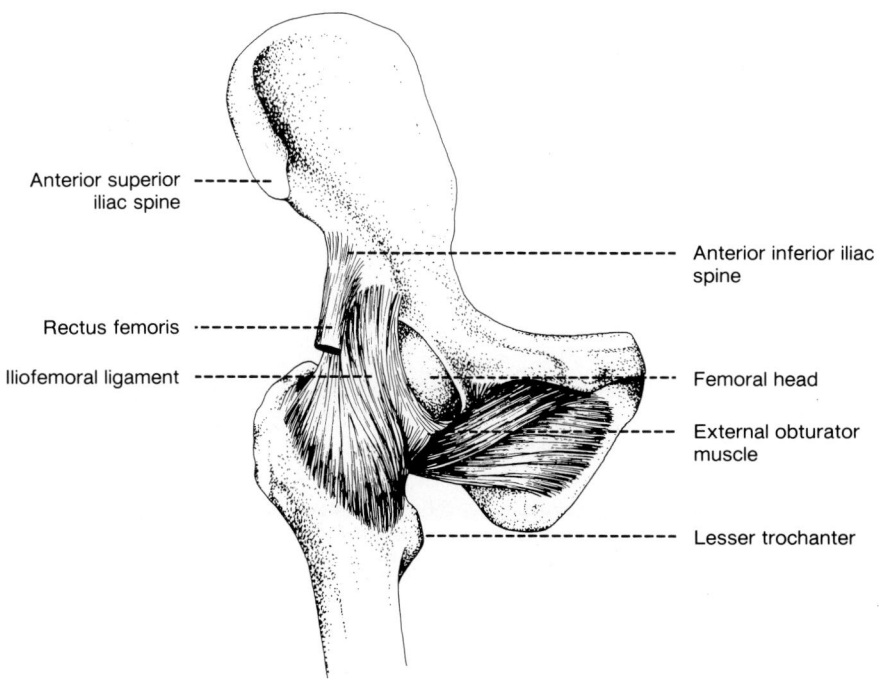

FIG. 7-2

by a thick intertrochanteric crest. Both trochanters as well as the intertrochanteric line and crest are important muscle attachment sites.

The femoral head is held to the acetabulum by five major ligaments: the capsular ligament, ligamentum teres, iliofemoral ligament, transverse ligament, and cotyloid ligament or acetabular labrum (Fig. 7-2). The capsular ligament is a strong, dense, fibrous band that extends from the margin of the acetabulum craniad over and surrounding the neck of the femur caudally. Its upper circumference is attached to the acetabulum, just external to the cotyloid ligament or labrum. Along the lower circumference of the acetabulum it is attached to the transverse ligament, as this ligament bridges the acetabular notch. The capsular ligament surrounds the neck of the femur and is attached to it. It is attached anteriorly to the anterior intertrochanteric line, posteriorly to the intertrochanteric crest, and craniad to the base of the neck of the femur. From these insertions the fibers are reflected upward over the neck of the femur forming a tubular sheath and a dense ligamentous joint capsule. While the external surface of the capsular ligament is rough and covered by numerous muscles, its inner surface is smooth, glistening, and lubricated by synovial fluid.

The iliofemoral ligament is a thick fibrous band that extends obliquely across the front or anterior aspect of the joint. It is intimately associated with the capsular ligament and serves to strengthen it. It is attached above to the lower portion of the anterior inferior spine of the ilium. Caudally it diverges to form two bands, one of which passes downward to insert on the anterior intertrochanteric line. The second band passes caudally and laterally and inserts on the upper portion of the intertrochanteric line adjacent to the neck and greater tuberosity of the femur.

The ligamentum teres, also called the ligamentum capitis femoris, is a strong triangular fibrous band that crosses the joint. The narrow apex of the ligament is attached to the femoral head at the fovea capitis femoris. The broad base of the ligament inserts into the acetabular fossa. Along its inferior portion the ligamentum teres blends into the cotyloid and transverse ligaments. The ligamentum teres is formed by connective tissue, but is surrounded by a tubular sheath of synovial membrane.

The cotyloid ligament or acetabular labrum is the fibrocartilaginous rim attached to the margin of the acetabulum. The function of the ligament is to deepen the acetabular fossa as well as to protect the edges of the acetabulum and to smooth the irregularities of its surface. On cross-section this ligament is prismoidal. The base which is attached to the margin of the acetabulum is thick, while its free edge is thin and sharp.

The transverse ligament bridges the caudal opening of the acetabulum between the acetabular notch. It forms a portion of the cotyloid ligament or acetabular labrum, although histologically it has a slightly different appearance. There is a small notch or opening at the lower portion of the acetabulum between the transverse ligament and the acetabulum itself. Through this small foramen passes nutrient vessels to the joint itself.

The synovial membrane of the joint is extensive. It covers all portions of the neck of the femur contained within the joint capsular ligament. From the neck it is reflected on the internal surface of the capsular ligament and covers both surfaces of the cotyloid ligament as well as the ligamentum teres.

The anatomical relations of the muscle of the hip can be best understood by dividing them into posterior, anterior, medial, and lateral groups. The posterior group, also known as the short rotators of the hip, consist of the piriformis, the obturator internus and externus, the two gemelli, and the quadratus femoris muscles (Fig. 7-3). The piriformis muscle is the most superior of this group, arising from the lateral mass of the sacrum. It extends laterally and inferiorly through the greater sciatic foramen to insert via a rounded tendon onto the upper medial surface of the greater trochanter of the femur. The internal obturator muscle arises from the deep inner surface of the obturator foramen and passes posteriorly through the lesser sciatic foramen and around the ischium where it turns laterally and extends to insert onto the greater trochanter of the femur just posterior and caudal to the piriformis muscle. The superior and inferior gemelli muscles arise from the ischial spine and ischial tuberosity, respectively, and travel along the superior and inferior aspect of the internal obturator muscle, converging laterally with the insertion of the internal obturator muscle. The external obturator muscle originates from the superficial surface of the obturator foramen and passes posteriorly and laterally beneath the hip joint. It inserts onto the posterior aspect of the greater trochanter below the obturator internus. The quadratus femoris muscle is the most inferior of this group. It arises from the lateral border of the ischial tuberosity and passes laterally to insert onto the posterior intertrochanter crest.

The lateral muscle group consists of the three gluteus muscles and the tensor fascia latae muscle. The gluteus minimus muscle is the deepest and most anterior gluteal muscle arising along the anterior lateral surface of the ilium. It extends inferiorly to insert on the anterior superior aspect of the greater trochanter. The gluteus medius muscle originates posterior and superior to the gluteus minimus. As it extends inferiorly, it covers the minimus and inserts on the posterior lateral surface of the greater trochanter. The gluteus maximus muscle is the largest and most superficial of the gluteal muscles. It originates from the posterior-most aspect of the ischium, the sacrum, and the sacrotuberous ligament. The gluteus maximus muscle extends inferiorly and laterally, with the bulk of the muscle inserting into the iliotibial tract. Approximately one quarter of the deep portion of the muscle inserts directly on the posterior superior aspect of the proximal

Anatomy and MRI of the Joints

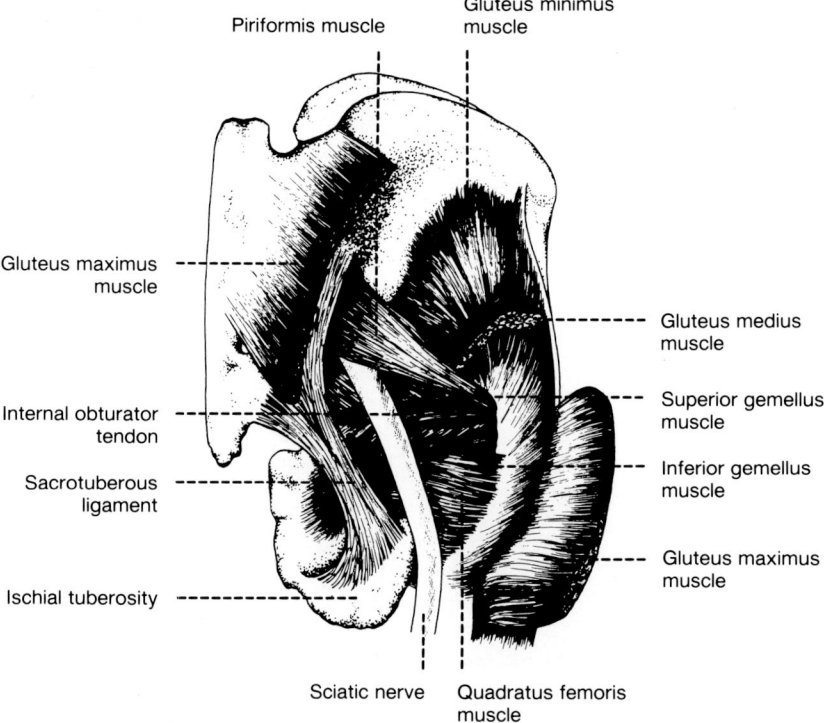

FIG. 7-3

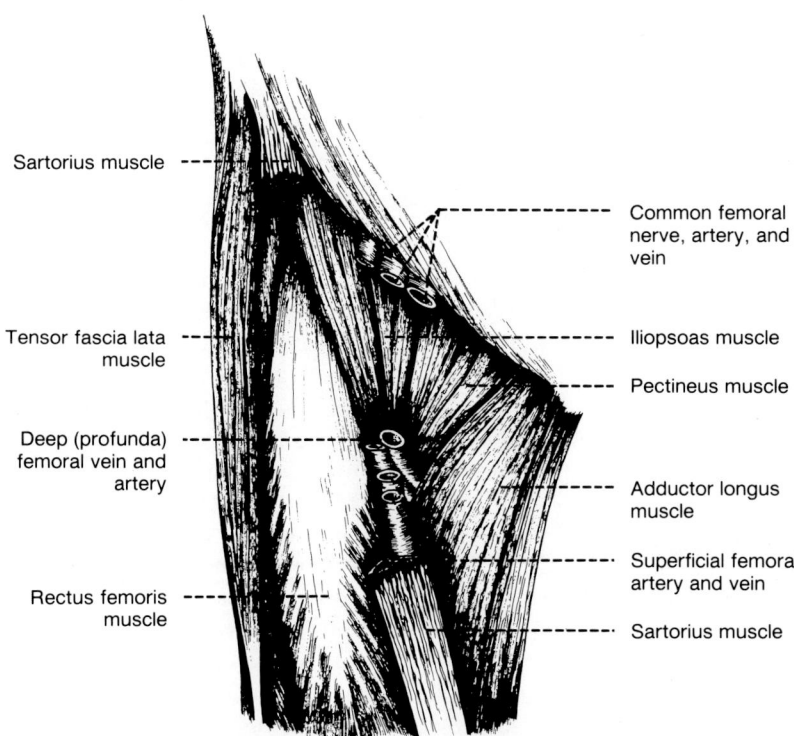

FIG. 7-4

femur. The tensor fascia latae muscle is a short strap-like muscle that originates anterior to the gluteus medius near the anterior superior iliac spine. It extends inferiorly to insert on the anterior aspect of the iliotibial tract.

The anterior muscles include the iliopsoas, sartorius, and rectus femoris muscles (Fig. 7-4). The iliopsoas muscle is the strongest flexor of the hip. At the level of the hip it passes deep to the inguinal ligament and crosses the anterior aspect of the joint. It inserts onto the lesser trochanter. The rectus femoris muscle is the most superior and superficial muscle of the quadriceps group and is the only muscle of this group that crosses the hip joint. It arises primarily as a thick tendon from the anterior inferior iliac spine, although a smaller tendon arises from the ilium immediately above the acetabulum. The sartorius muscle is the longest muscle in the body and travels as the most superficial muscle of the anterior thigh. It arises from the anterior superior iliac spine and travels inferiorly and medially toward the knee.

The medial muscle group includes the pectineus, the adductors, and the gracilis muscles. Although all of these muscles act on the hip, only the pectineus muscle is well seen in images of the hip. It arises from the anterior aspect of the superior pubic ramus and extends inferiorly and laterally over the external obturator muscle to insert onto the posterior aspect of the upper femur.

Several large neurovascular structures can be identified in cross-sectional views of the hip. The femoral nerve, artery, and vein travel vertically along the anterior aspect of the hip. They are located superficial to the iliopsoas muscle and deep to the inguinal ligament. The common femoral artery bifurcates into the superficial femoral and deep (profunda) femoral arteries approximately 3 cm below the inguinal ligament. The medial and lateral femoral circumflex arteries are branches of the deep femoral artery which provide blood supply to the hip joint.

The sciatic nerve is the largest peripheral nerve in the body. It originates from the lumbosacral trunk and the sacral plexus anterior to the piriformis muscle. It exits the pelvis through the greater sciatic foramen between the piriformis muscle and the sacrospinous ligament. Outside the pelvis the sciatic nerve runs dorsal to the internal obturator and gemelli muscles and deep to the gluteus maximus muscle.

THE HIP

AXIAL
    Cryomicrotomes.........................FIGS. 7–5 to 7–10
    MR Images.............................FIGS. 7–11 to 7–18

SAGITTAL
    Cryomicrotomes.........................FIGS. 7–19 to 7–24
    MR Images.............................FIGS. 7–25 to 7–32

CORONAL
    Cryomicrotomes.........................FIGS. 7–33 to 7–40
    MR Images.............................FIGS. 7–41 to 7–48

Anatomy and MRI of the Joints

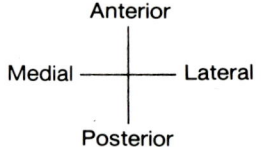

FIG. 7-5

AXIAL

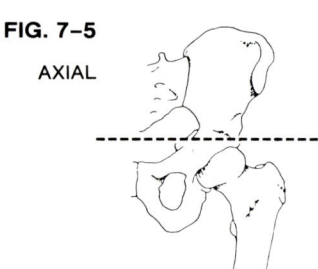

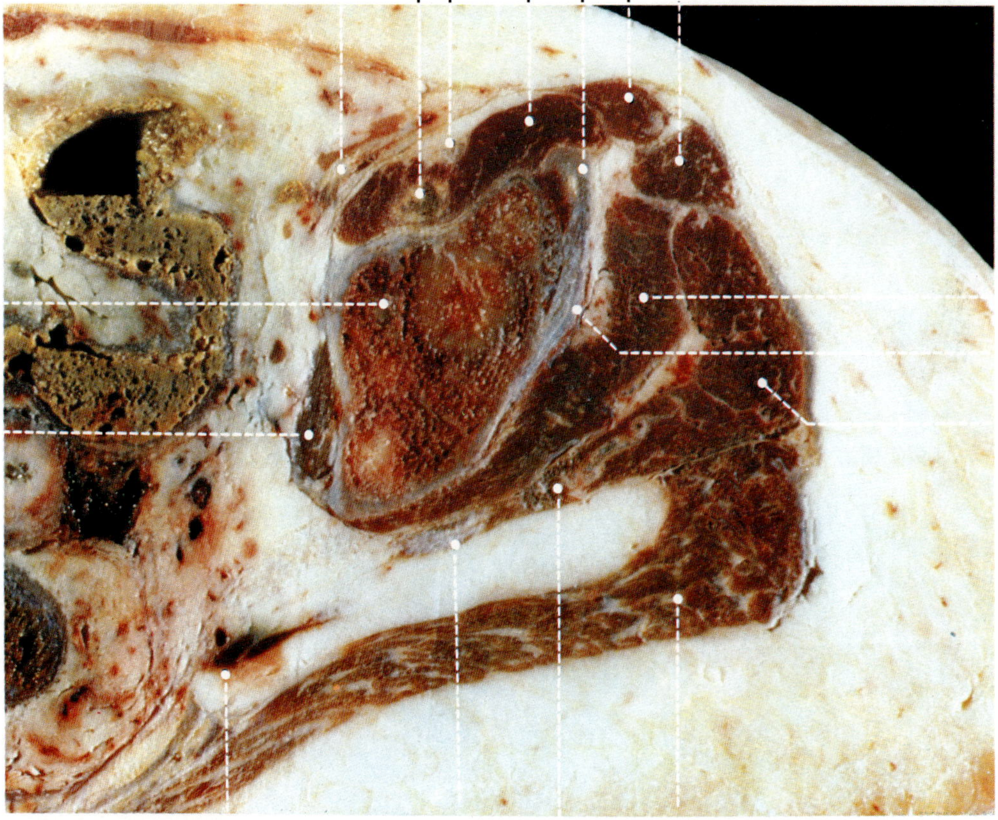

Labels (clockwise):
- Area of common femoral artery and vein
- Femoral nerve
- Iliopsoas tendon
- Iliopsoas muscle
- Tendon insertion for rectus femoris muscle
- Sartorius muscle
- Tensor fascia latae muscle
- Gluteus minimus muscle
- Capsular ligament insertion
- Gluteus medius muscle
- Gluteus maximus muscle
- Piriformis tendon
- Sciatic nerve
- Inferior gluteal artery and vein
- Internal obturator muscle
- Ilium

Anterior

Medial — Lateral

Posterior

FIG. 7–6

AXIAL

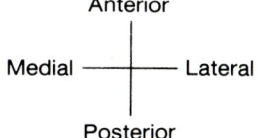

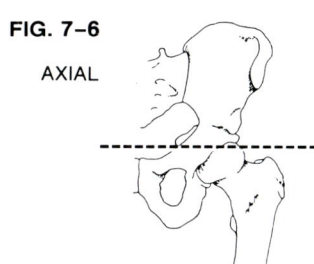

Femoral nerve
Tendon for ilopsoas muscle
Common femoral artery and vein
Labrum of acetabulum (cotyloid ligament)
Iliopsoas muscle
Rectus femoris muscle
Sartorius muscle
Tensor fascia latae muscle
Femoral head
Labrum of acetabulum (cotyloid ligament)
Internal obturator muscle
Iliofemoral ligament
Gluteus minimus muscle
Tendon for gluteus minimus muscle
Gluteus medius muscle
Inferior gluteal artery and vein
Sciatic nerve
Capsular ligament
Gluteus maximus muscle
Tendon for piriformis muscle

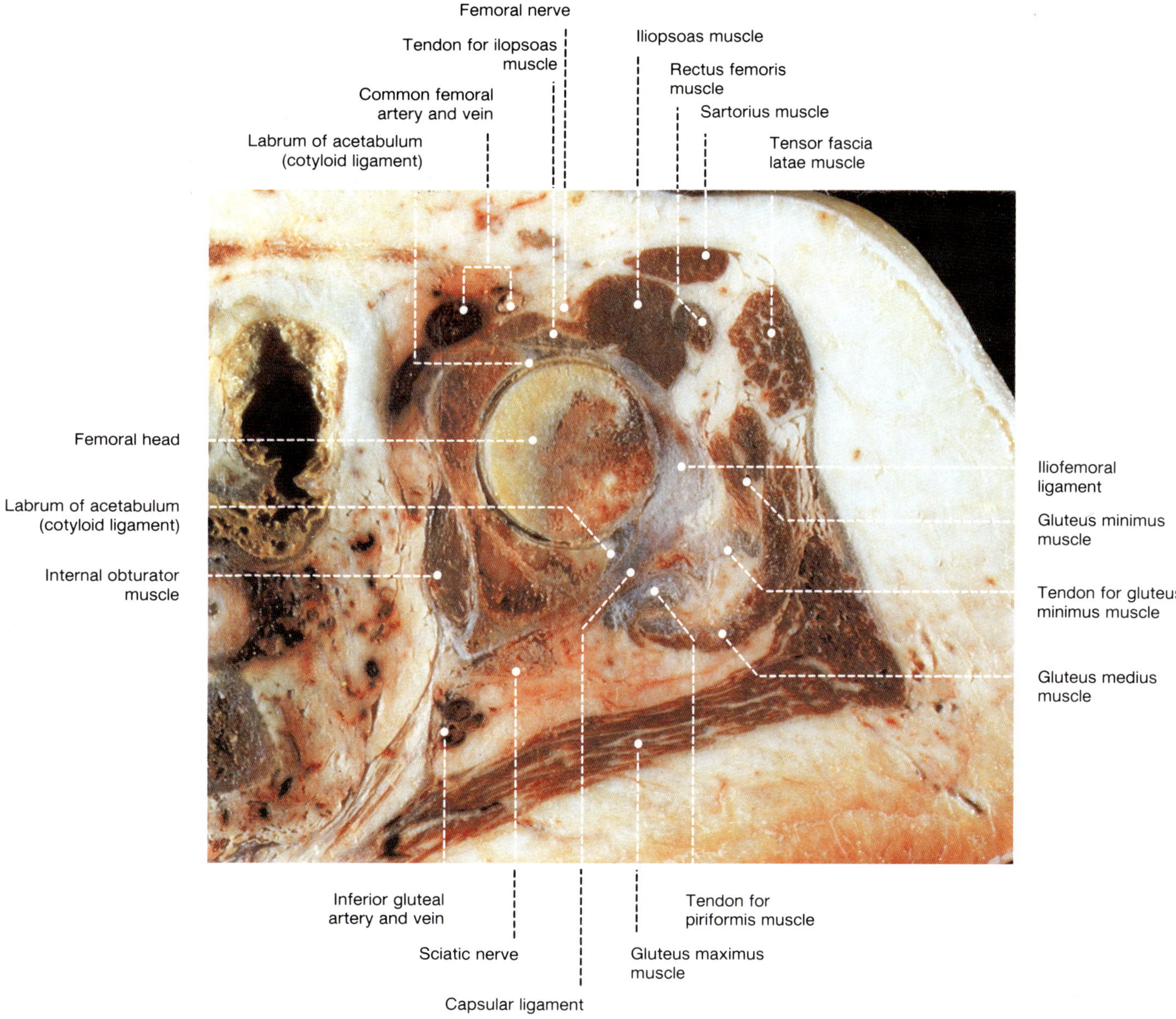

Anatomy and MRI of the Joints 162

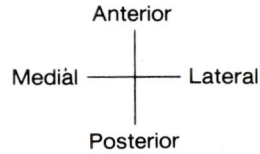

FIG. 7-7
AXIAL

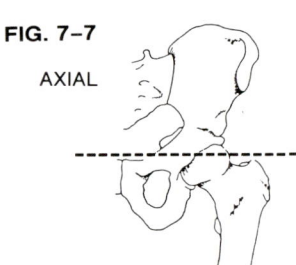

Figure 7-7. Axial section through the hip joint showing: Pectineus muscle, Common femoral artery and vein, Femoral nerve, Iliopsoas muscle, Tendon for rectus femoris muscle, Sartorius muscle, Tensor fascia latae muscle, Iliofemoral and capsular ligaments, Fascia latae, Gluteus minimus muscle, Gluteus medius muscle, Tendon for piriformis muscle, Tendon for gluteus medius muscle, Tendon for internal obturator muscle, Labrum of acetabulum (cotyloid ligament), Superior gemellus muscle, Sciatic nerve, Gluteus maximus muscle, Ischial spine, Sacrospinous ligament, Internal obturator muscle, Ligamentum teres, Pubis.

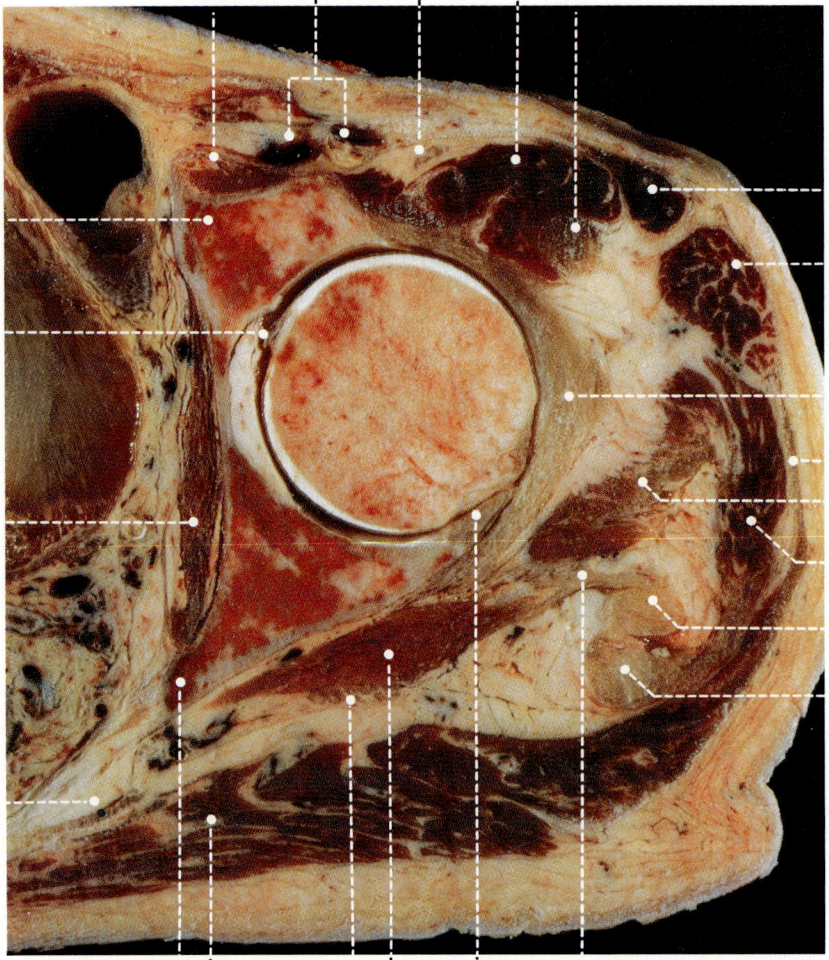

Anterior
Medial
Lateral
Posterior

FIG. 7–8

AXIAL

Common femoral artery and vein
Head of femur
Labrum of acetabulum
Iliopsoas muscle
Pectineus muscle
Sartorius muscle
Pubis
Rectus femoris muscle
Tensor fascia latae muscle
Internal obturator muscle
Iliofemoral and capsular ligament
Acetabular fossa
Neck of femur
Tendon of vastus lateralis muscle
Labrum of acetabulum (cotyloid ligament)
Gluteus minimus muscle
Capsular ligament
Tendon of external obturator muscle
Ischial tuberosity
Gluteus maximus muscle
Greater trochanter of femur
Sacrotuberous ligament (great sacrosciatic ligament)
Quadratus femoris muscle
Internal obturator muscle
Inferior gemellus muscle
Gluteus maximus muscle
Sciatic nerve

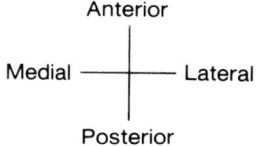

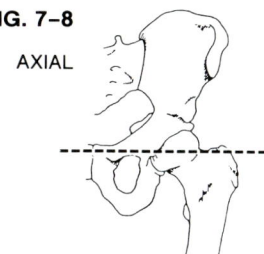

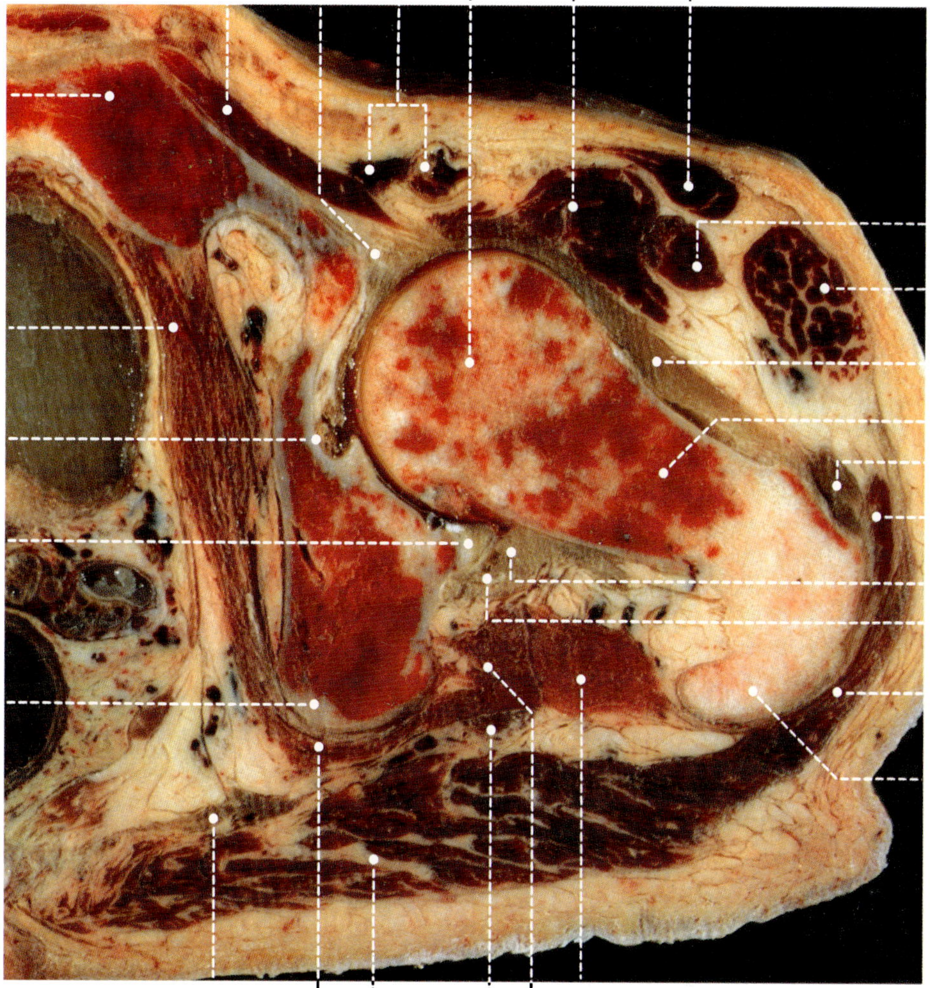

Anatomy and MRI of the Joints

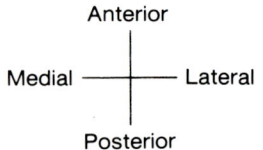

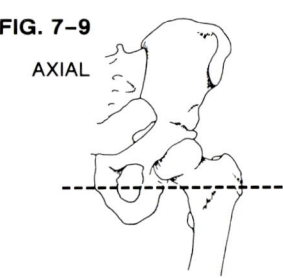

FIG. 7-9
AXIAL

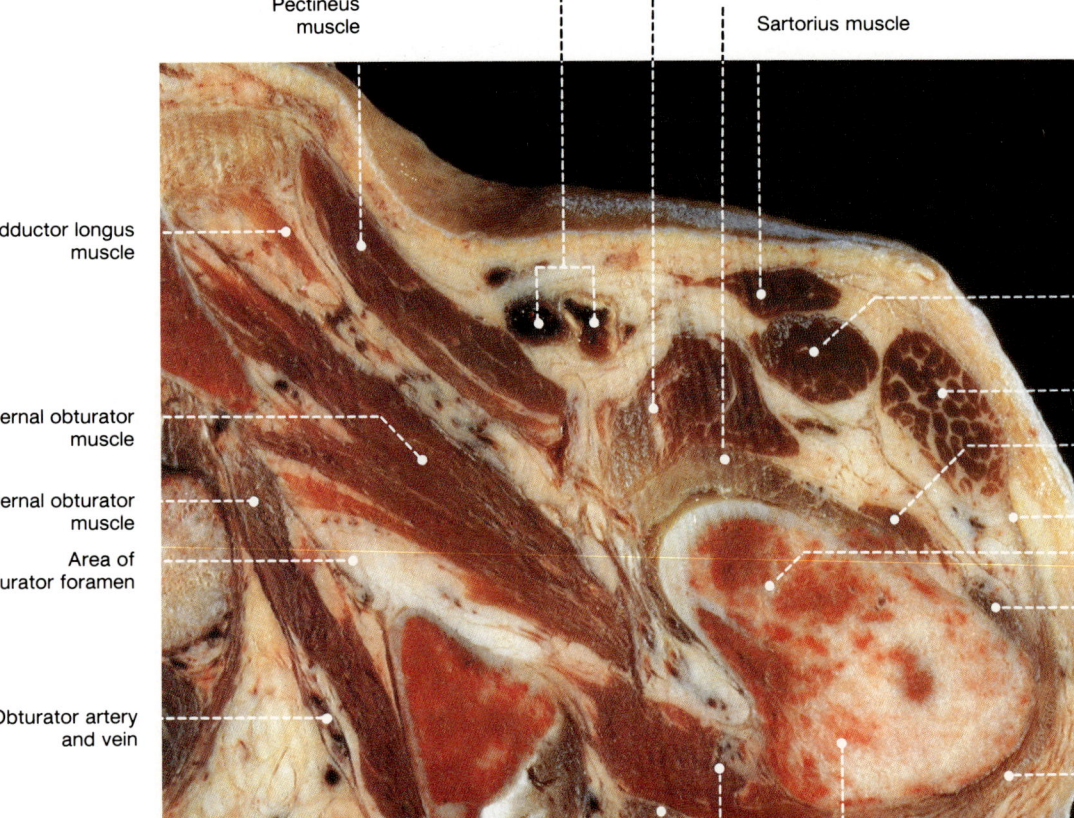

165 THE HIP

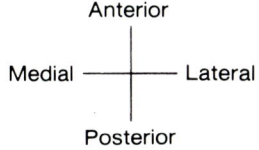

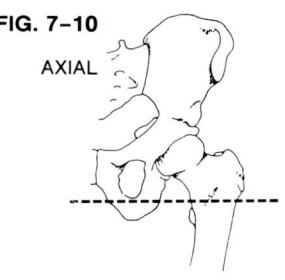

FIG. 7-10
AXIAL

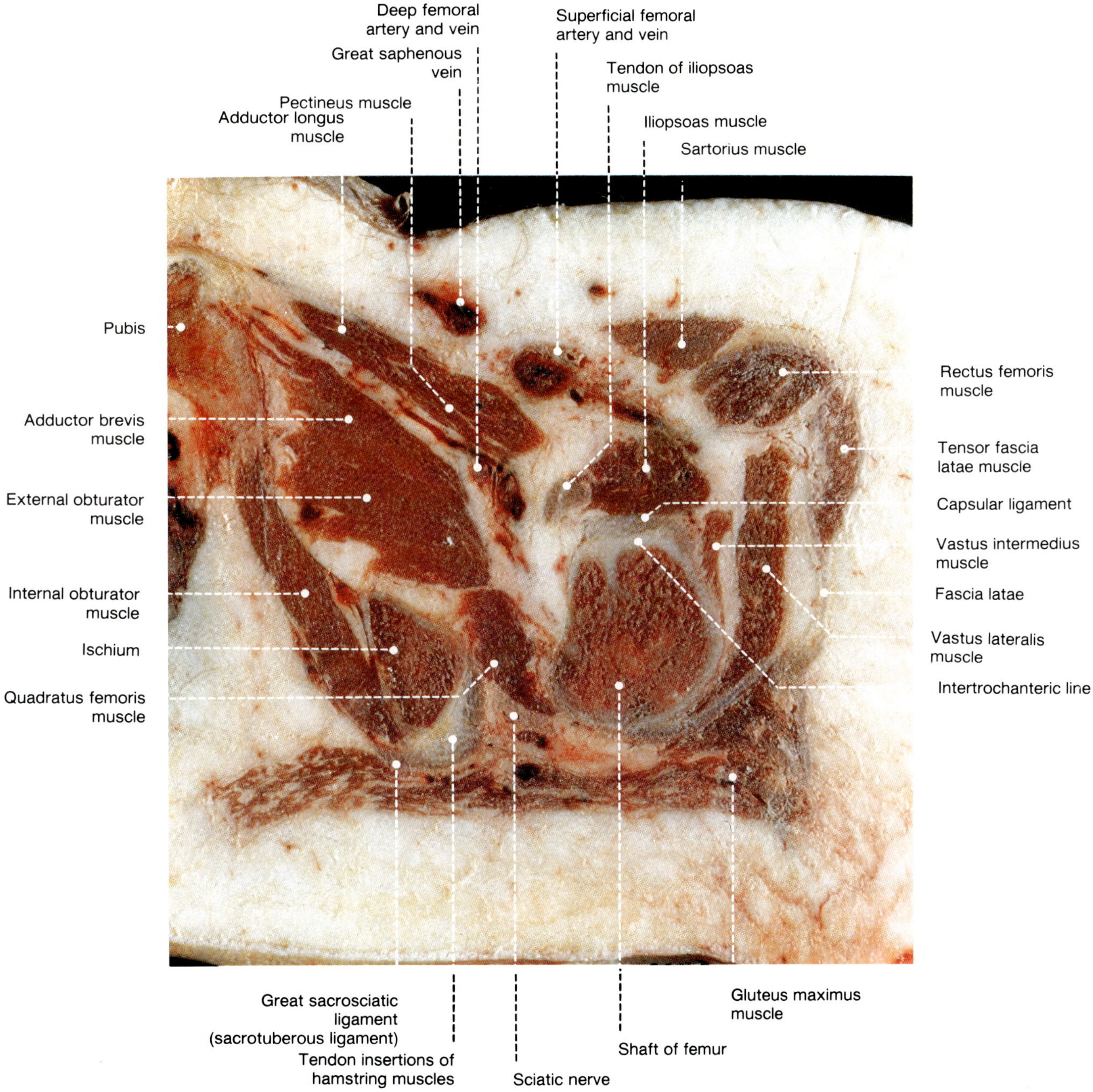

Labels (clockwise from top):
- Deep femoral artery and vein
- Great saphenous vein
- Superficial femoral artery and vein
- Tendon of iliopsoas muscle
- Iliopsoas muscle
- Sartorius muscle
- Rectus femoris muscle
- Tensor fascia latae muscle
- Capsular ligament
- Vastus intermedius muscle
- Fascia latae
- Vastus lateralis muscle
- Intertrochanteric line
- Gluteus maximus muscle
- Shaft of femur
- Sciatic nerve
- Tendon insertions of hamstring muscles
- Great sacrosciatic ligament (sacrotuberous ligament)
- Quadratus femoris muscle
- Ischium
- Internal obturator muscle
- External obturator muscle
- Adductor brevis muscle
- Pubis
- Pectineus muscle
- Adductor longus muscle

Anatomy and MRI of the Joints

FIG. 7–11
AXIAL

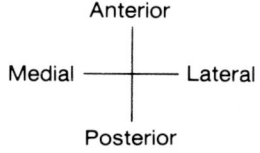

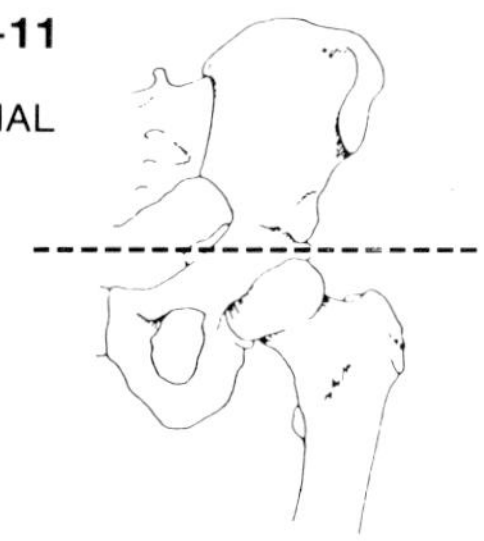

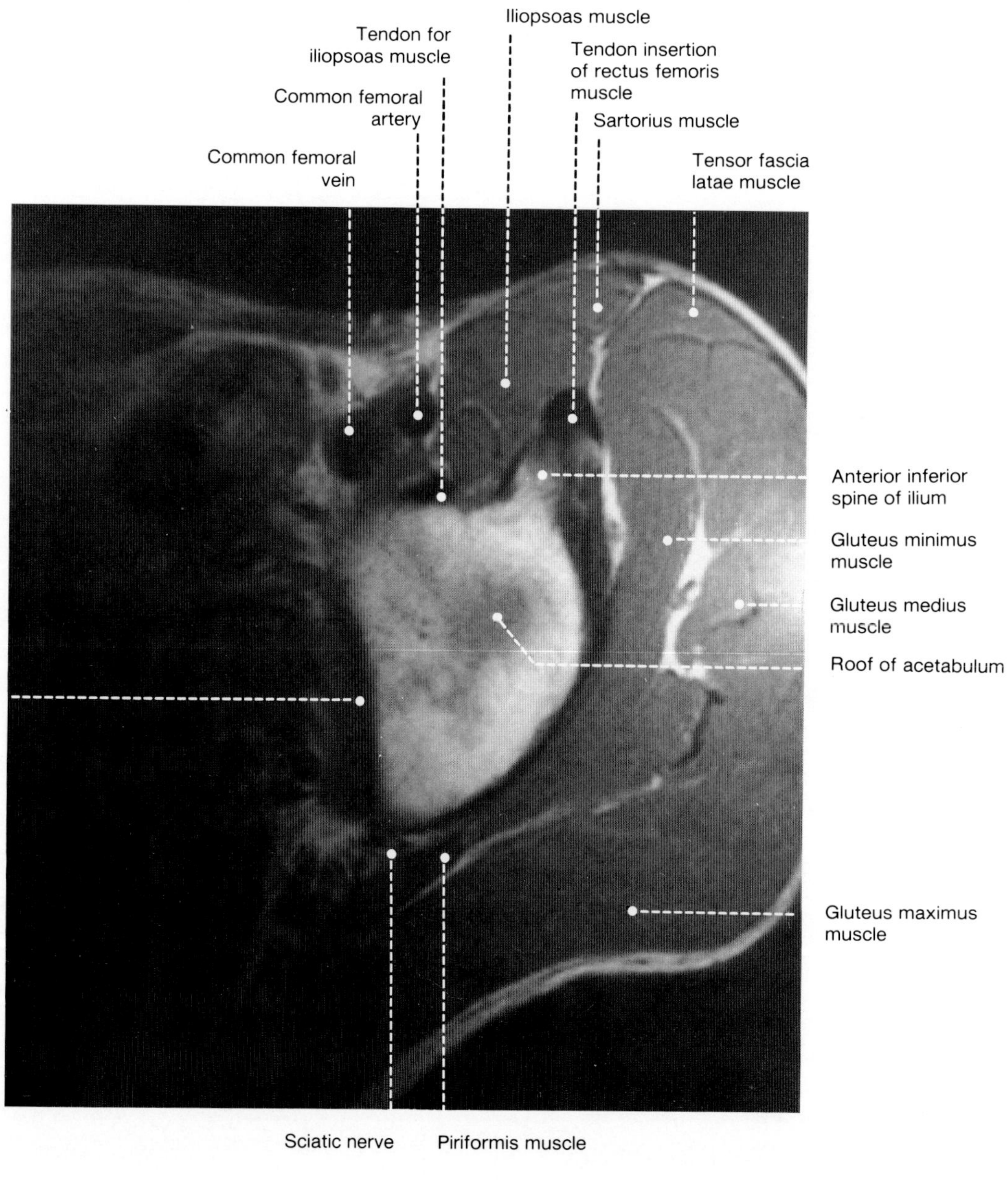

THE HIP

FIG. 7-12
AXIAL

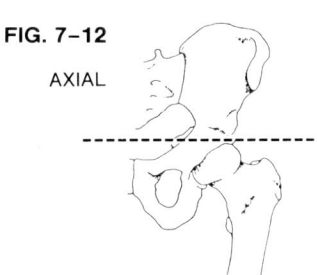

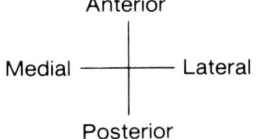

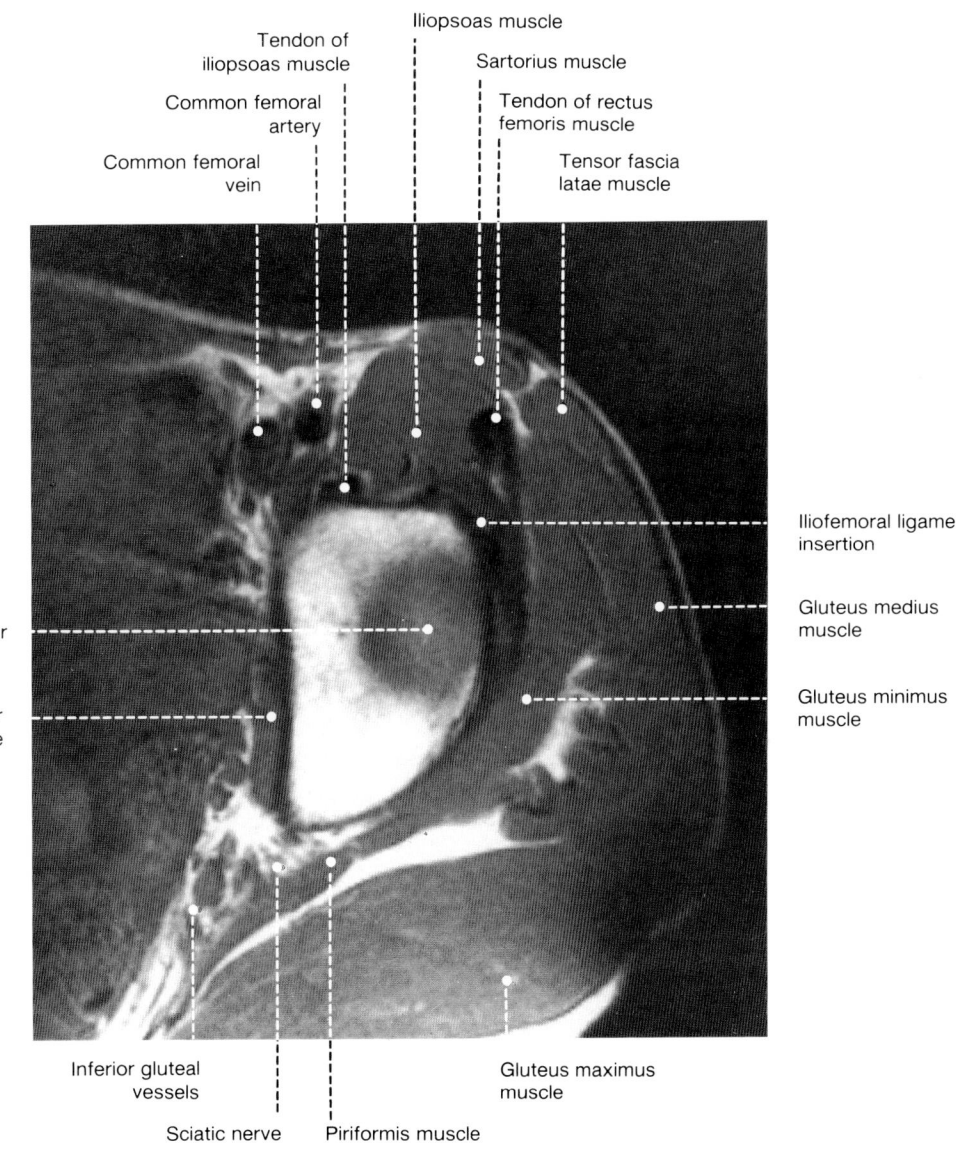

Anatomy and MRI of the Joints 168

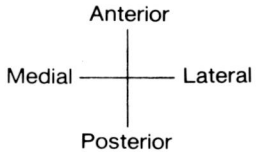

FIG. 7-13

AXIAL

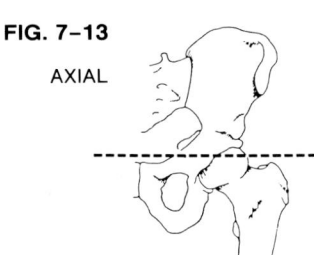

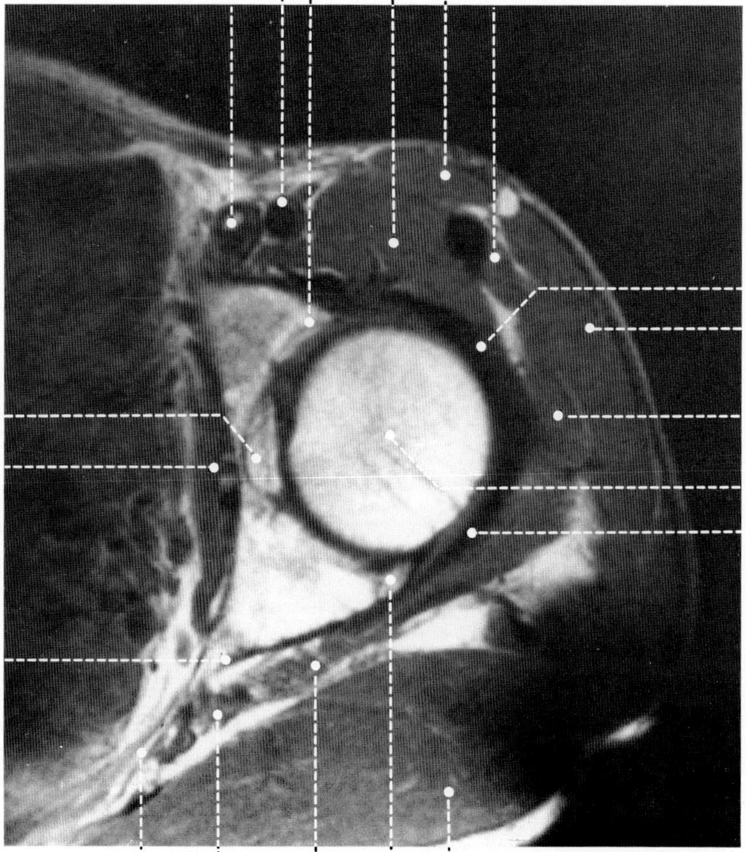

Rim of acetabulum
Common femoral artery
Common femoral vein
Iliopsoas muscle
Sartorius muscle
Rectus femoris muscle and tendon
Iliofemoral ligament
Gluteus medius muscle
Acetabular fossa
Internal obturator muscle
Gluteus minimus muscle
Head of femur
Capsular ligament
Spine of ischium
Sacrospinous ligament
Sciatic nerve
Superior gemellus muscle
Gluteus maximus muscle
Rim of acetabulum

Anterior
Medial
Lateral
Posterior

FIG. 7–14

AXIAL

Iliopsoas muscle
Common femoral artery
Sartorius muscle
Common femoral vein
Rectus femoris muscle and ligament
Labrum of acetabulum (cotyloid ligament)
Rim of acetabulum
Head of femur
Ligamentum teres
Acetabular fossa
Internal obturator muscle
Spine of ischium
Tensor fascia latae muscle
Iliofemoral ligament
Gluteus medius muscle
Gluteus minimus muscle
Capsular ligament
Greater trochanter of femur
Sacrospinous ligament
Sciatic nerve
Superior gemellus muscle
Tendon of interior obturator muscle
Gluteus maximus muscle

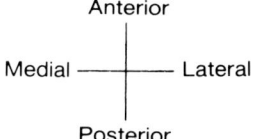

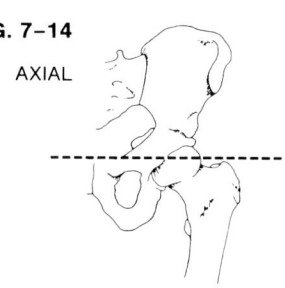

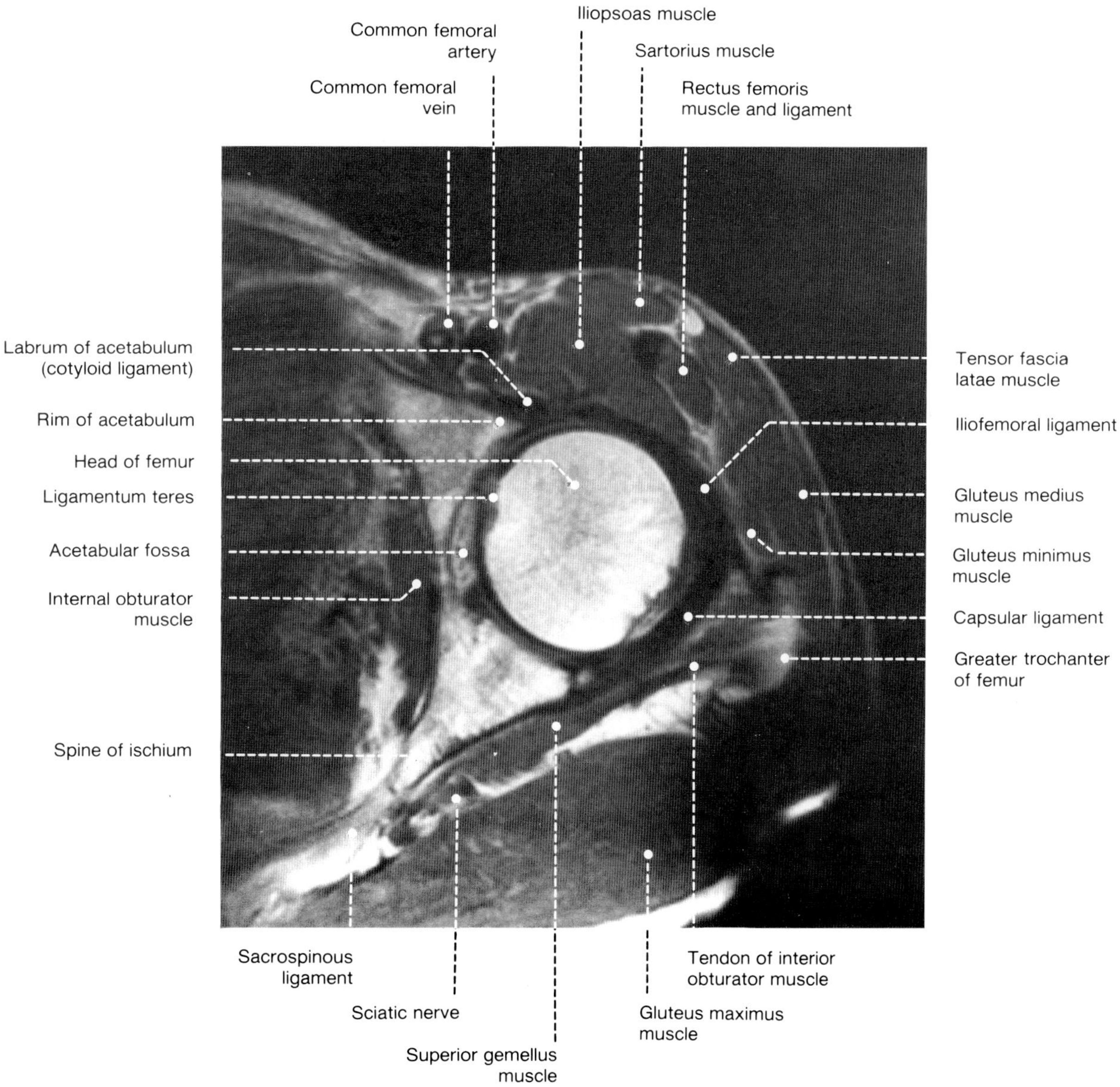

Anatomy and MRI of the Joints

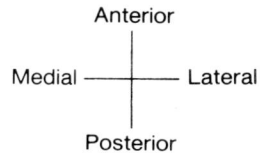

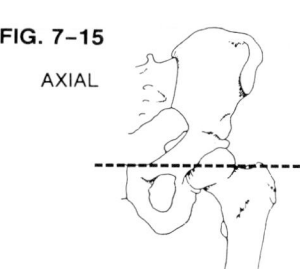

FIG. 7–15
AXIAL

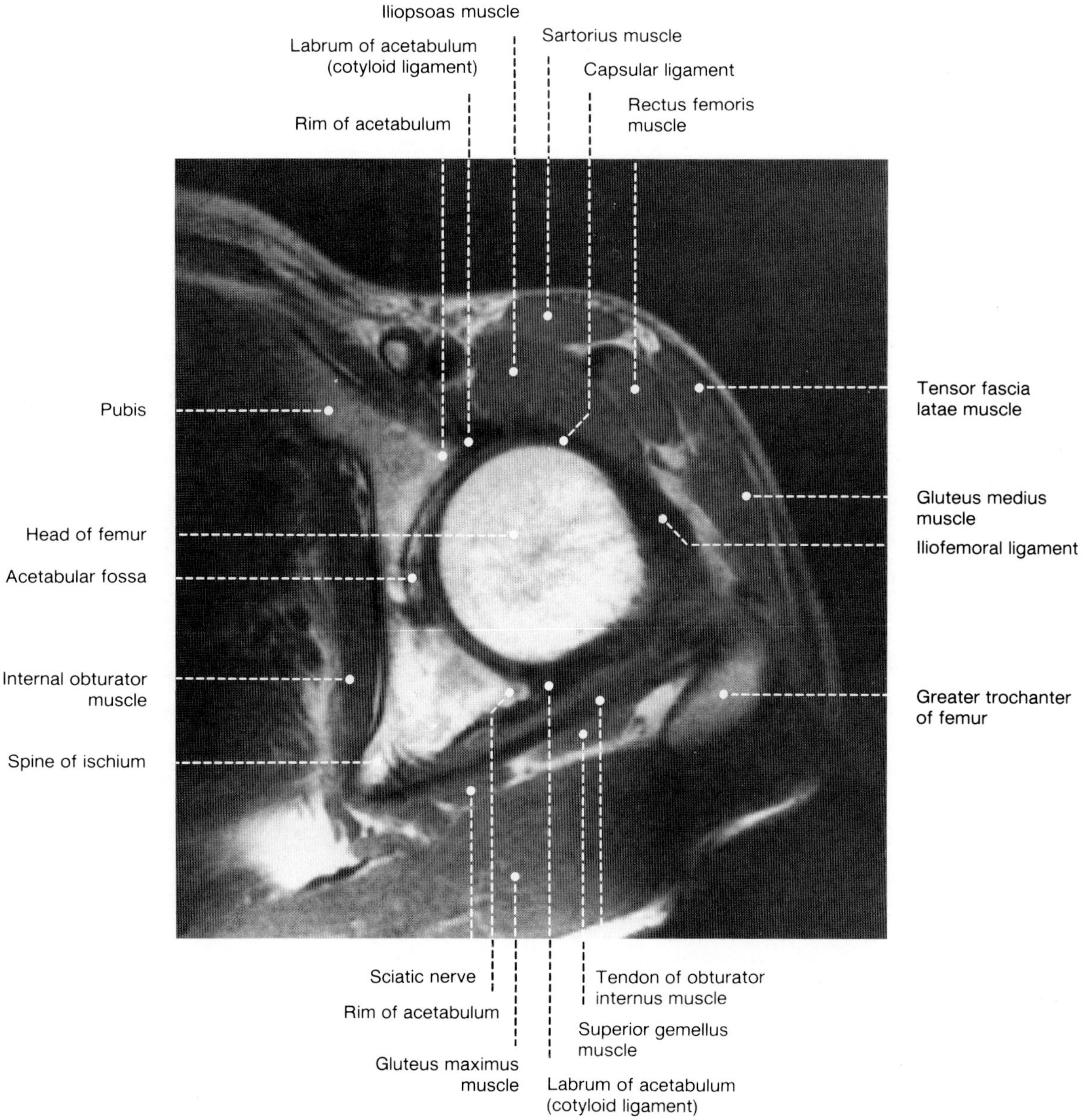

Anterior
Medial
Lateral
Posterior

FIG. 7–16

AXIAL

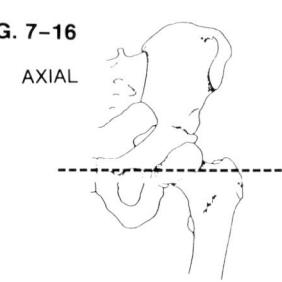

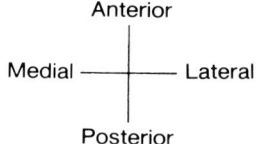

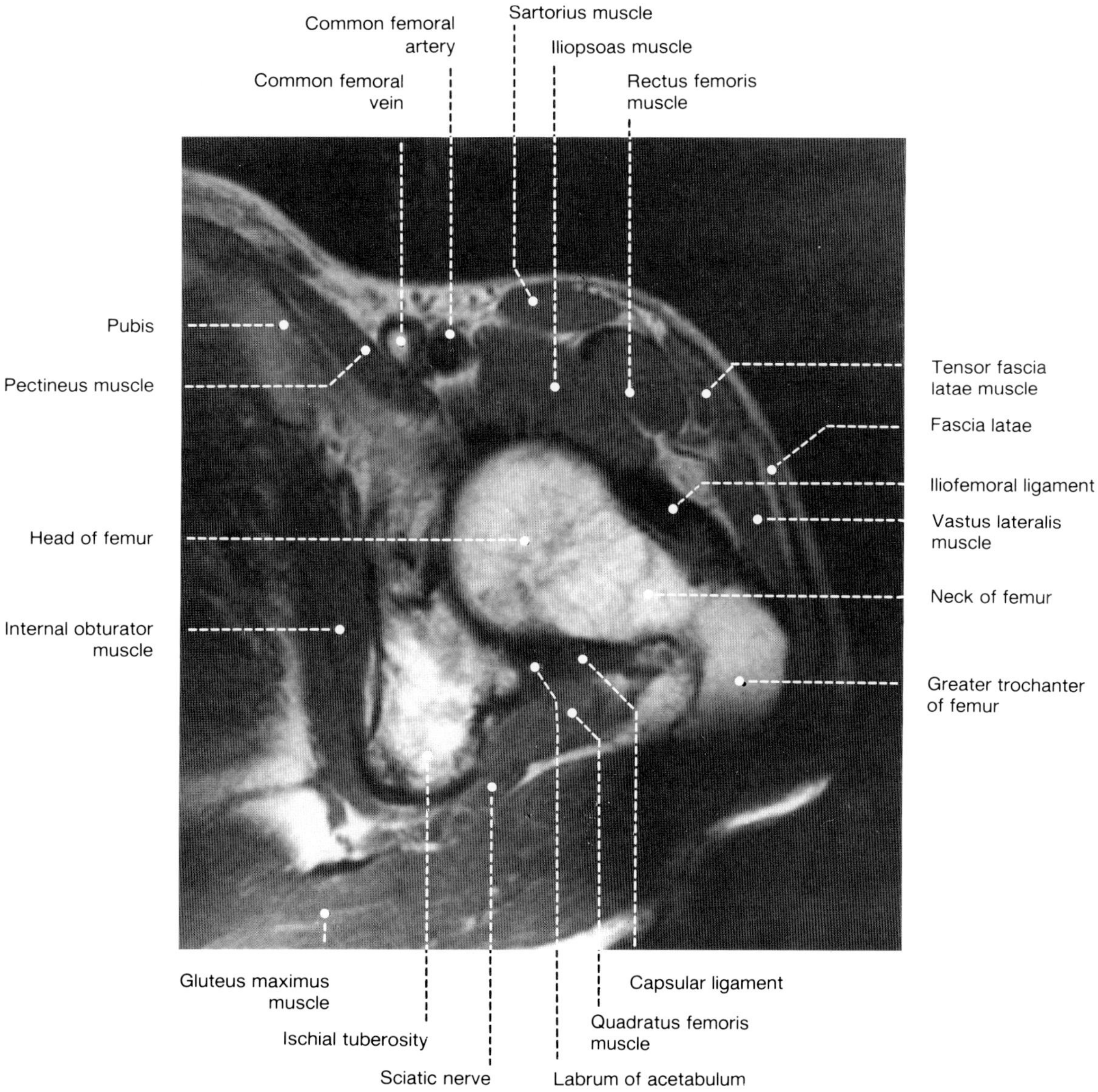

Common femoral artery
Sartorius muscle
Iliopsoas muscle
Common femoral vein
Rectus femoris muscle
Pubis
Pectineus muscle
Head of femur
Internal obturator muscle
Tensor fascia latae muscle
Fascia latae
Iliofemoral ligament
Vastus lateralis muscle
Neck of femur
Greater trochanter of femur
Gluteus maximus muscle
Ischial tuberosity
Sciatic nerve
Capsular ligament
Quadratus femoris muscle
Labrum of acetabulum

Anatomy and MRI of the Joints   172

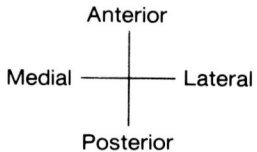

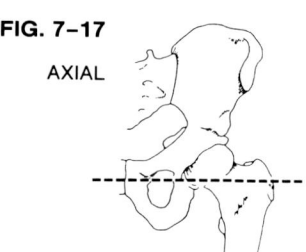

FIG. 7-17
AXIAL

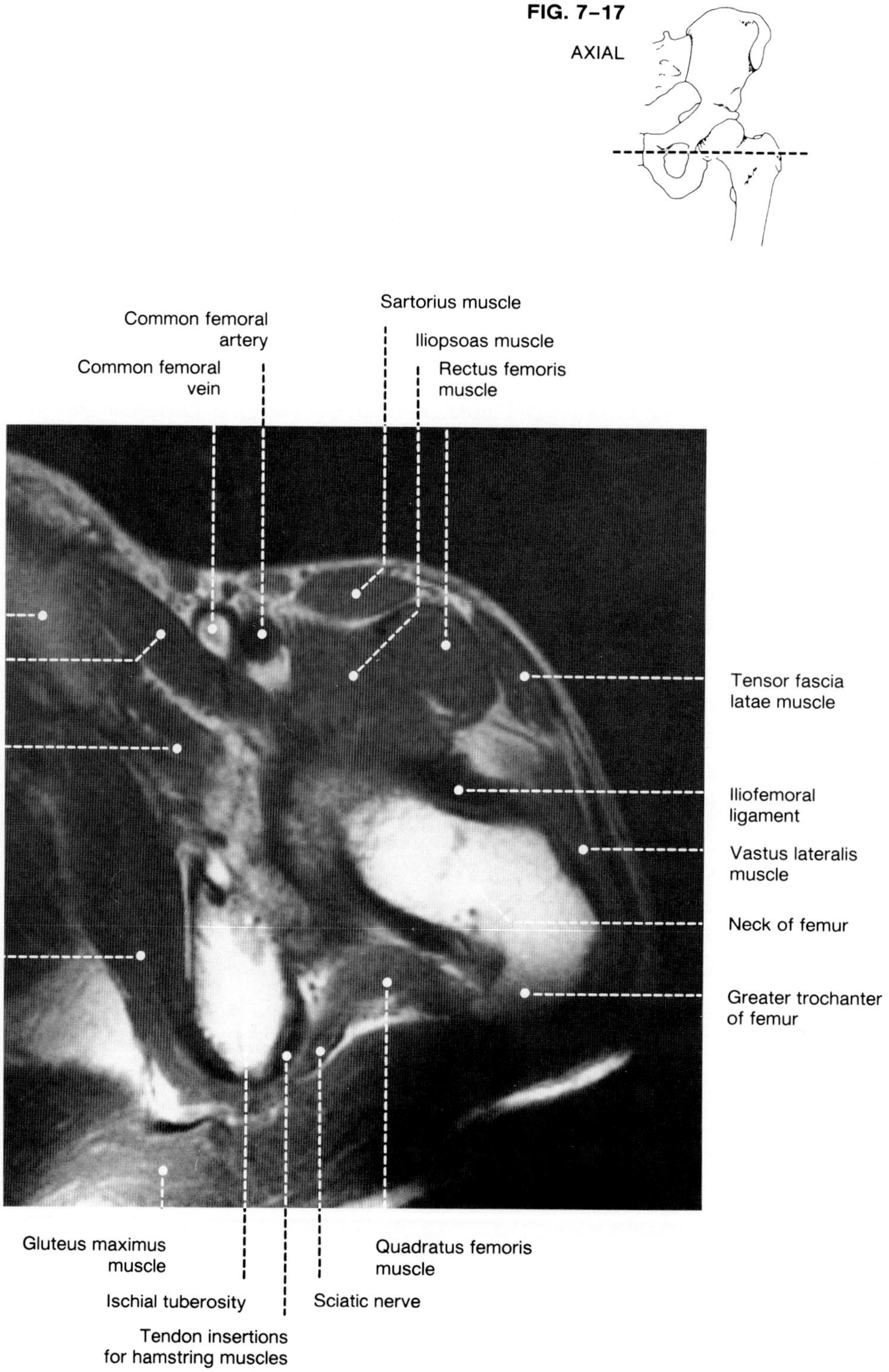

Anterior
Medial — Lateral
Posterior

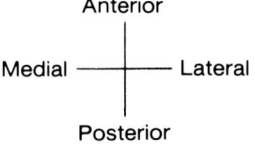

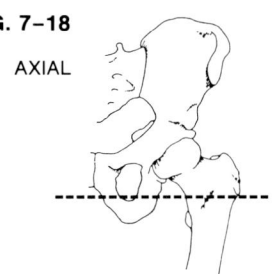

FIG. 7–18

AXIAL

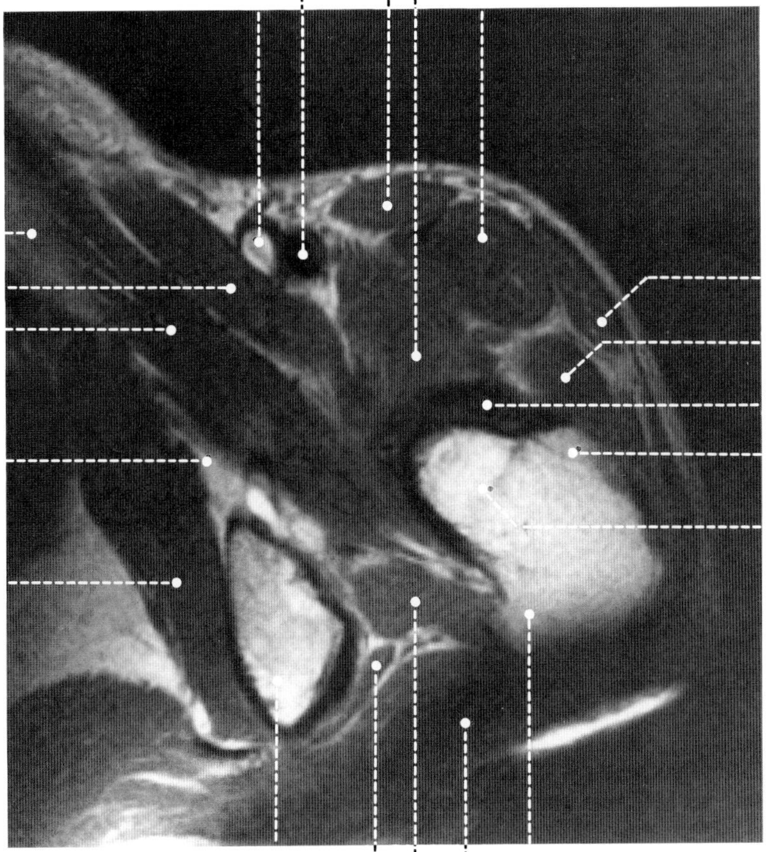

Anatomy and MRI of the Joints

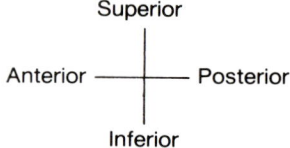

FIG. 7-19
SAGITTAL

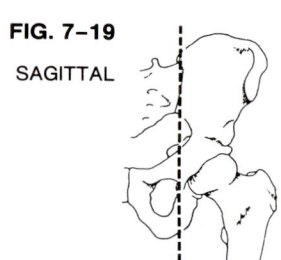

- Iliopsoas muscle
- Sacrum
- Sacroiliac joint
- Ilium
- Branches of internal iliac artery and vein
- Sciatic plexus
- Piriformis muscle
- External iliac artery
- Sciatic nerve
- Gluteus maximus muscle
- Internal obturator muscle
- Iliopectineal imminence (iliopubic imminence)
- Ischial spine
- Internal obturator and gemelli muscle complex
- Pectineus muscle
- External obturator muscle
- Ischial tuberosity
- Sartorius muscle
- Adductor longus muscle
- Adductor brevis muscle
- Tendon insertion of hamstring muscles

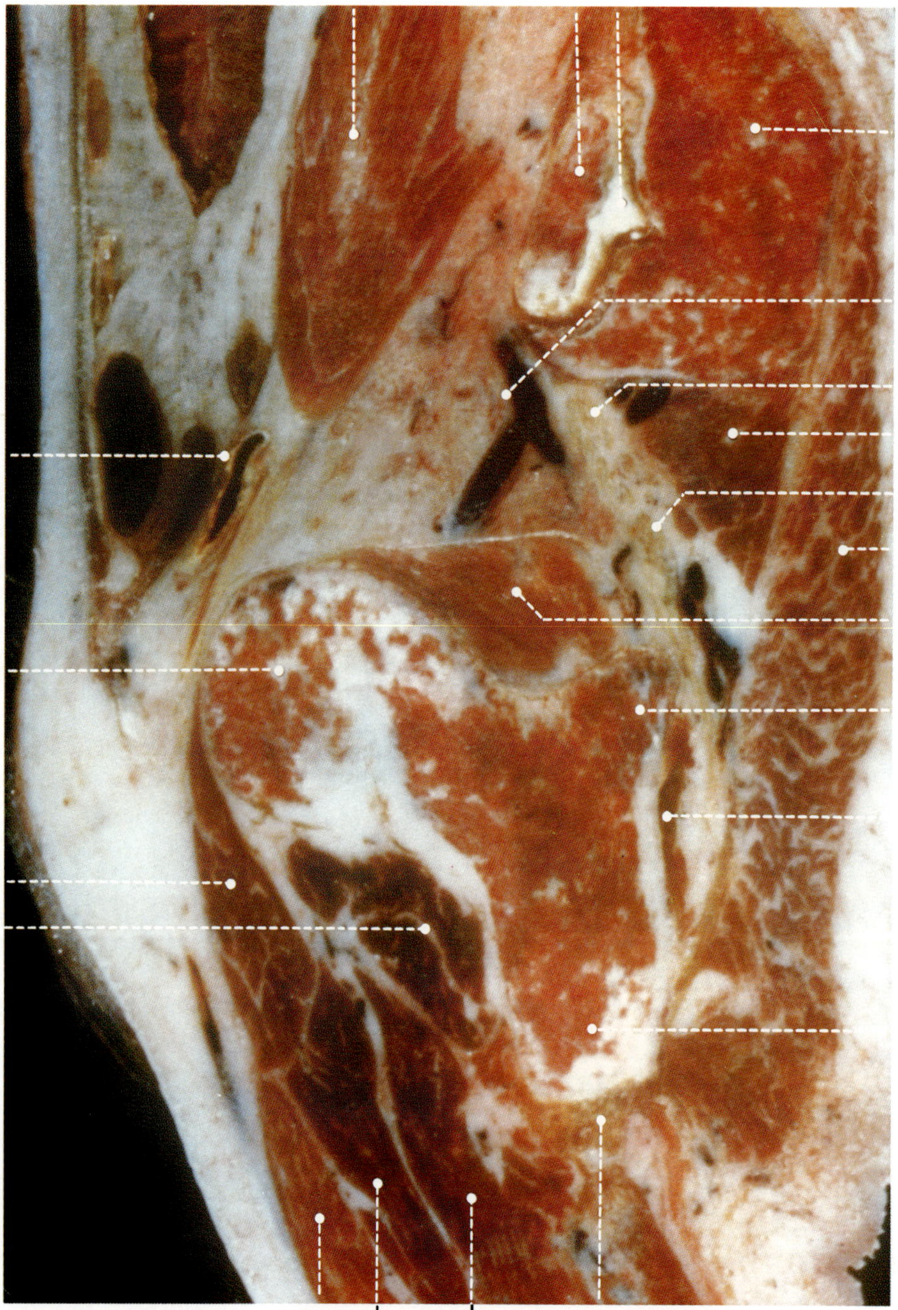

Superior
Anterior
Posterior
Inferior

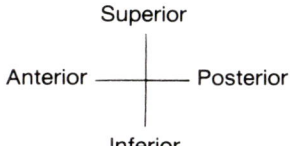

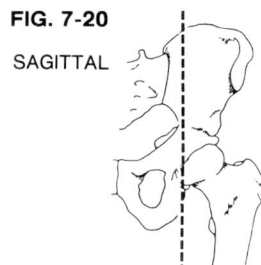

FIG. 7-20

SAGITTAL

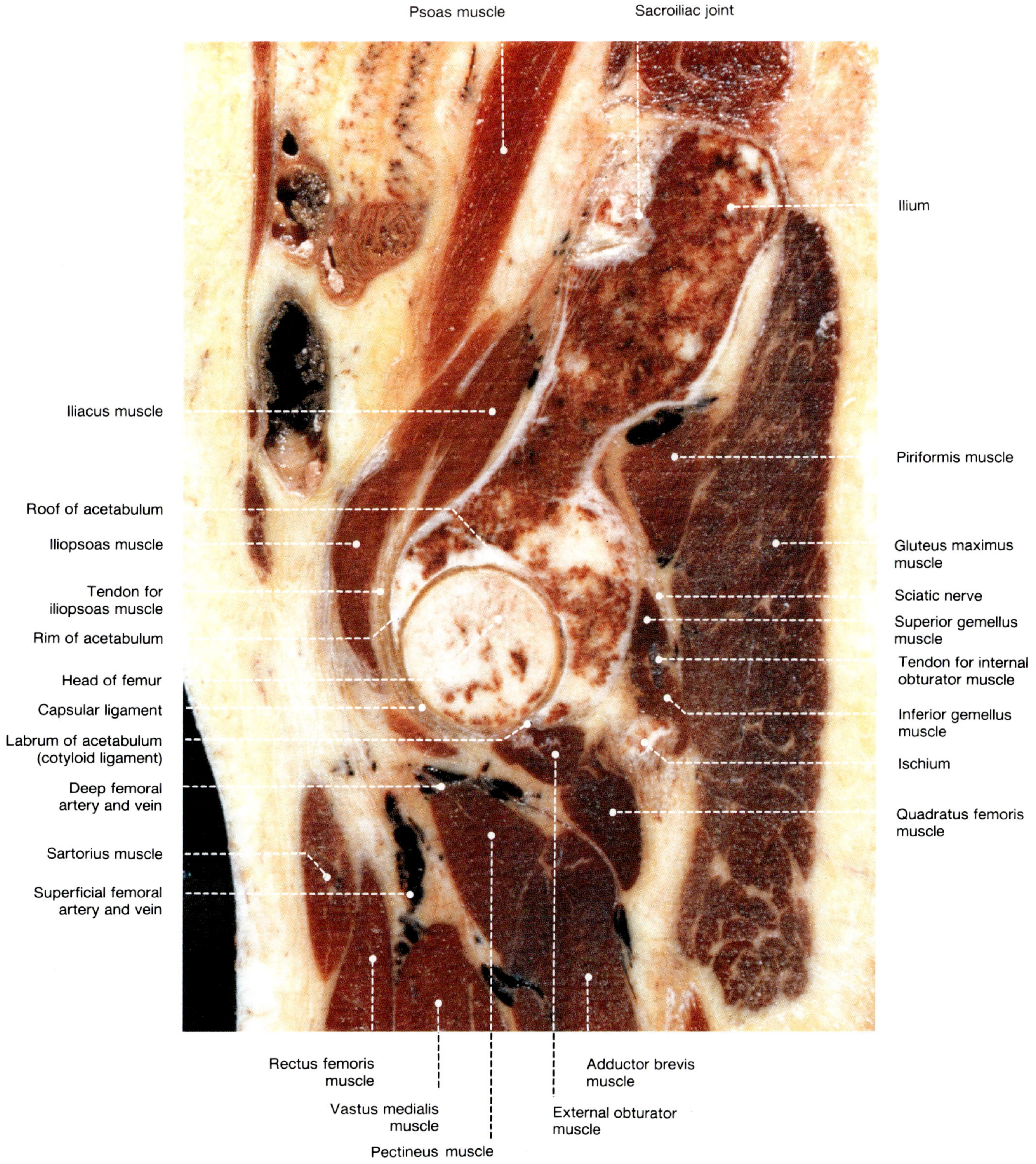

Psoas muscle
Sacroiliac joint
Ilium
Iliacus muscle
Piriformis muscle
Roof of acetabulum
Iliopsoas muscle
Gluteus maximus muscle
Tendon for iliopsoas muscle
Sciatic nerve
Superior gemellus muscle
Rim of acetabulum
Tendon for internal obturator muscle
Head of femur
Capsular ligament
Inferior gemellus muscle
Labrum of acetabulum (cotyloid ligament)
Ischium
Deep femoral artery and vein
Quadratus femoris muscle
Sartorius muscle
Superficial femoral artery and vein
Rectus femoris muscle
Adductor brevis muscle
Vastus medialis muscle
External obturator muscle
Pectineus muscle

Anatomy and MRI of the Joints 176 FIG. 7-21
SAGITTAL

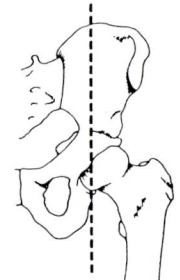

THE HIP

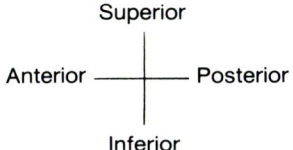

FIG. 7-22

SAGITTAL

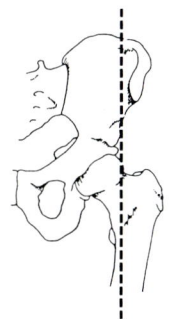

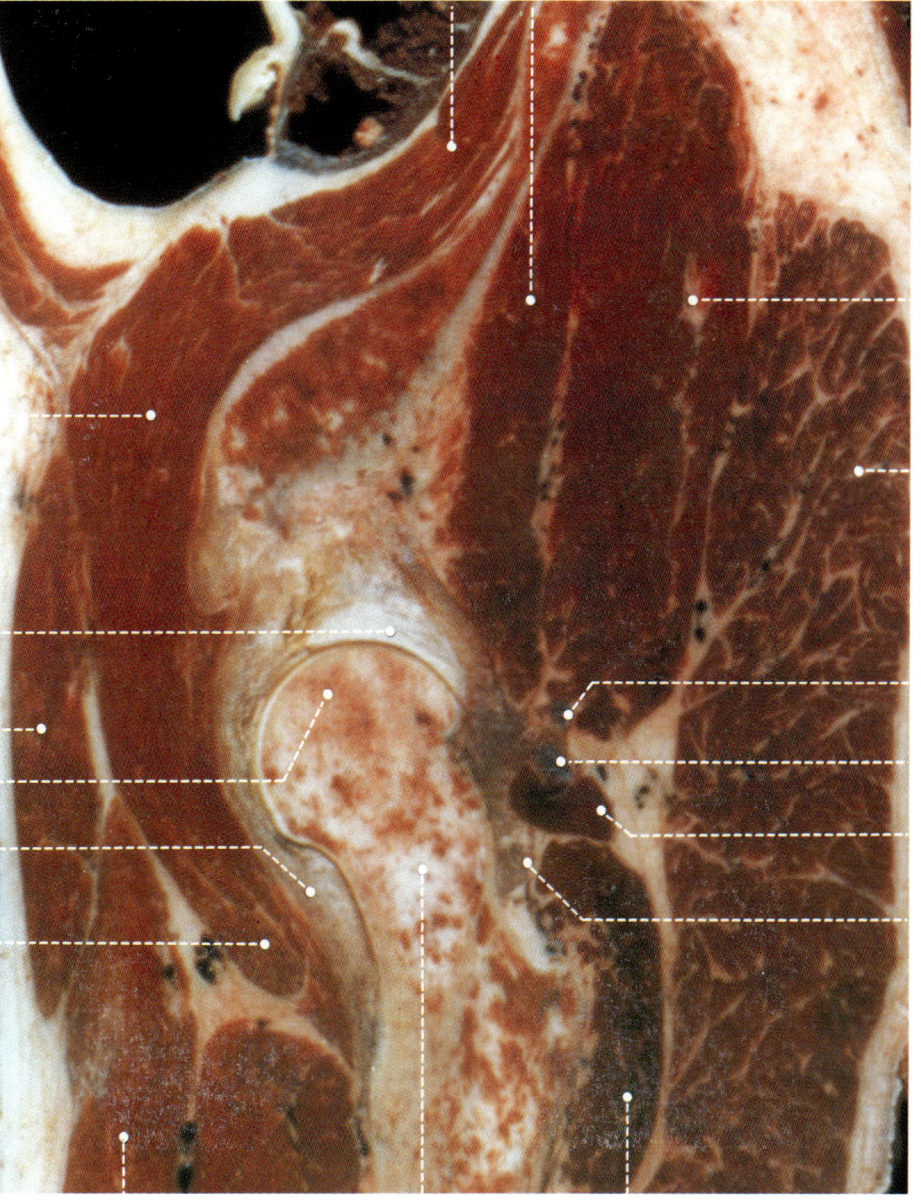

Anatomy and MRI of the Joints

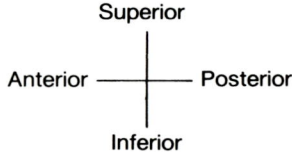

FIG. 7-23

SAGITTAL

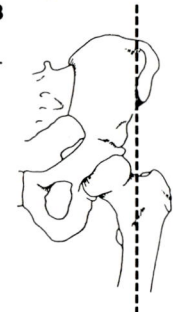

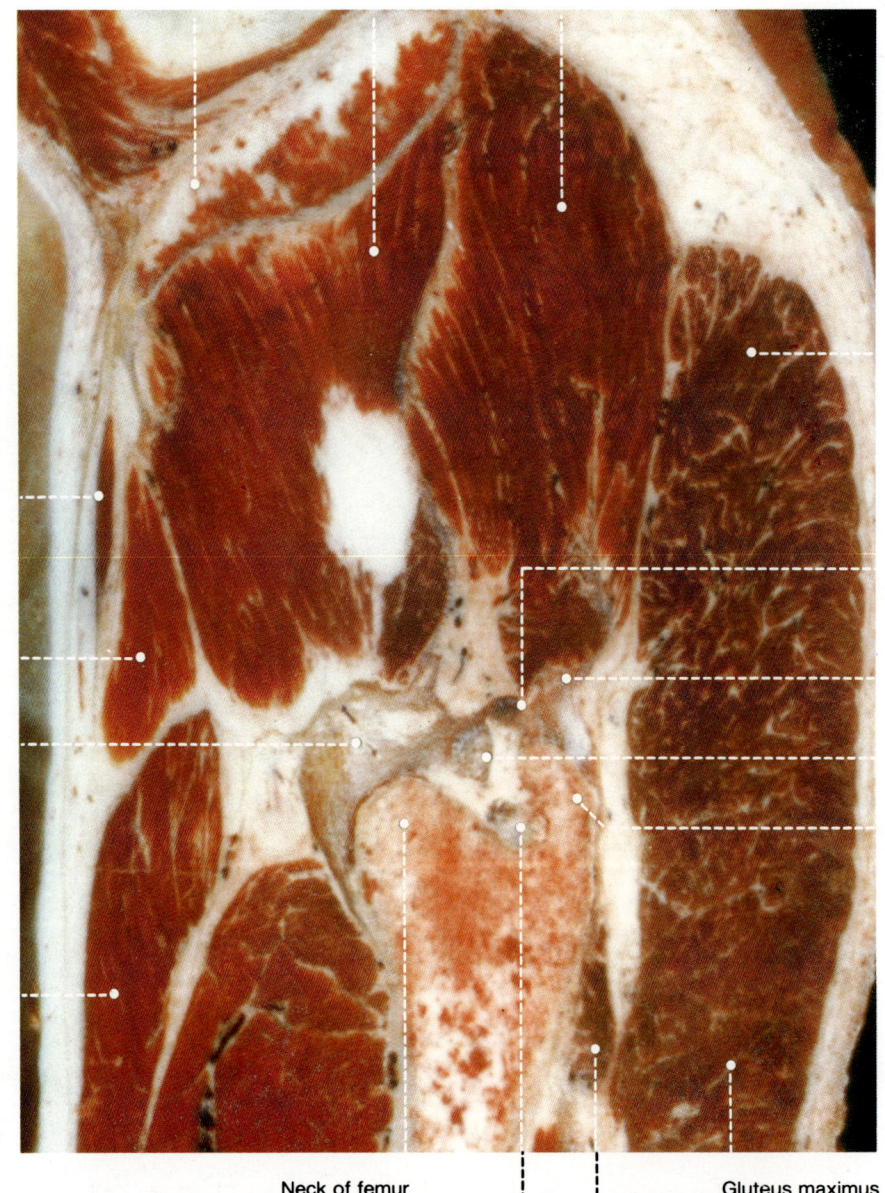

179 THE HIP

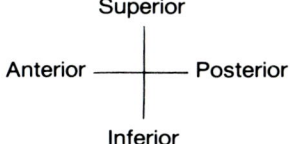

FIG. 7-24
SAGITTAL

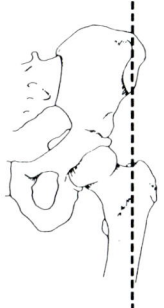

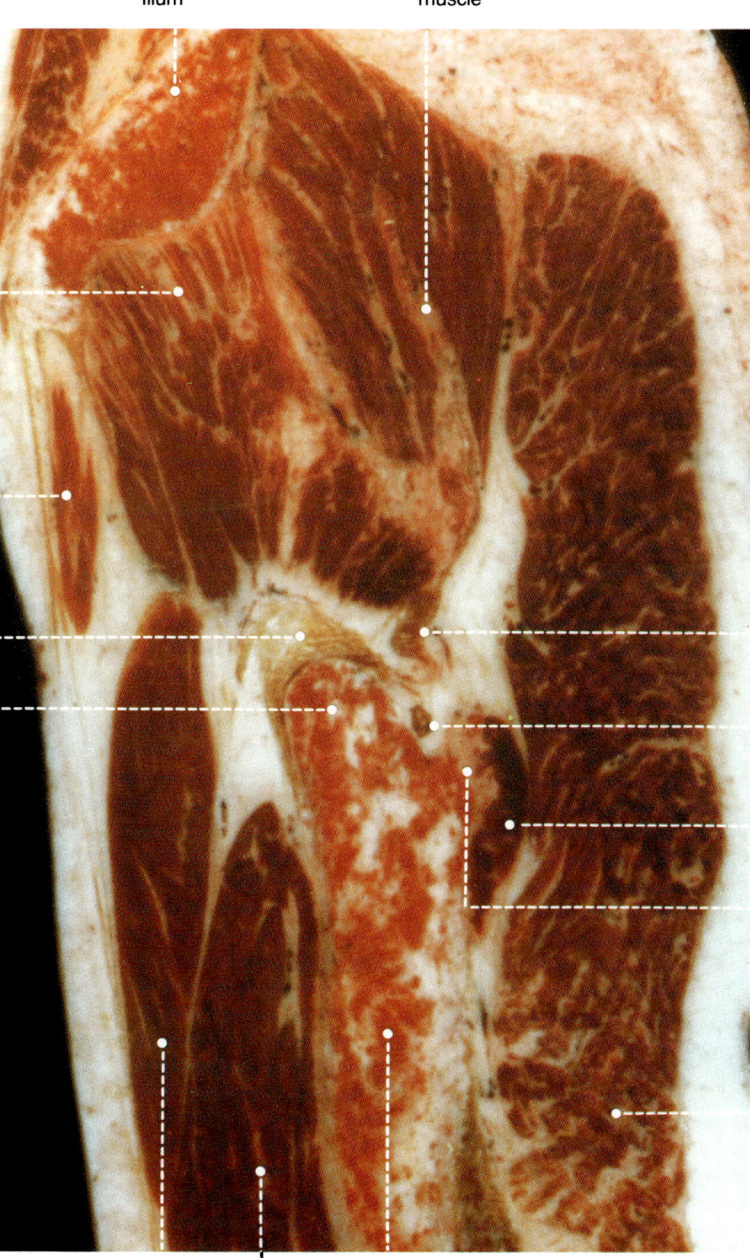

Anatomy and MRI of the Joints

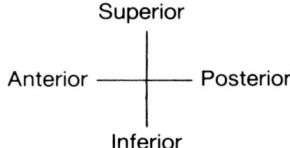

FIG. 7-25
SAGITTAL

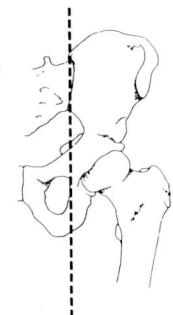

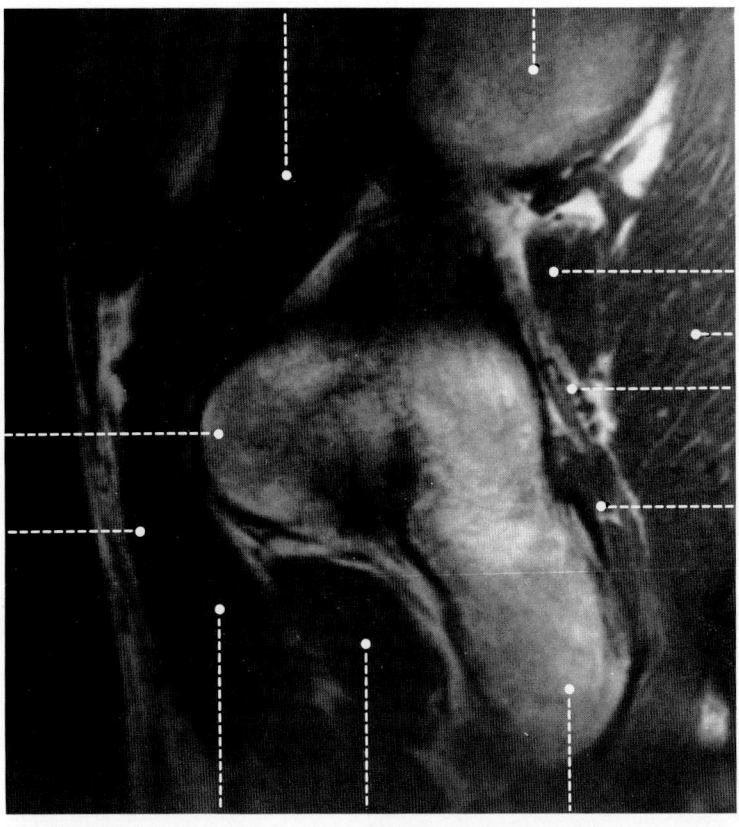

THE HIP

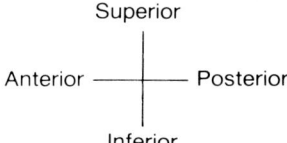

FIG. 7-26

SAGITTAL

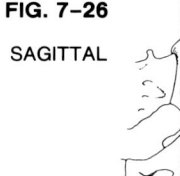

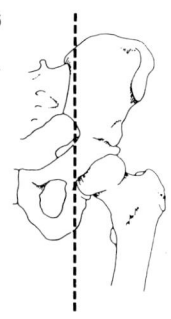

Anatomy and MRI of the Joints

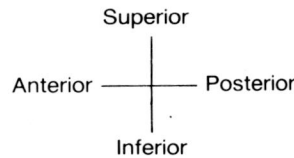

FIG. 7-27

SAGITTAL

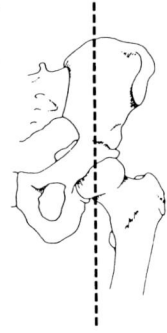

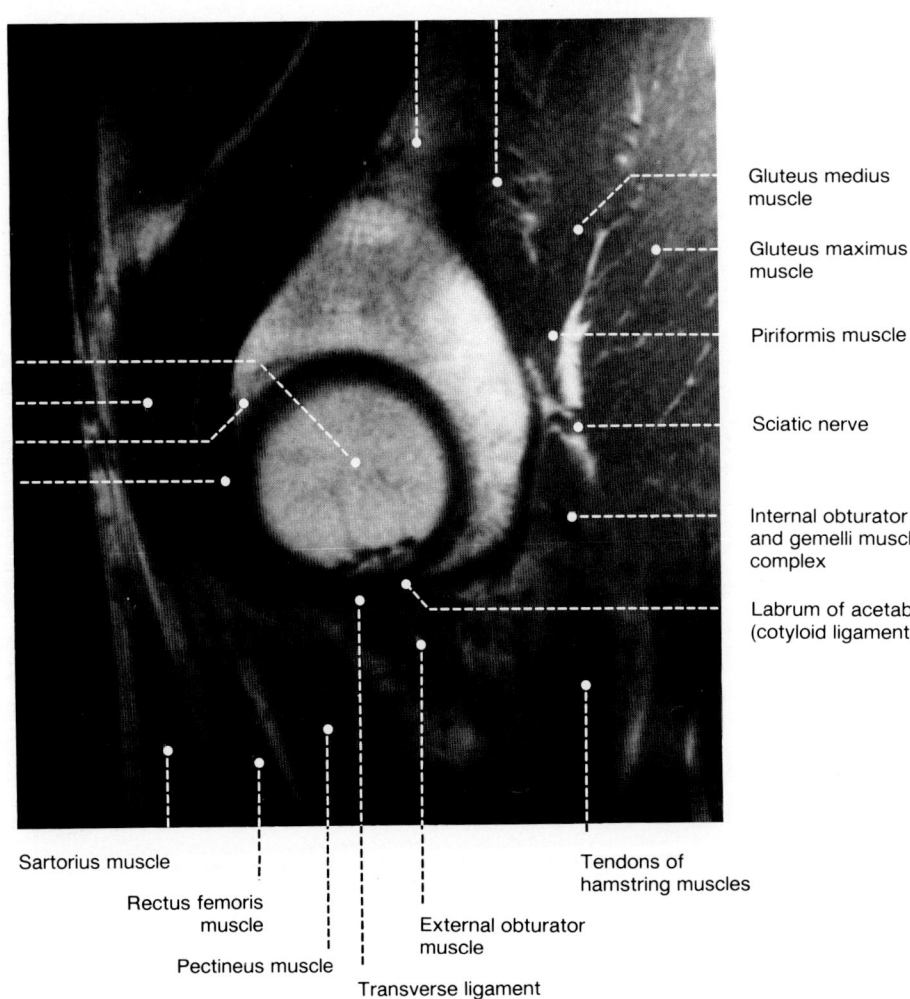

Labels: Ilium; Gluteus minimus muscle; Gluteus medius muscle; Gluteus maximus muscle; Piriformis muscle; Sciatic nerve; Internal obturator and gemelli muscle complex; Labrum of acetabulum (cotyloid ligament); Head of femur; Iliopsoas muscle; Rim of acetabulum; Iliofemoral ligament; Sartorius muscle; Rectus femoris muscle; Pectineus muscle; External obturator muscle; Transverse ligament; Tendons of hamstring muscles

183 THE HIP

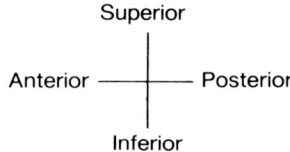

FIG. 7–28
SAGITTAL

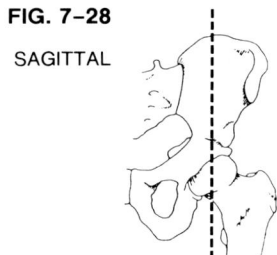

- Gluteus minimus muscle
- Gluteus medius muscle
- Iliopsoas muscle
- Gluteus maximus muscle
- Head of femur
- Rim of acetabulum
- Labrum of acetabulum (cotyloid ligament)
- Superior gemellus muscle
- Capsular ligament
- Tendon of internal obturator muscle
- Inferior gemellus muscle
- Sartorius muscle
- Iliopsoas muscle
- Rectus femoris muscle
- Quadratus femoris muscle
- External obturator muscle
- Transverse ligament

Anatomy and MRI of the Joints

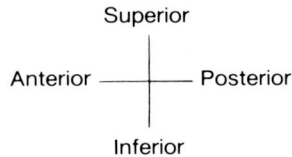

FIG. 7–29

SAGITTAL

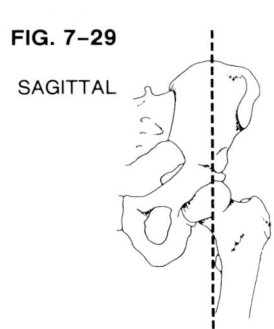

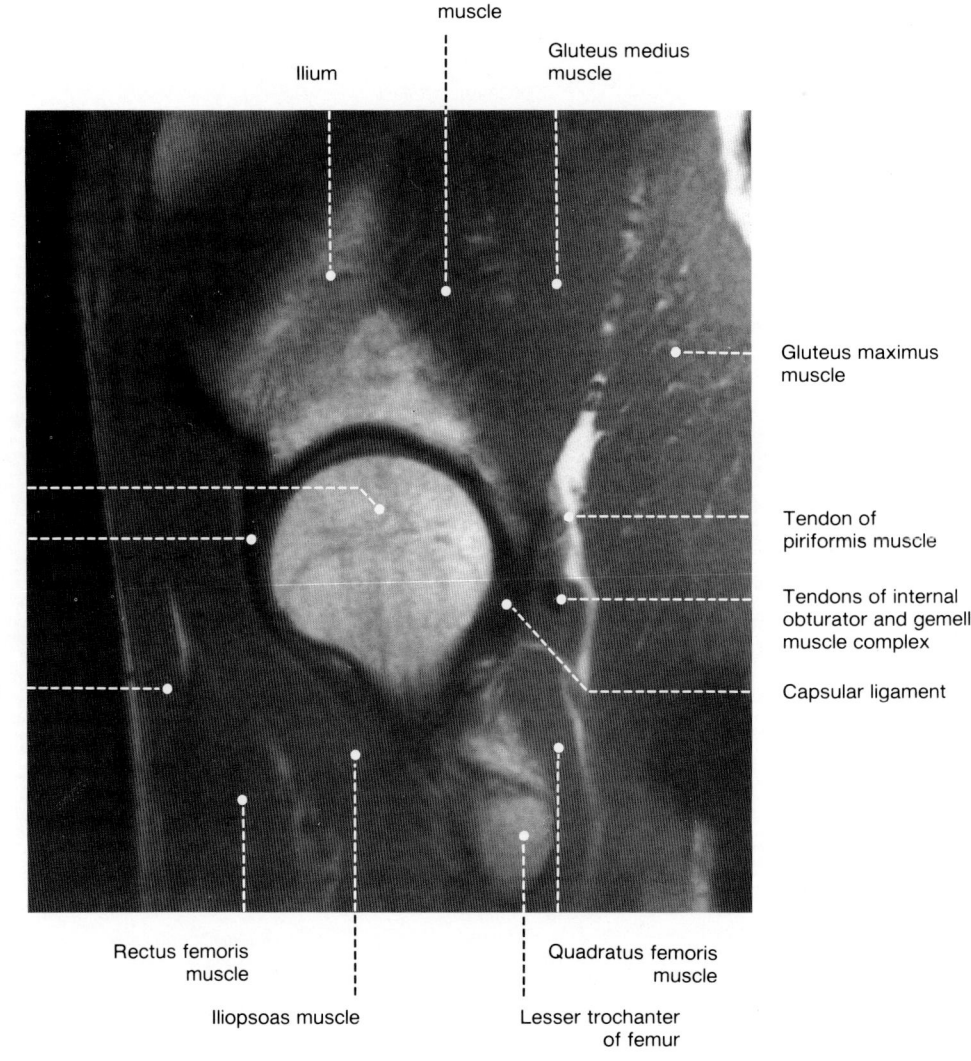

185 THE HIP

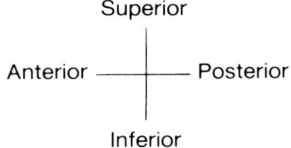

FIG. 7-30

SAGITTAL

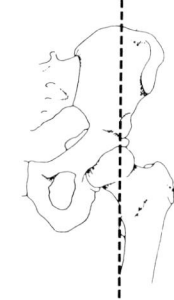

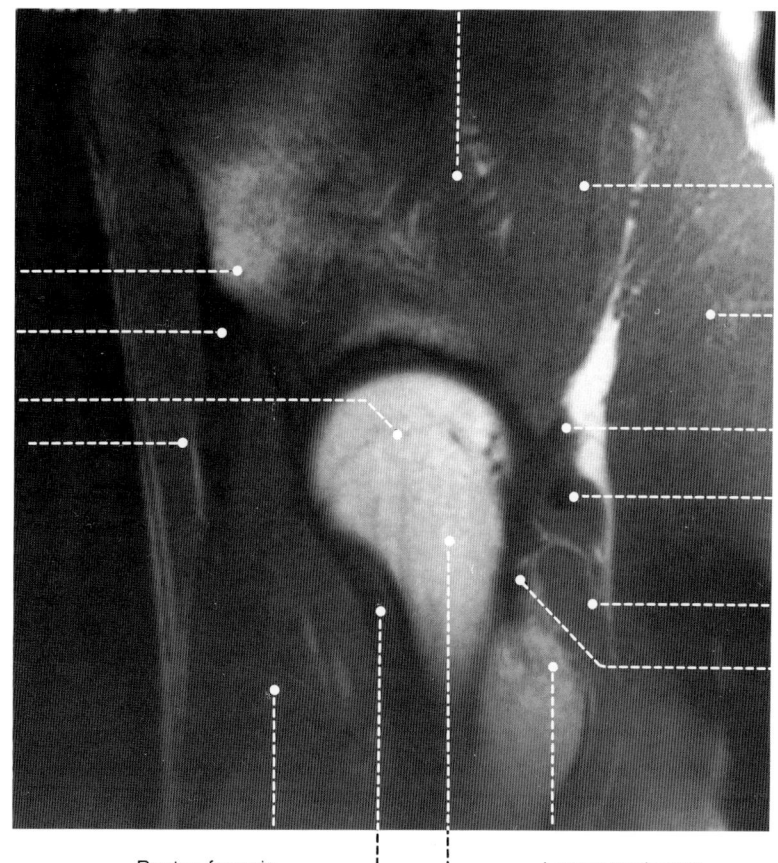

Gluteus minimus muscle

Gluteus medius muscle

Anterior inferior iliac spine

Tendon of rectus femoris muscle

Head of femur

Sartorius muscle

Gluteus maximus muscle

Tendon of piriformis muscle

Tendon of internal obturator and gemelli muscle complex

Quadratus femoris muscle

Tendon of external obturator muscle

Rectus femoris muscle

Lesser trochanter of femur

Iliofemoral ligament

Neck of femur

Anatomy and MRI of the Joints 186

Superior — Anterior — Posterior — Inferior

FIG. 7–31
SAGITTAL

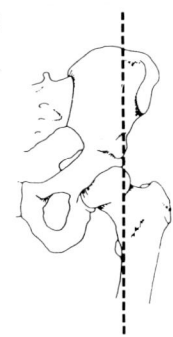

- Gluteus minimus muscle
- Anterior superior iliac spine
- Gluteus medius muscle
- Gluteus maximus muscle
- Sartorius muscle
- Tendon of piriformis muscle
- Internal obturator and gemelli muscle complex
- Rectus femoris muscle
- Iliofemoral ligament
- Neck of femur
- Greater trochanter of femur
- Tendon of external obturator muscle

THE HIP

FIG. 7-32

SAGITTAL

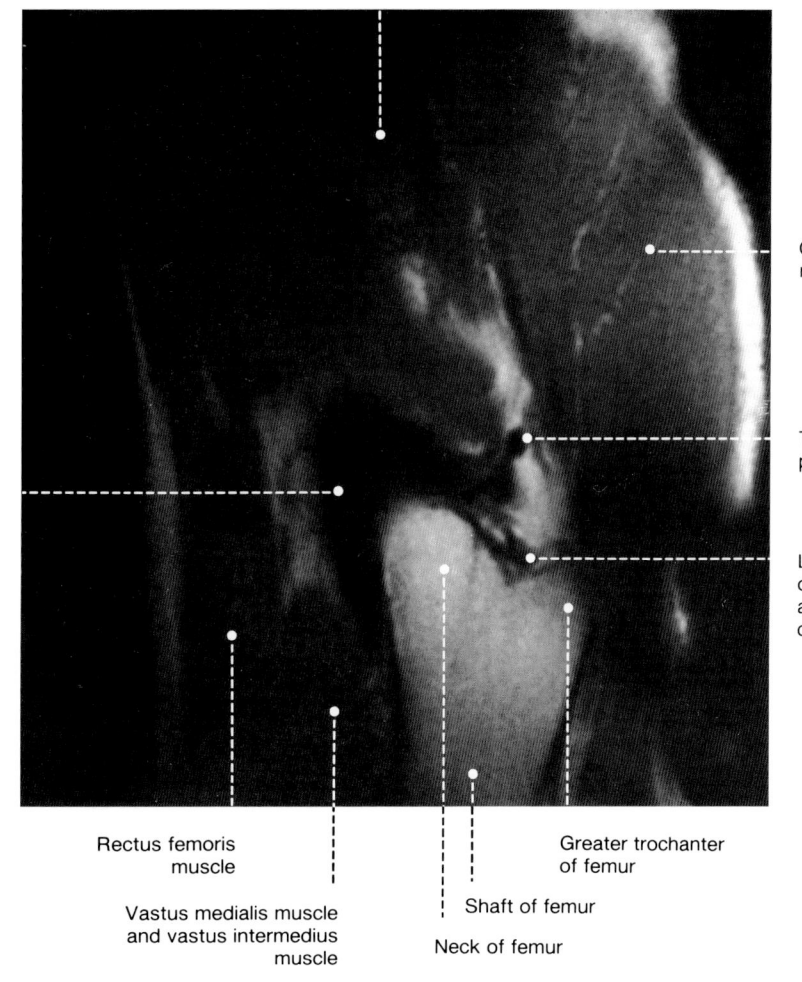

Anatomy and MRI of the Joints

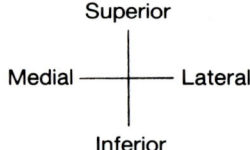

FIG. 7-33
CORONAL

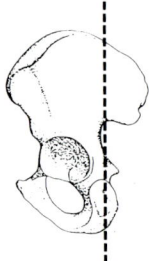

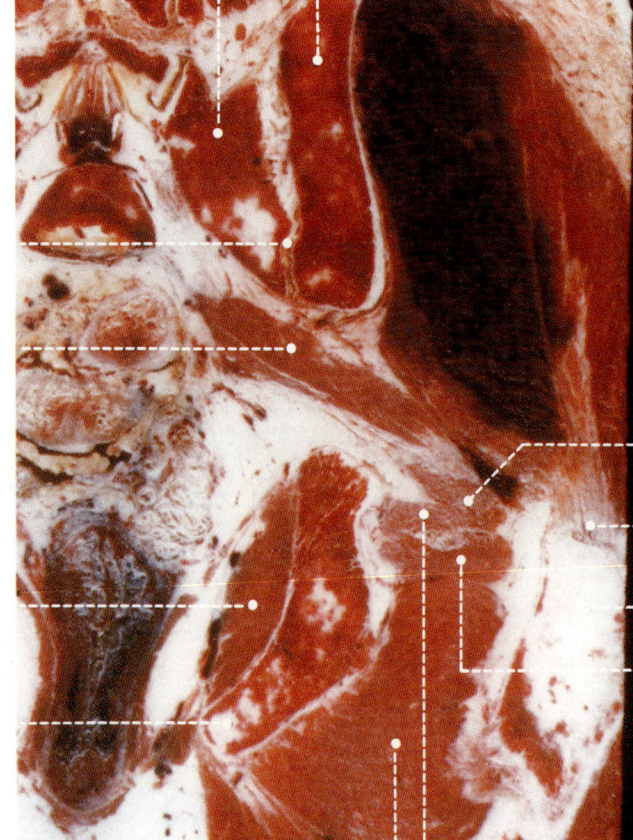

THE HIP

FIG. 7-34

CORONAL

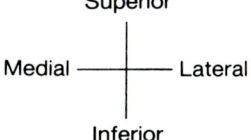
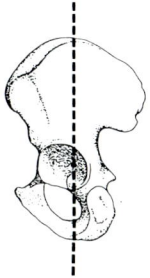
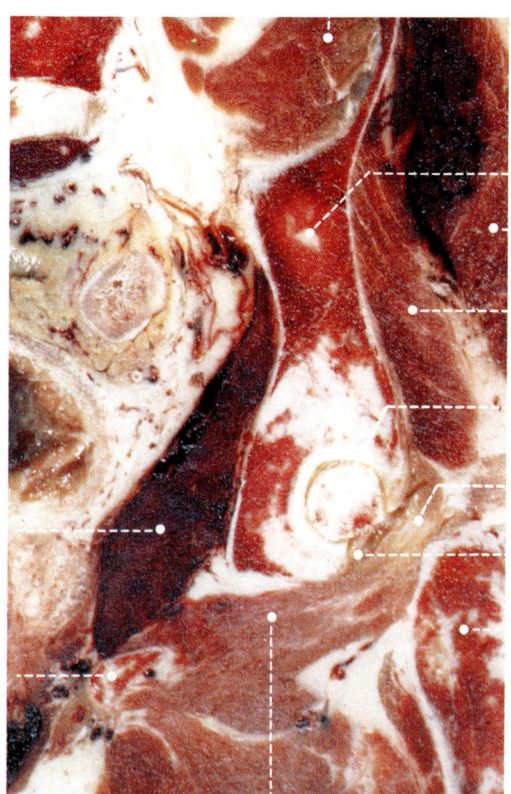

Iliacus muscle

Ilium

Gluteus medius muscle

Gluteus minimus muscle

Femoral head

External obturator tendon

Capsular ligament

Femur

Internal obturator muscle

Pubis

External obturator muscle

Anatomy and MRI of the Joints 190

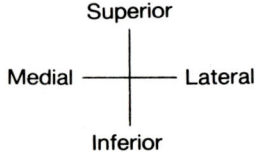

FIG. 7–35
CORONAL

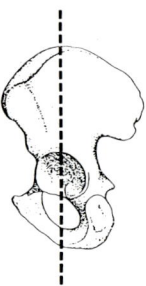

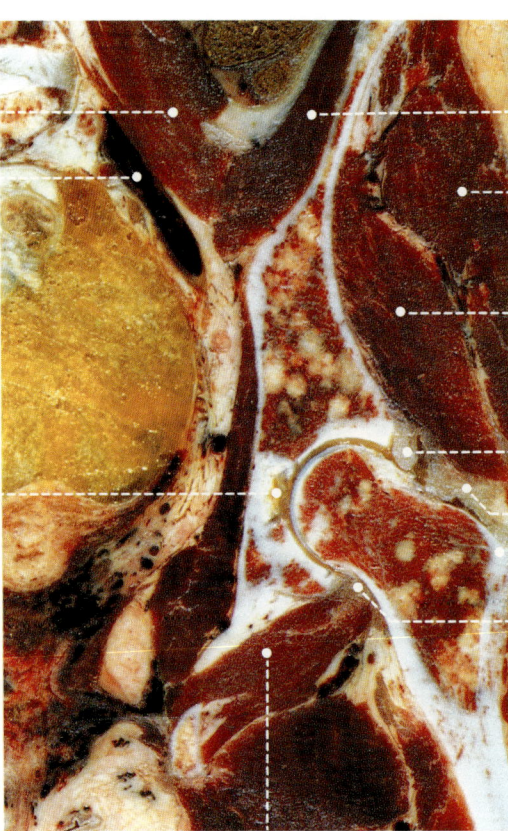

- Psoas muscle
- Common iliac vein
- Acetabular fossa
- Iliacus muscle
- Gluteus medius muscle
- Gluteus minimus muscle
- Labrum of actabulum (cotyloid ligament)
- Capsular ligament
- Greater trochanter of femur
- Transverse ligaments
- External obturator muscle

THE HIP

FIG. 7-36

CORONAL

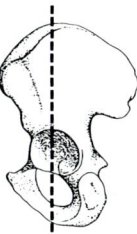

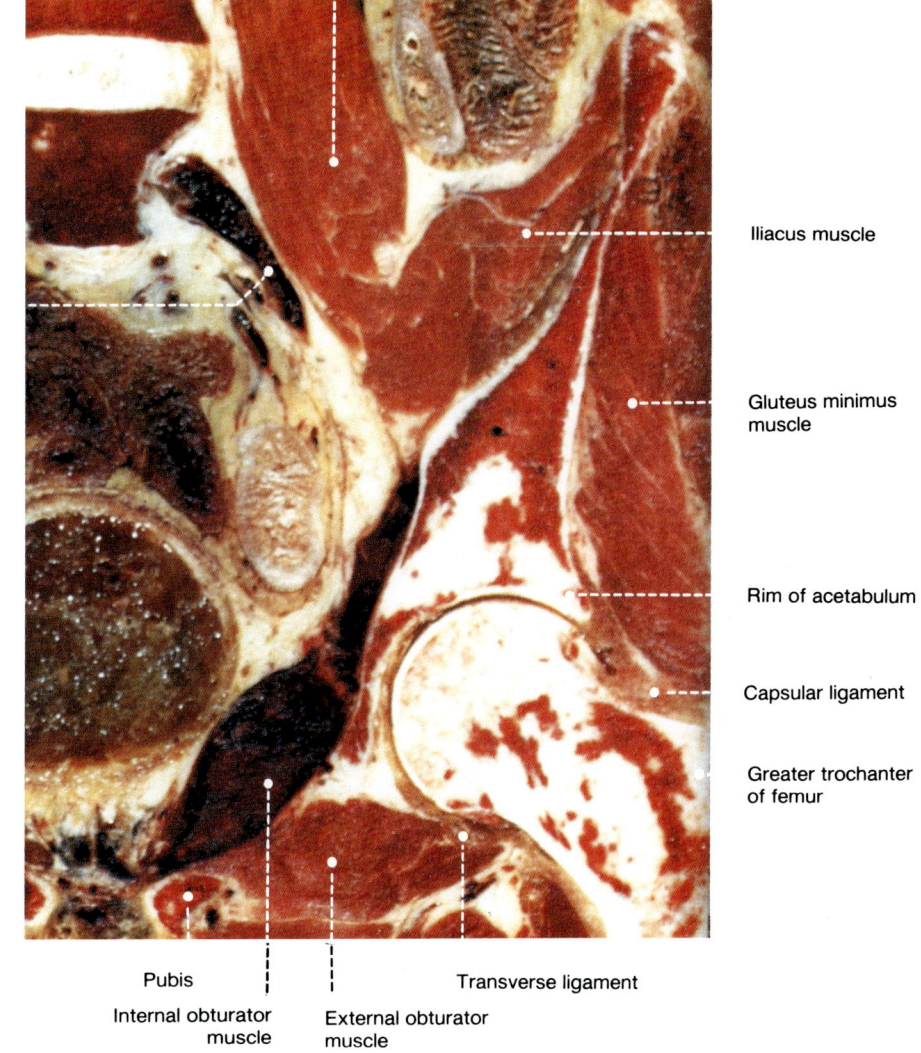

Anatomy and MRI of the Joints   192

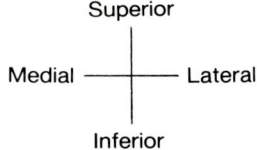

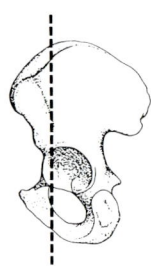

FIG. 7-37
CORONAL

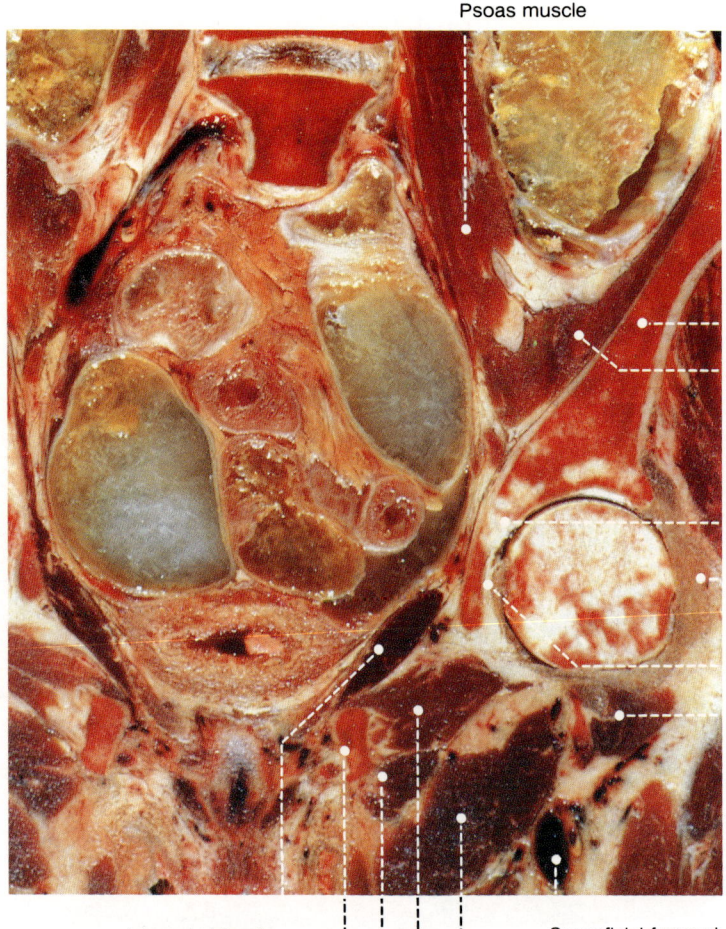

Psoas muscle

Iliac wing

Iliacus muscle

Rim of acetabulum and labrum

Capsular and iliofemoral ligament

Ligamentum teres

Iliopsoas muscle

Internal obturator muscle

Pubis

Adductor brevis muscle

External obturator muscle

Adductor magnus muscle

Superficial femoral artery and vein

THE HIP

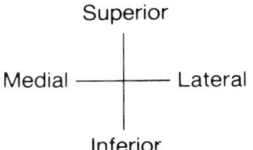

FIG. 7-38

CORONAL

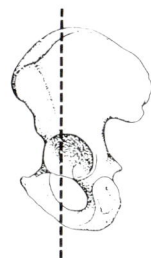

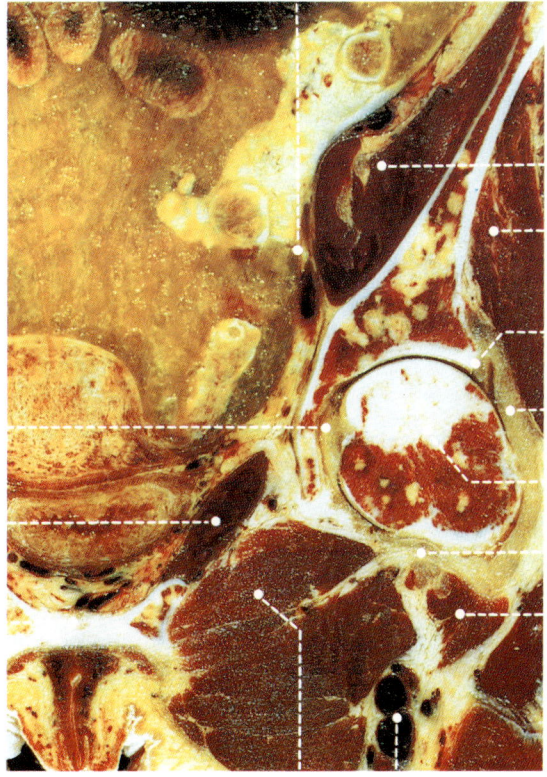

Anatomy and MRI of the Joints 194

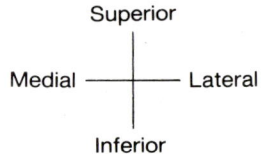

FIG. 7–39
CORONAL

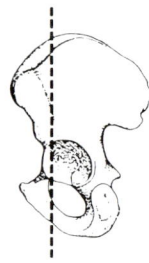

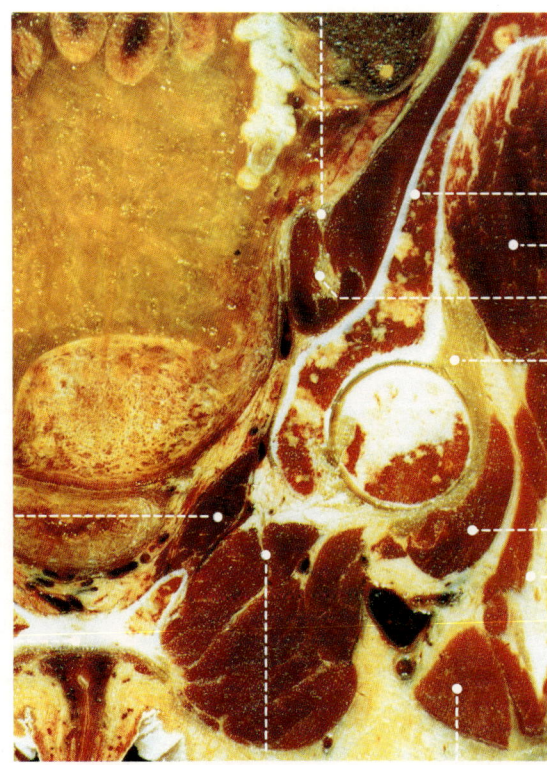

Femoral nerve
Ilium
Gluteus minimus muscle
Tendon of iliopsoas muscle
Capsular and iliofemoral ligament
Iliopsoas muscle
Rectus femoris muscle
Internal obturator muscle
Pubic symphysis
External obturator muscle
Vastus intermedius muscle

THE HIP

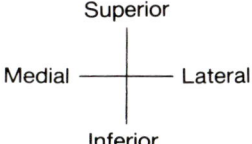

FIG. 7-40
CORONAL

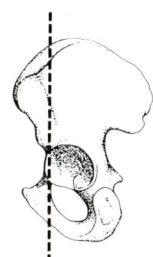

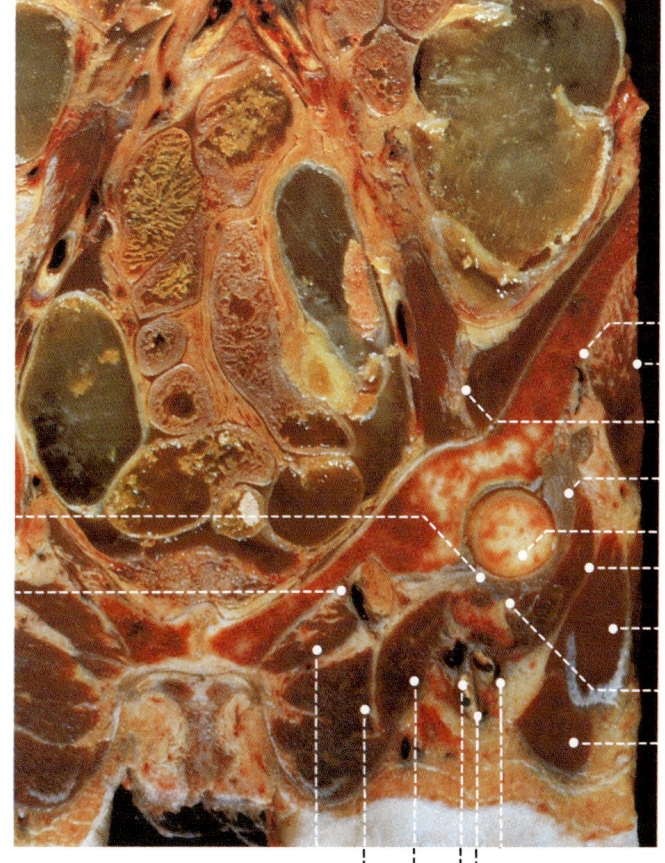

- Iliac wing
- Gluteus minimus muscle
- Tendon of iliopsoas muscle
- Iliofemoral ligament
- Head of femur
- Iliopsoas muscle
- Rectus femoris muscle
- Capsular ligament
- Vastus intermedius muscle

- Labrum of acetabulum (cotyloid ligament)
- Superior pubic ramus

- Obturator externus muscle
- Adductor brevis muscle
- Pectineus muscle
- Deep femoral artery
- Superficial femoral artery
- Common femoral vein

Anatomy and MRI of the Joints

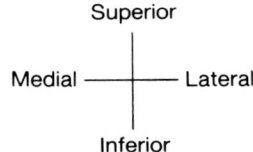

FIG. 7–41
CORONAL

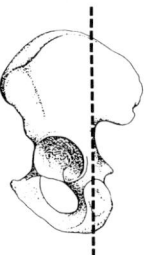

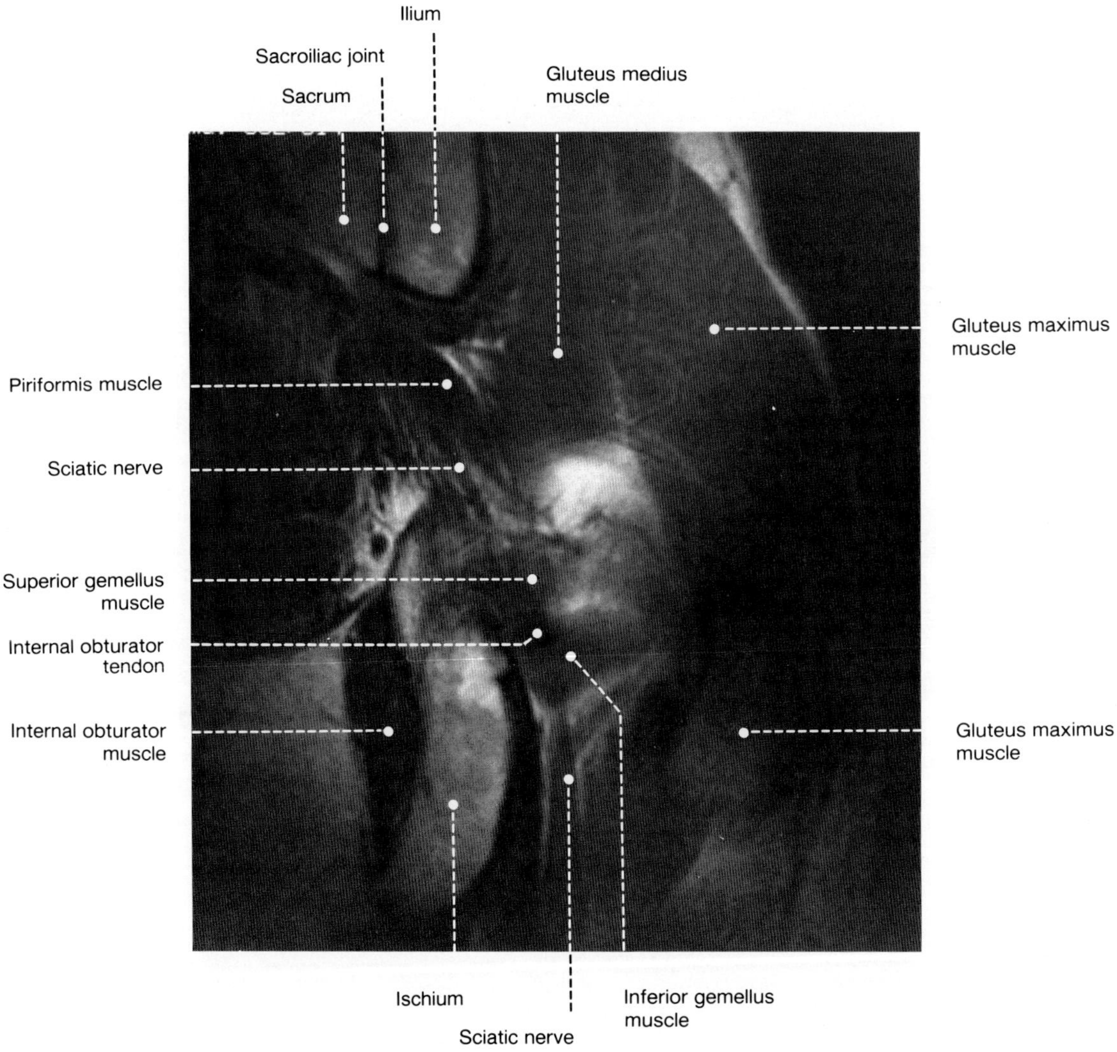

THE HIP

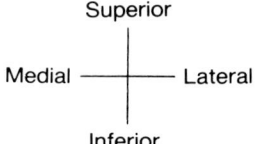

FIG. 7-42
CORONAL

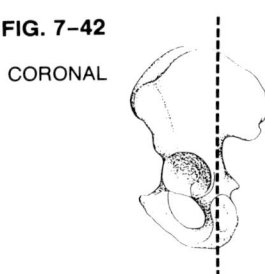

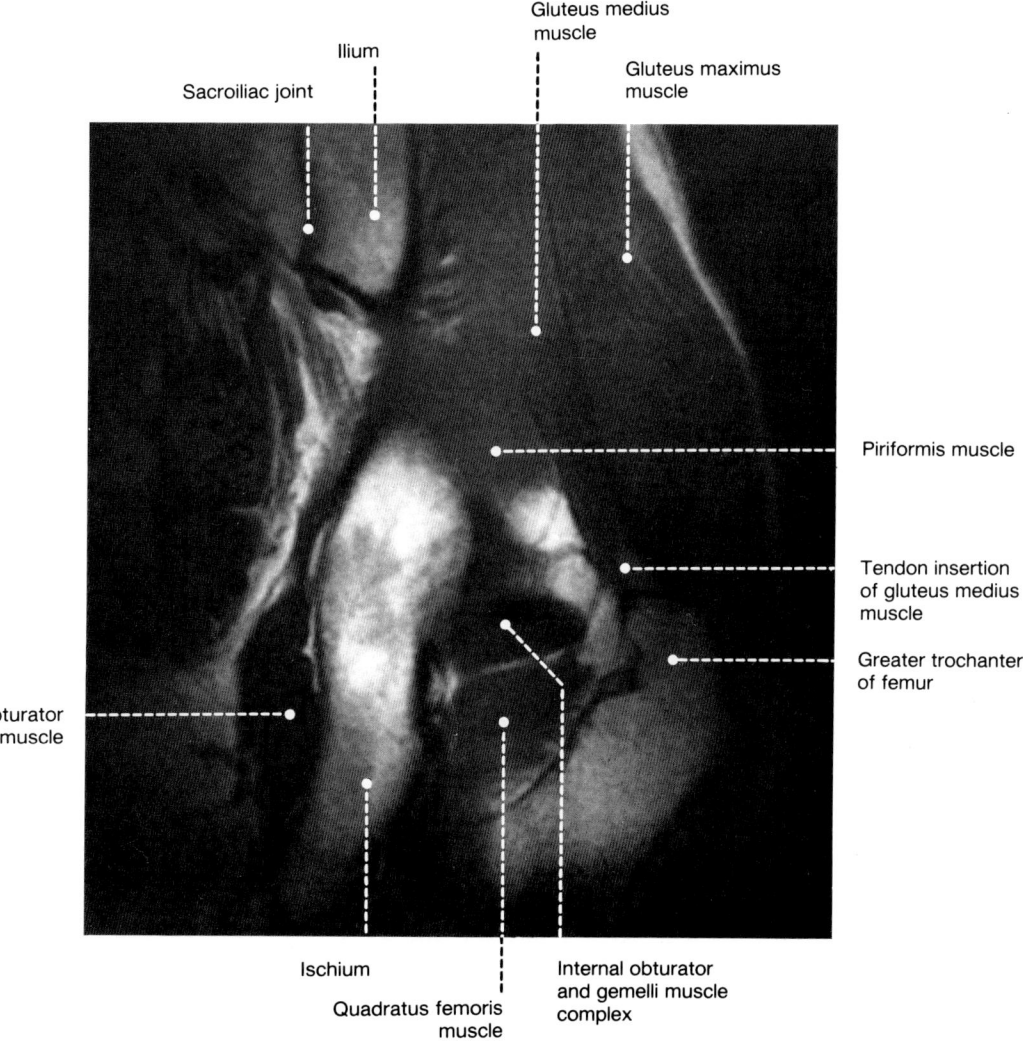

Anatomy and MRI of the Joints

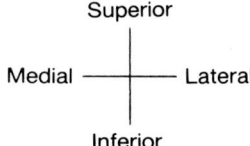

FIG. 7-43
CORONAL

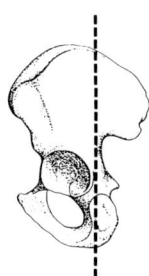

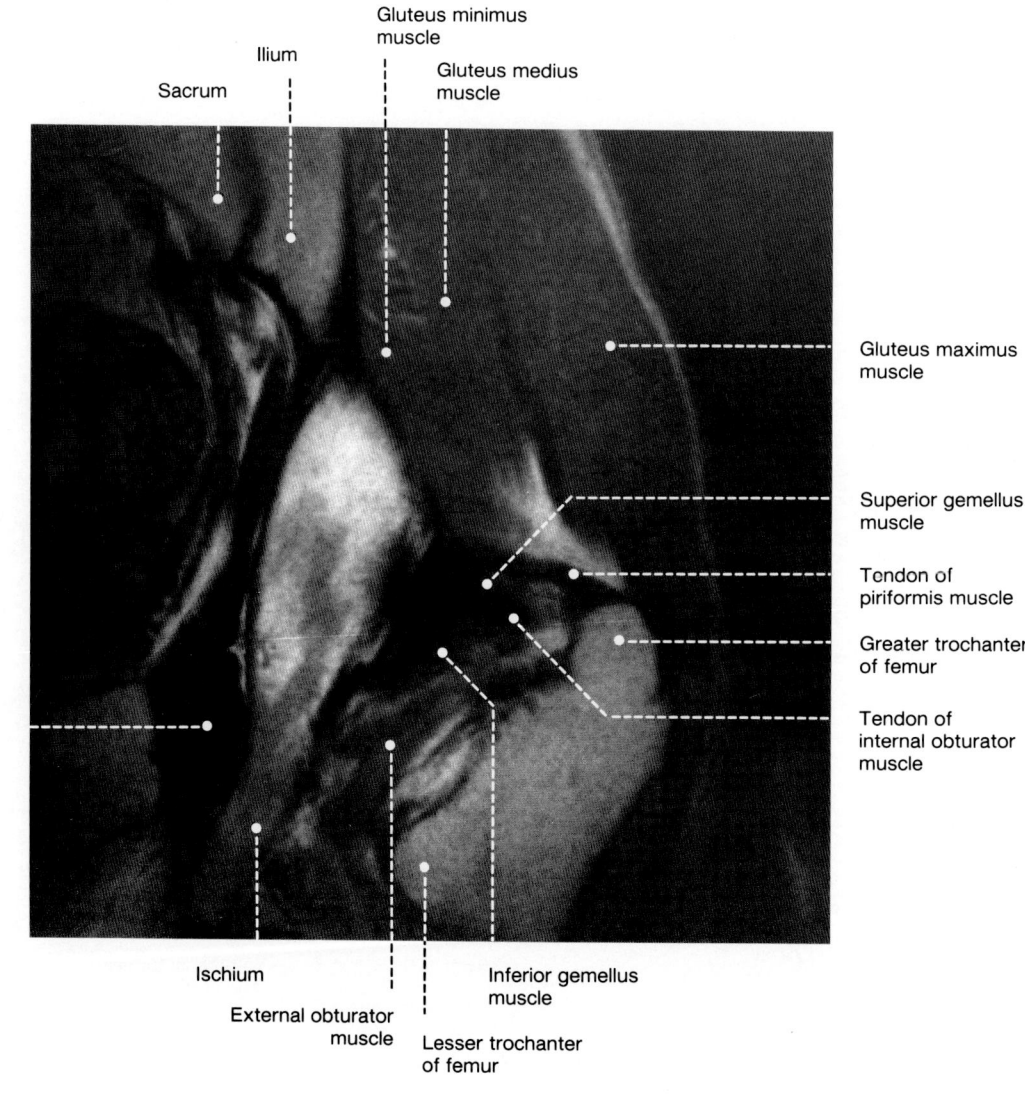

Superior
Medial — Lateral
Inferior

FIG. 7–44
CORONAL

Ilium
Sacroiliac joint
Gluteus medius muscle
Gluteus maximus muscle
Gluteus minimus muscle
Capsular ligament
Tendon of piriformis muscle
Greater trochanter of femur
Tendon insertion of gemelli muscle complex
Head of femur
Internal obturator muscle
Rim of acetabulum
Neck of femur
External obturator muscle
Transverse ligament

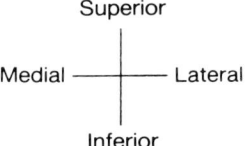

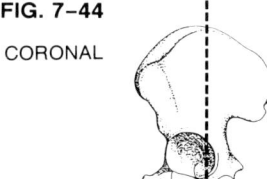

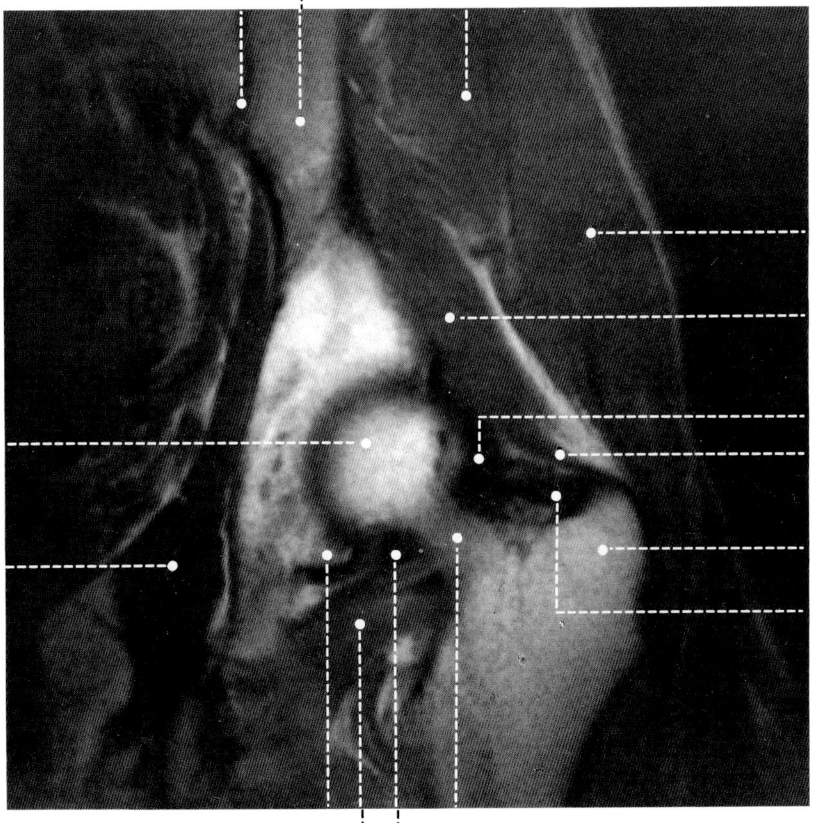

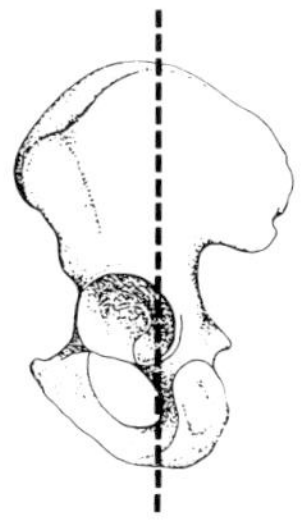

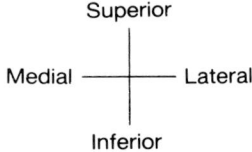
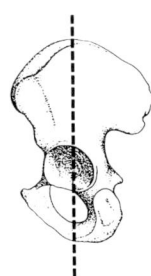

FIG. 7-45
CORONAL

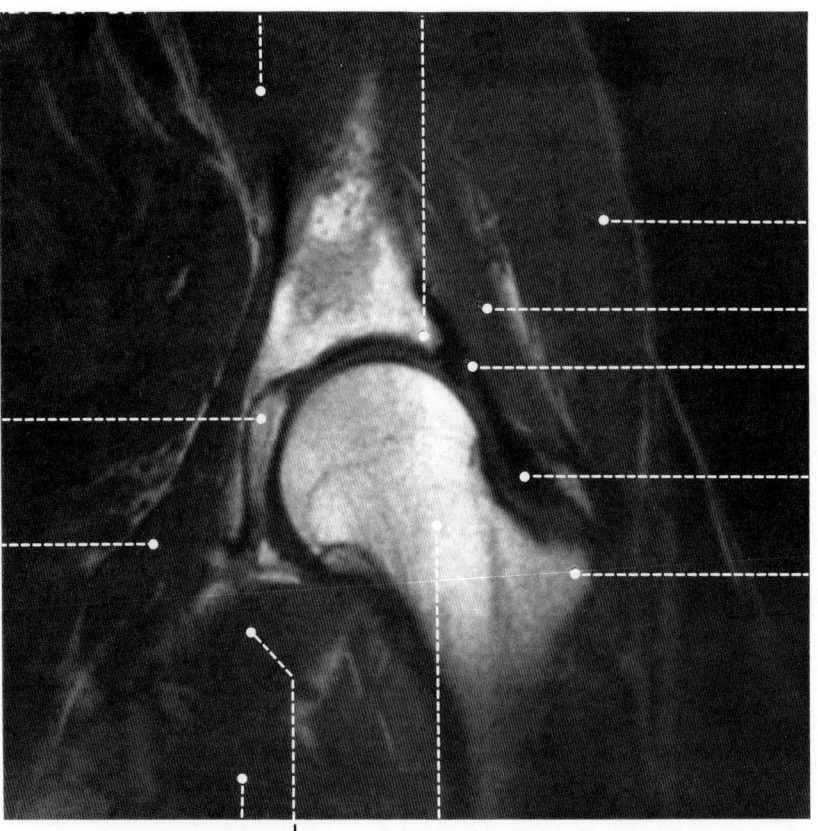

THE HIP

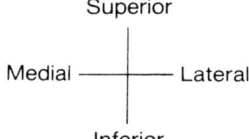

FIG. 7-46
CORONAL

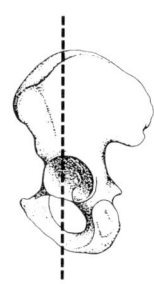

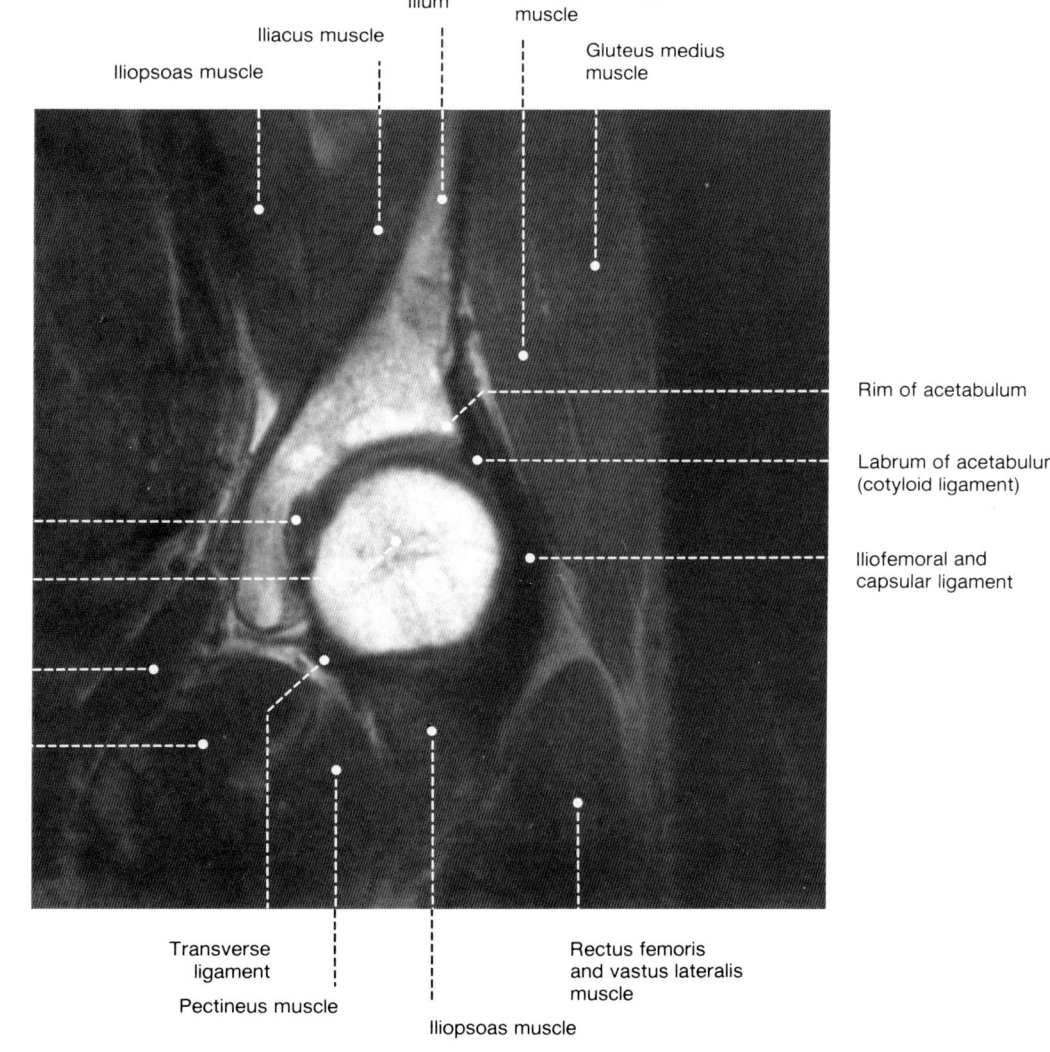

Iliopsoas muscle
Iliacus muscle
Ilium
Gluteus minimus muscle
Gluteus medius muscle

Rim of acetabulum
Labrum of acetabulum (cotyloid ligament)
Iliofemoral and capsular ligament

Fossa of acetabulum and ligamentum teres
Head of femur
Internal obturator muscle
External obturator muscle

Transverse ligament
Pectineus muscle
Iliopsoas muscle
Rectus femoris and vastus lateralis muscle

Anatomy and MRI of the Joints   202

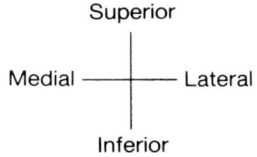

FIG. 7-47

CORONAL

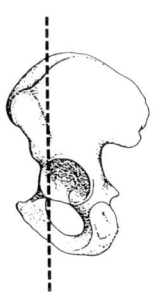

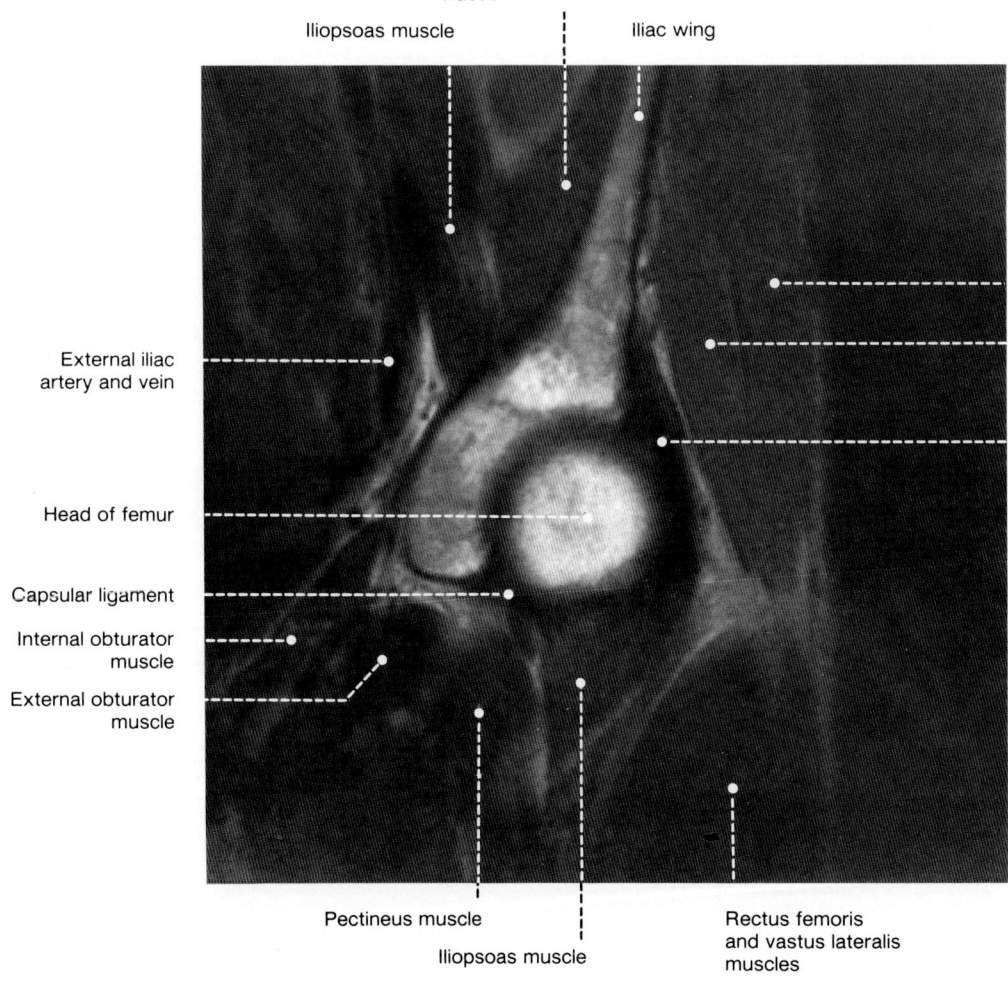

THE HIP

FIG. 7-48
CORONAL

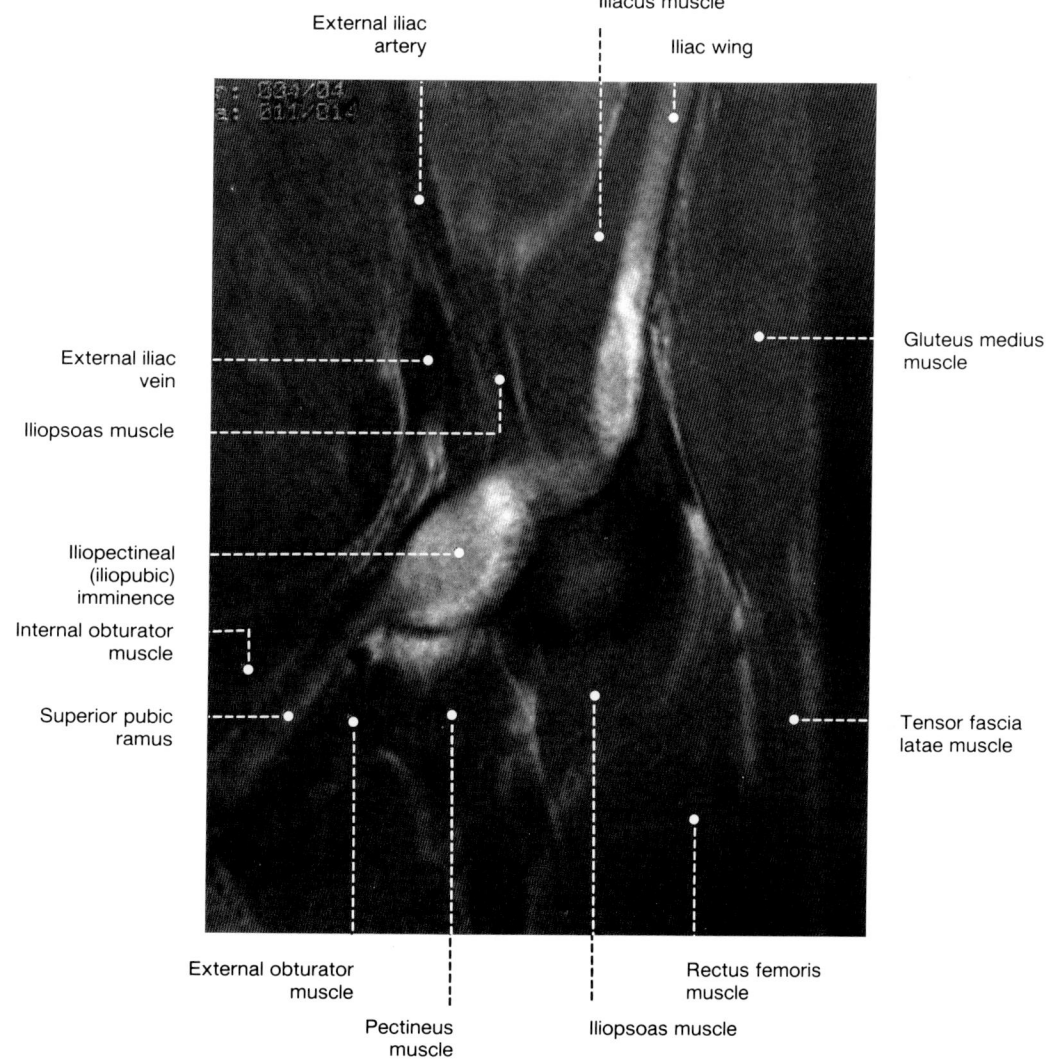

CHAPTER 8

THE KNEE

Gary W. Hinson, M.D. and William D. Middleton, M.D.

The knee is a complex hinge joint that must accommodate a variety of stresses. A supporting array of ligaments, tendons, crossing muscles, and menisci operate in concert to meet the functional demands of the knee. These structures, as well as intimately related neurovascular structures, are well depicted in cross-sectional images and anatomic sections. Precise understanding of cross-sectional anatomy is necessary for careful examination of cross-sectional images of the knee.

The three osseous structures of the knee are the patella, the distal femoral condyle, and the proximal tibial plateaus. These structures form three articular compartments. The medial and lateral femoral condyles articulate with their respective tibial plateaus to form the medial and lateral articular compartments. Anteriorly, the patella lies between the femoral condyles to form the patello-femoral articular compartment. A small medial patellar facet and a larger lateral patellar facet articulate with the femoral condyles.

Separating the rather flat medial and lateral tibial plateaus is the intercondylar eminence with its medial and lateral intercondylar tubercles. The cruciate ligaments and menisci have attachment sites just anterior and posterior to the intercondylar eminence.

The medial and lateral menisci are crescent-shaped fibrocartilaginous structures which separate the femoral condyles from the tibial plateaus (Fig. 8-1). Anterior and posterior to the intercondylar eminence the anterior and posterior horns of the medial meniscus have firm attachments to the tibia. The peripheral border of the medial meniscus is firmly attached to the medial capsule and through the coronary ligaments to the upper border of the tibia. The inner border of the medial meniscus is thin, concave, and free of attachment.

The anterior horn of the lateral meniscus inserts into the tibia anterior to the intercondylar eminence. Insertion of the posterior horn of the lateral meniscus is into the posterior aspect of the intercondylar eminence. The posterior horn of the lateral meniscus is often further anchored to the femoral condyle by the ligament of Humphrey or the ligament of Wrisberg. The lateral meniscus is loosely attached to the tibia peripherally via its coronary ligament. The popliteus tendon perforates the coronary ligament and travels obliquely adjacent to the posterior lateral aspect of the lateral meniscus. This tendon separates the posterior lateral edge of the lateral meniscus from the joint capsule and the lateral collateral ligament (Fig. 8-2).

The capsule of the knee is a fibrous sleeve that has its anterior margin at the patella and patellar ligament and extends posteriorly to circumferentially encompass the knee. The middle region of the medial capsule is reinforced by thickened fibers that have been referred to as the deep layer of the medial or tibial collateral ligament. This capsular segment originates from the femoral condyle and epicondyle and inserts just below the tibial articular margin. There is a meniscofemoral and a meniscotibial division of the thickened mid-medial capsule. The meniscotibial division extends as the coronary ligament of the meniscus to its tibial insertion. The medial capsule may be further divided into anteromedial and posteromedial regions. Similarly, the lateral capsule may be divided into anterolateral, mid-lateral, and posterolateral regions. The mid-lateral capsule is not as well defined anatomically as the medial capsule.

The tibial or medial collateral ligament originates on the medial femoral condyle and inserts approximately 8 to 10 cm below the joint line on the posterior half of the medial surface of the tibial metaphysis (Figs. 8-2 and 8-3). The fibular or lateral collateral ligament has its proximal attachment to the lateral femoral condyle and its distal attachment to the fibular head (Figs. 8-2 and 8-4).

The anterior and posterior cruciate ligaments are the central ligaments of the knee (Fig. 8-1). The anterior cruciate ligament extends obliquely from a fossa on the me-

Anatomy and MRI of the Joints

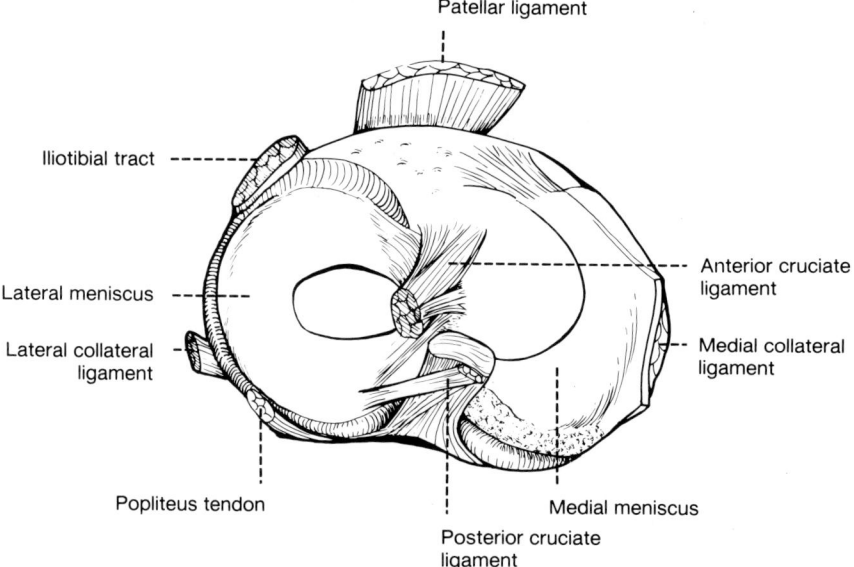

FIG. 8–1

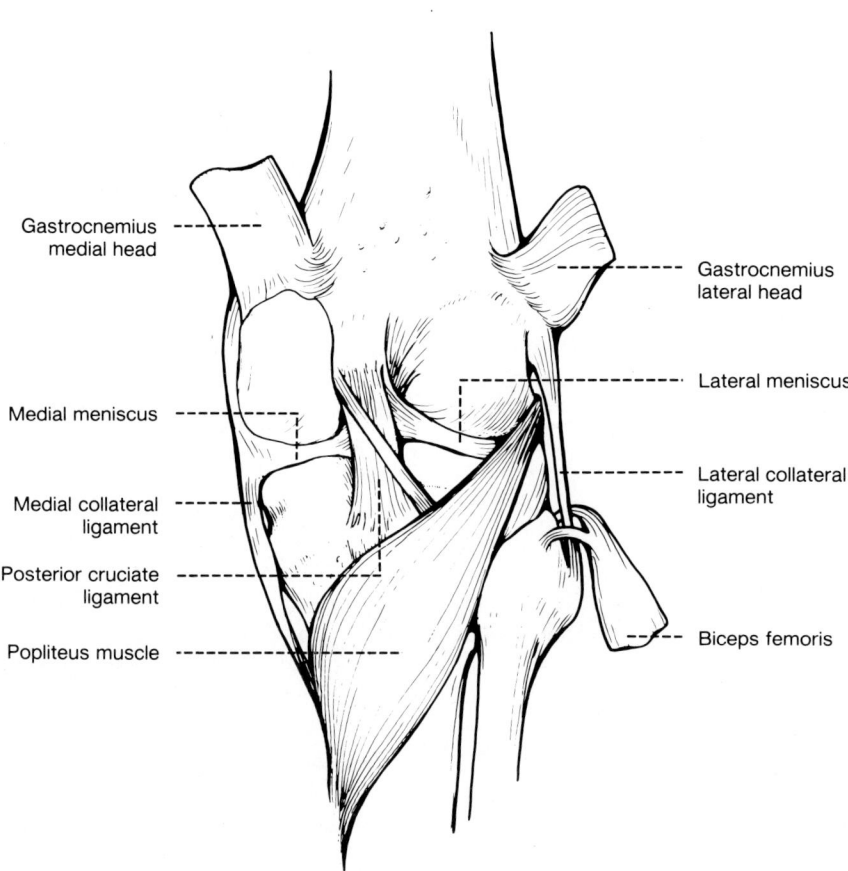

FIG. 8–2

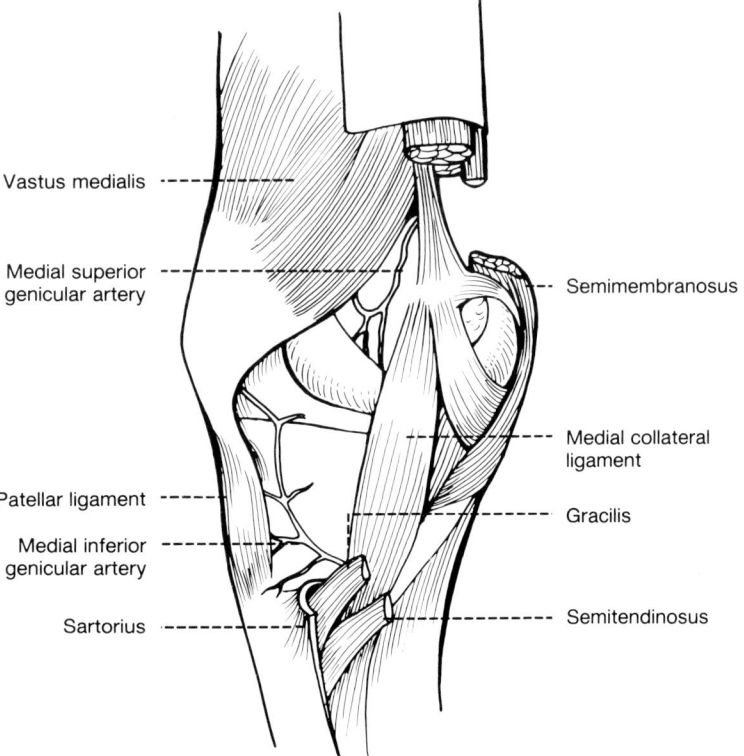

FIG. 8-3

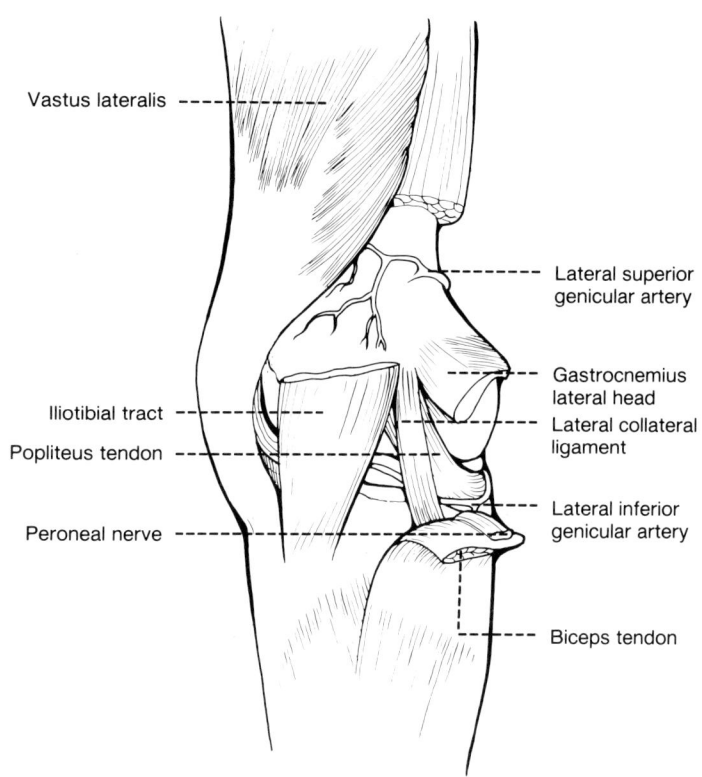

FIG. 8-4

dial posterior aspect of the lateral femoral condyle to the tibial surface just anterior to the medial tubercle of the intercondyle eminence. The posterior cruciate ligament originates as a broad, flat band from the posterior part of the tibia and inserts anteriorly on the lateral surface of the medial femoral condyle.

The transverse ligament traverses between the anterior horns of both the medial and lateral meniscus and can often be followed from medial to lateral meniscus on sagittal images.

The important muscle units of the knee are the quadriceps group, the medial and lateral hamstring groups, the popliteus muscle, and the gastrocnemius muscle.

The quadriceps muscle group consists of the rectus femoris, vastus medialis, vastus lateralis, and vastus intermedius muscles. These muscles form a trilaminar quadriceps tendon which inserts into the proximal pole of the patella. The patellar ligament originates from the distal pole of the patella and inserts into the tibial tuberosity (Fig. 8-3).

Fibers from the aponeurosis of the vastus medialis insert directly into the medial border of the patella and patellar ligament to form the medial retinaculum. Similarly, the lateral retinaculum is an extension of the vastus lateralis. The lateral retinaculum is also attached to the anterior margin of the iliotibial band.

The gastrocnemius muscle consists of two heads that arise posteriorly from the medial and lateral femoral condyles and span the posterior aspect of the knee in close proximity to the posterior capsule (Fig. 8-2). The plantaris muscle is a small and functionally unimportant muscle that originates with the lateral head of the gastrocnemius and rapidly tapers into a long, string-like tendon.

The medial hamstring muscles include the semimembranosus, semitendinosus, gracilis, and sartorius (Fig. 8-3). The sartorius is the largest muscle in the body. It runs superficially in the thigh from the anterior superior iliac spine to the medial aspect of the knee. At the level of the knee it becomes thin and flat. It remains muscular throughout most of its course, and muscle components are always seen at the level of the knee.

The gracilis muscle originates with the adductors from the anterior aspect of the pubis. At the level of the knee it runs deep to the sartorius. Unlike the sartorius, it becomes entirely tendinous prior to the level of the knee.

The semitendinosus originates from the ischial tuberosity and runs superficial to the semimembranosus. It is completely tendinous at the knee level. Together with the gracilis and sartorius it inserts on the medial aspect of the proximal tibia. The pes anserinus is the common insertion of the tendons of the sartorius, gracilis, and semitendinosus muscles on the medial aspect of the proximal tibia.

The semimembranosus originates from the ischial tuberosity with the semitendinosus. It inserts on the back of the medial tibial condyle. Unlike the semitendinosus, the semimembranosus remains muscular at the knee level.

The two heads of the biceps form the lateral hamstring. They unite into a single tendon that inserts distally into the fibular head (Fig. 8-2). Muscular components do extend to the level of the knee.

Superficially along the lateral aspects of the knee there is a dense fascial sheath termed the iliotibial track (Fig. 4). The iliotibial track inserts proximally into the lateral femoral condyle and distally into the lateral tibial tubercle (Gerdy's tubercle). This dense fascial band is contiguous anteriorly with the vastus lateralis and is contiguous posteriorly with the biceps femoris muscle.

There are four major neurovascular structures in the popliteal fossa. Their relationship from medial to lateral is: popliteal artery, popliteal vein, tibial nerve, and common peroneal nerve. The three more medial structures parallel one another and are closely aligned.

At the level of the popliteal fossa, the sciatic nerve has already divided into the more laterally directed common peroneal nerve and the tibial nerve. The tibial nerve gives off muscular branches that innervate the medial and lateral heads of the gastrocnemius muscle. The medial sural nerve is also a branch of the tibial nerve. The lateral sural nerve branches form the common peroneal nerve.

Within the popliteal fossa, the popliteal artery usually gives rise to five genicular arteries: two superior (lateral and medial), one middle, and two inferior (lateral and medial). These vessels course around the bones of the knee joint and supply the joint itself. There are also sural arteries that branch from the popliteal artery and supply the medial and lateral heads of the gastrocnemius muscle.

THE KNEE

AXIAL
    Cryomicrotomes .... FIGS. 8–5 to 8–11
    MR Images .... FIGS. 8–12 to 8–17

SAGITTAL
    Cryomicrotomes .... FIGS. 8–18 to 8–24
    MR Images .... FIGS. 8–25 to 8–31

CORONAL
    Cryomicrotomes .... FIGS. 8–32 to 8–38
    MR Images .... FIGS. 8–39 to 8–45

Anatomy and MRI of the Joints   210

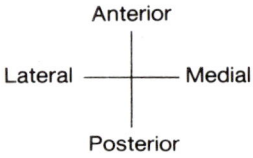

FIG. 8-5

AXIAL

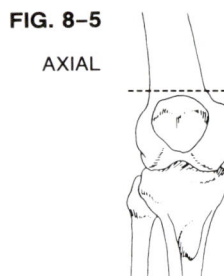

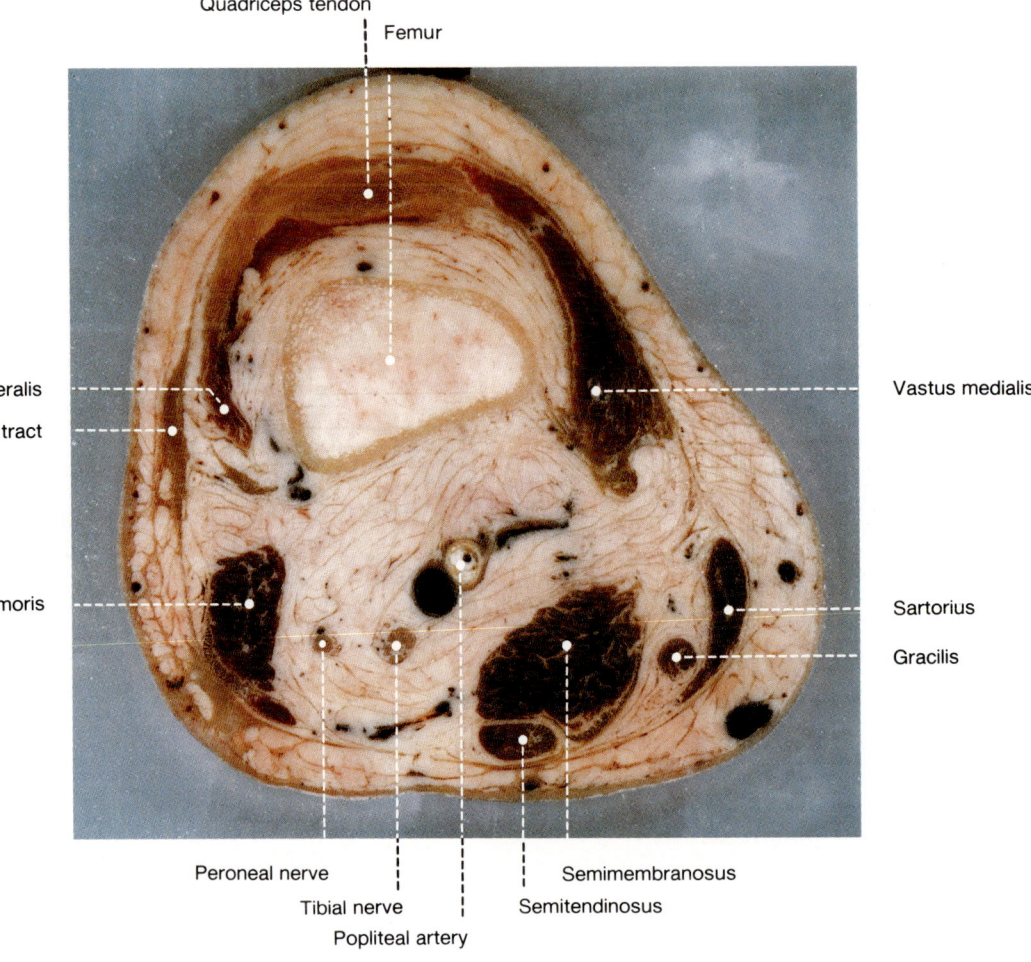

Anterior
Lateral
Medial
Posterior

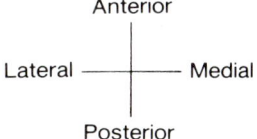

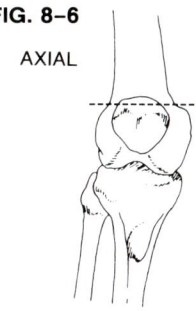

FIG. 8–6

AXIAL

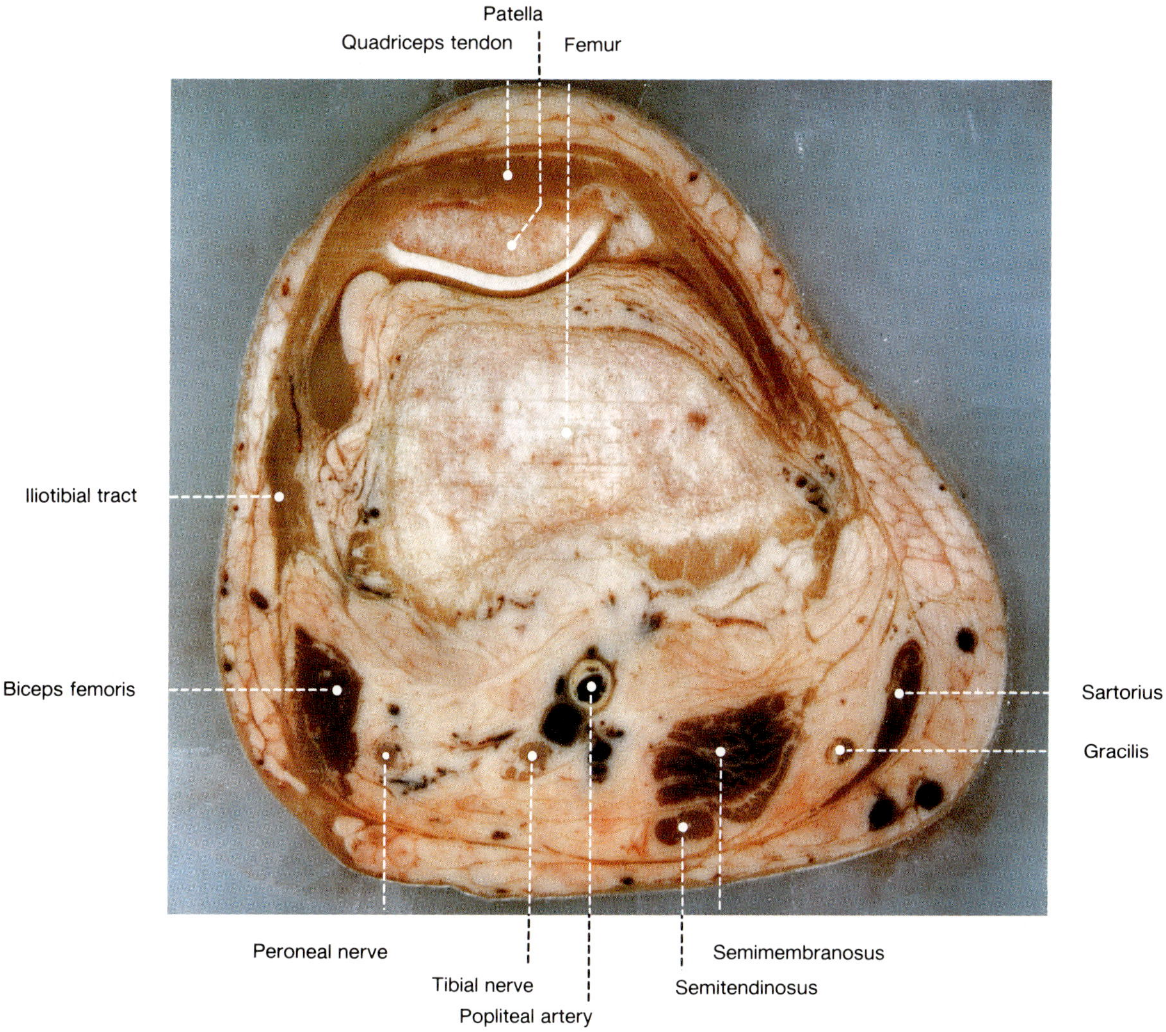

Patella
Quadriceps tendon
Femur
Iliotibial tract
Biceps femoris
Sartorius
Gracilis
Peroneal nerve
Tibial nerve
Popliteal artery
Semimembranosus
Semitendinosus

Anatomy and MRI of the Joints   212

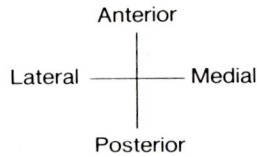

FIG. 8-7

AXIAL

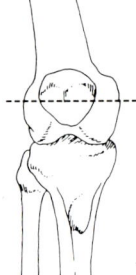

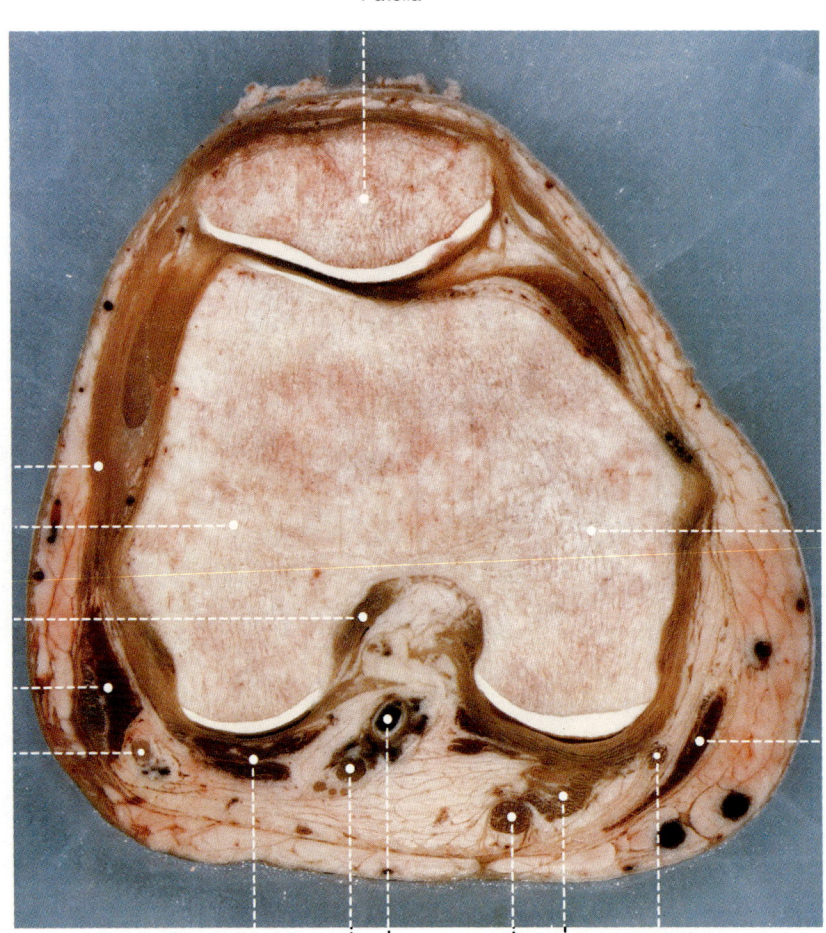

Anatomy and MRI of the Joints   213   THE KNEE

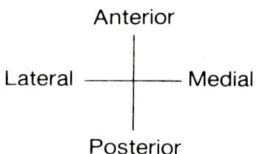

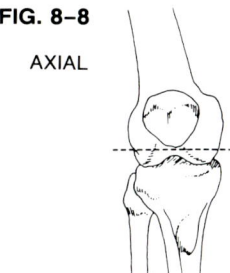

FIG. 8-8
AXIAL

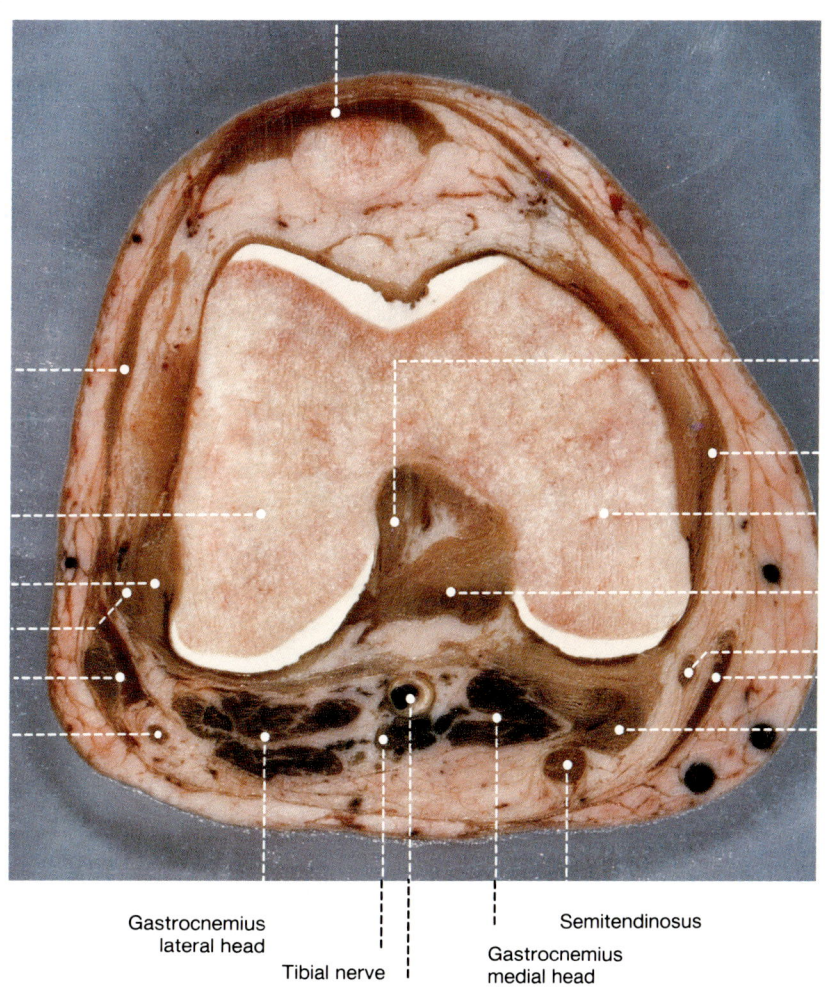

Anatomy and MRI of the Joints 214

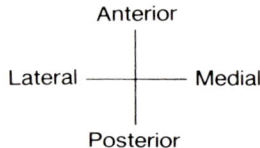

FIG. 8–9
AXIAL

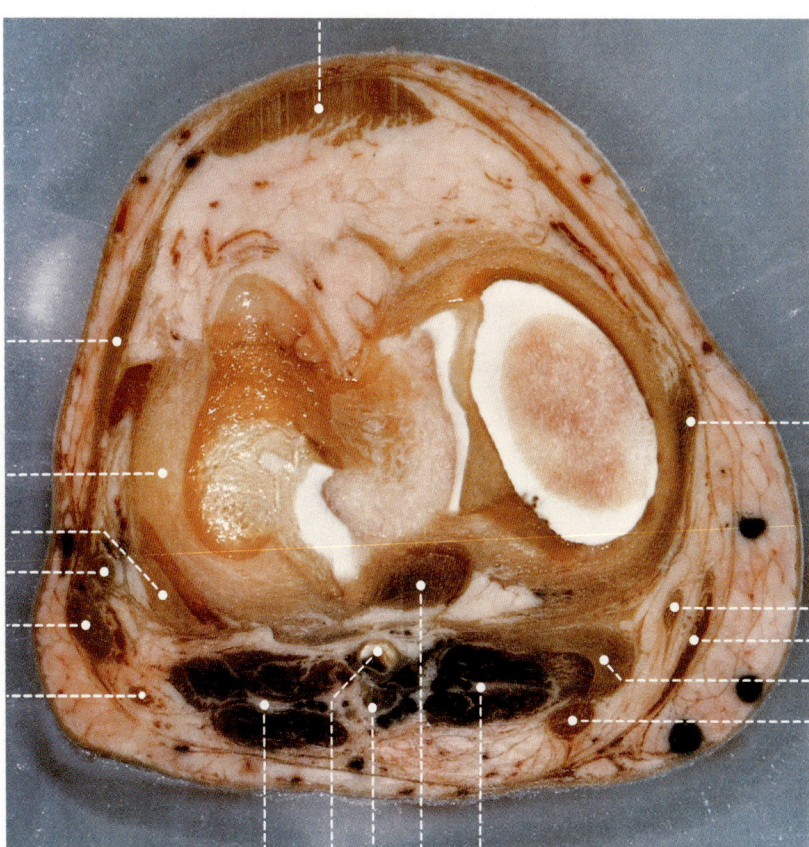

THE KNEE

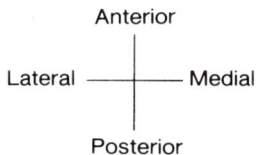

FIG. 8–10

AXIAL

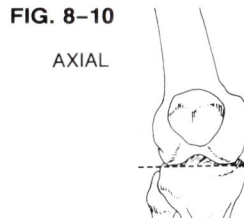

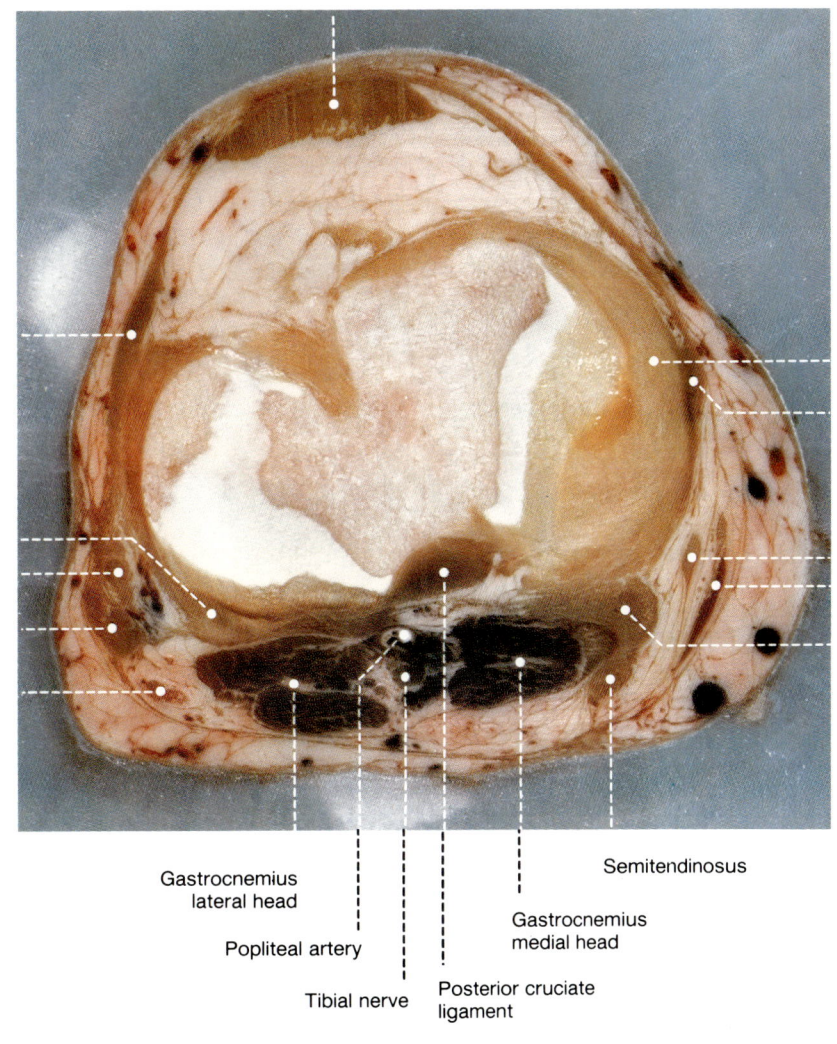

Patellar tendon

Iliotibial tract

Popliteus tendon
Lateral collateral ligament
Biceps femoris
Peroneal nerve

Medial meniscus
Medial collateral ligament

Gracilis
Sartorius
Semimembranosus

Gastrocnemius lateral head
Popliteal artery
Tibial nerve
Posterior cruciate ligament
Gastrocnemius medial head
Semitendinosus

Anatomy and MRI of the Joints

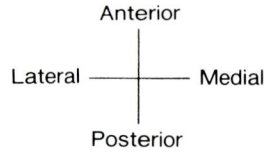

FIG. 8-11
AXIAL

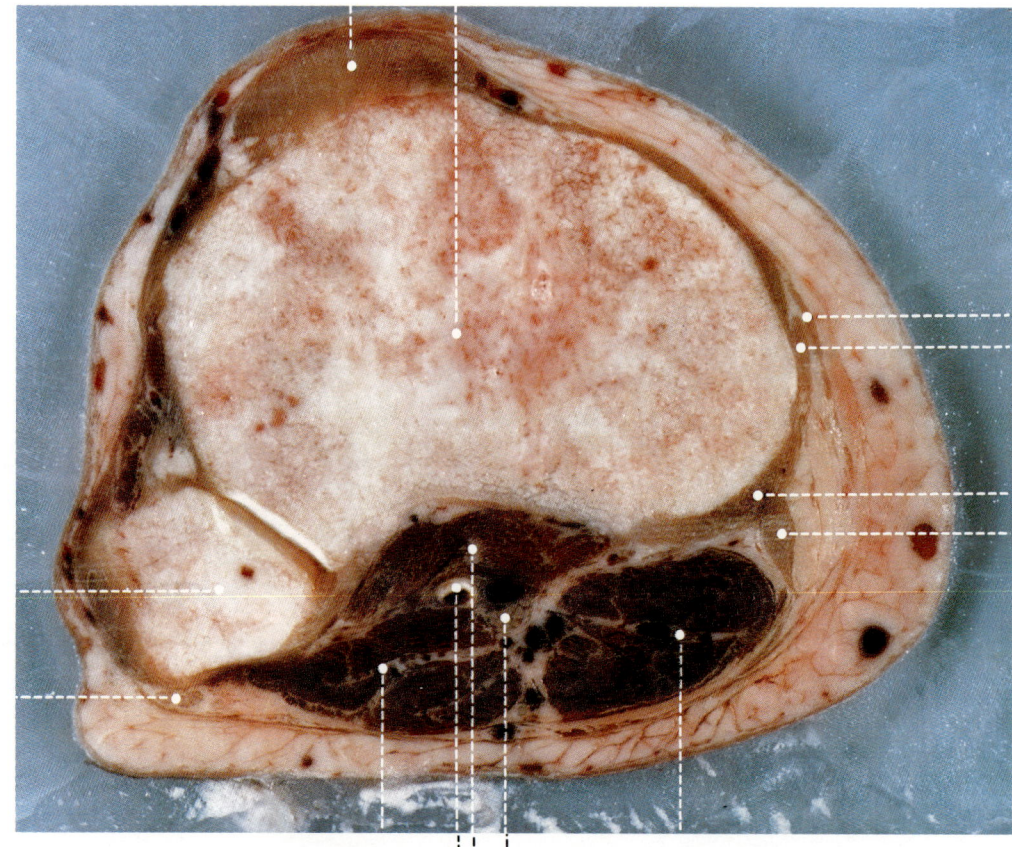

Anterior

Lateral — Medial

Posterior

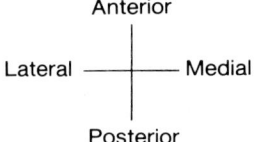

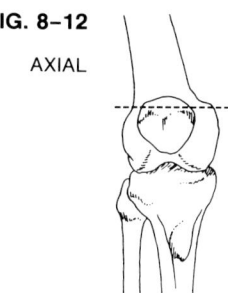

FIG. 8–12

AXIAL

Quadriceps tendon
Distal femur
Patella
Vastus lateralis
Iliotibial tract
Biceps femoris
Vastus medialis
Sartorius
Peroneal nerve
Tibial nerve
Popliteal artery
Gastrocnemius medial head
Semimembranosus
Semitendinosus
Gracilis

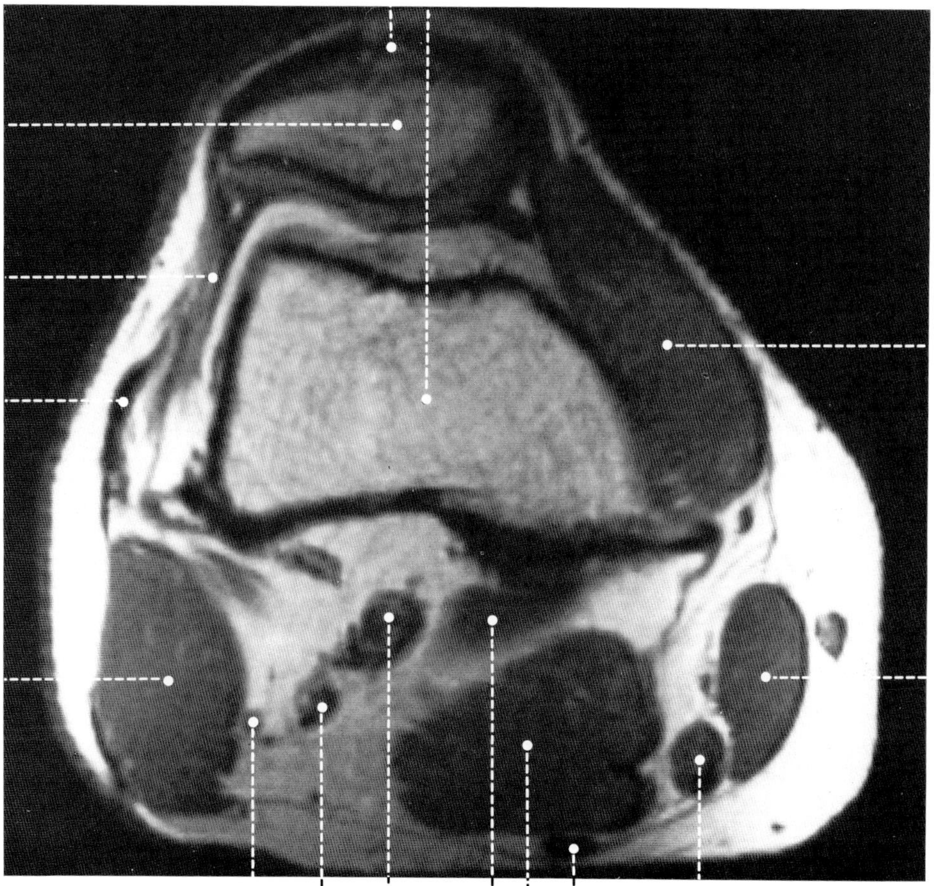

Anatomy and MRI of the Joints 218

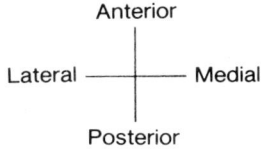

FIG. 8-13
AXIAL

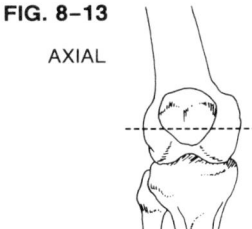

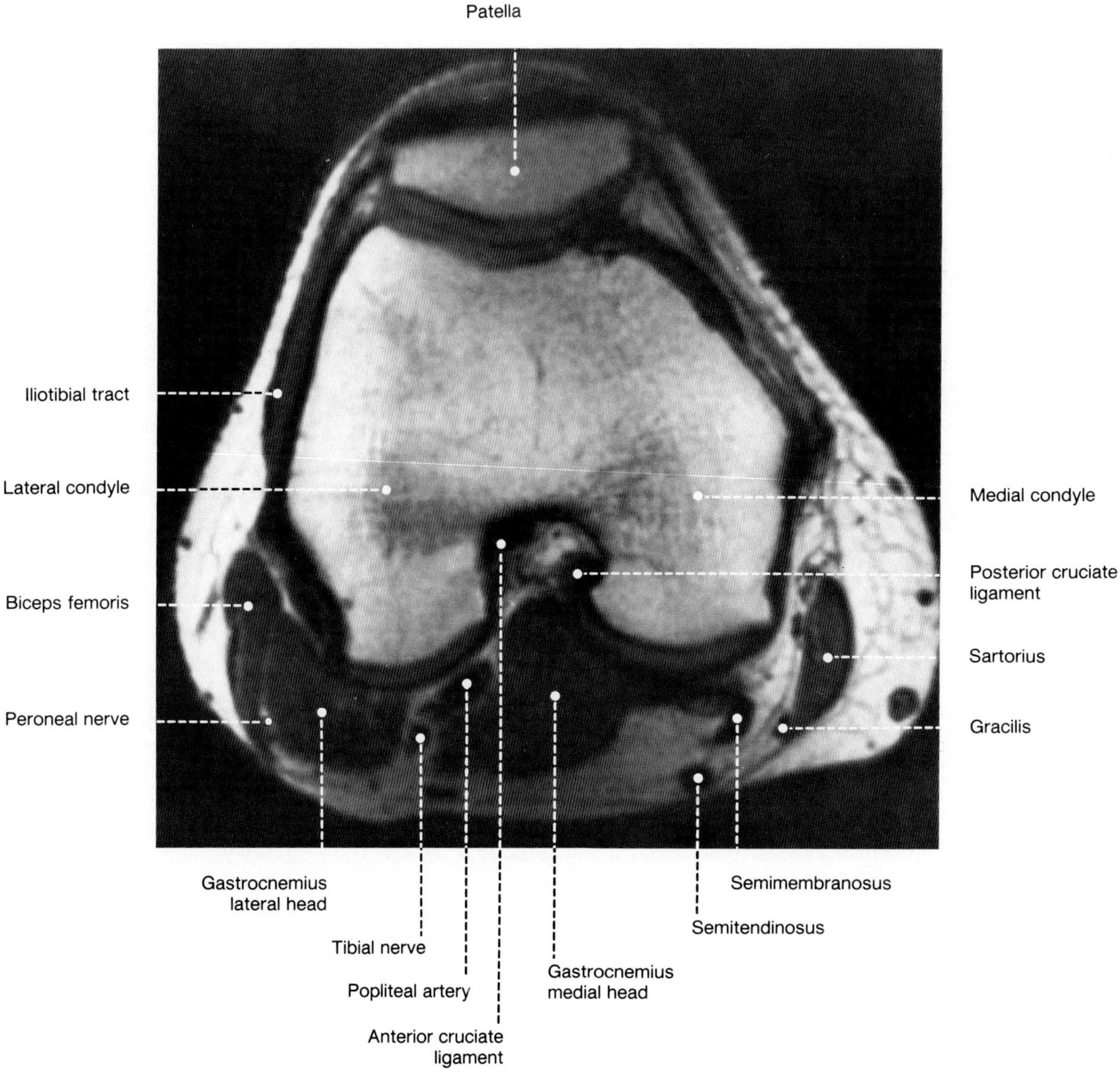

Patella

Iliotibial tract
Lateral condyle
Biceps femoris
Peroneal nerve

Medial condyle
Posterior cruciate ligament
Sartorius
Gracilis

Gastrocnemius lateral head
Tibial nerve
Popliteal artery
Anterior cruciate ligament
Gastrocnemius medial head
Semitendinosus
Semimembranosus

219 THE KNEE

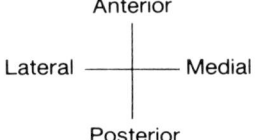

FIG. 8-14

AXIAL

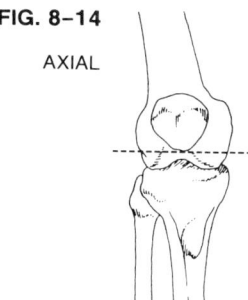

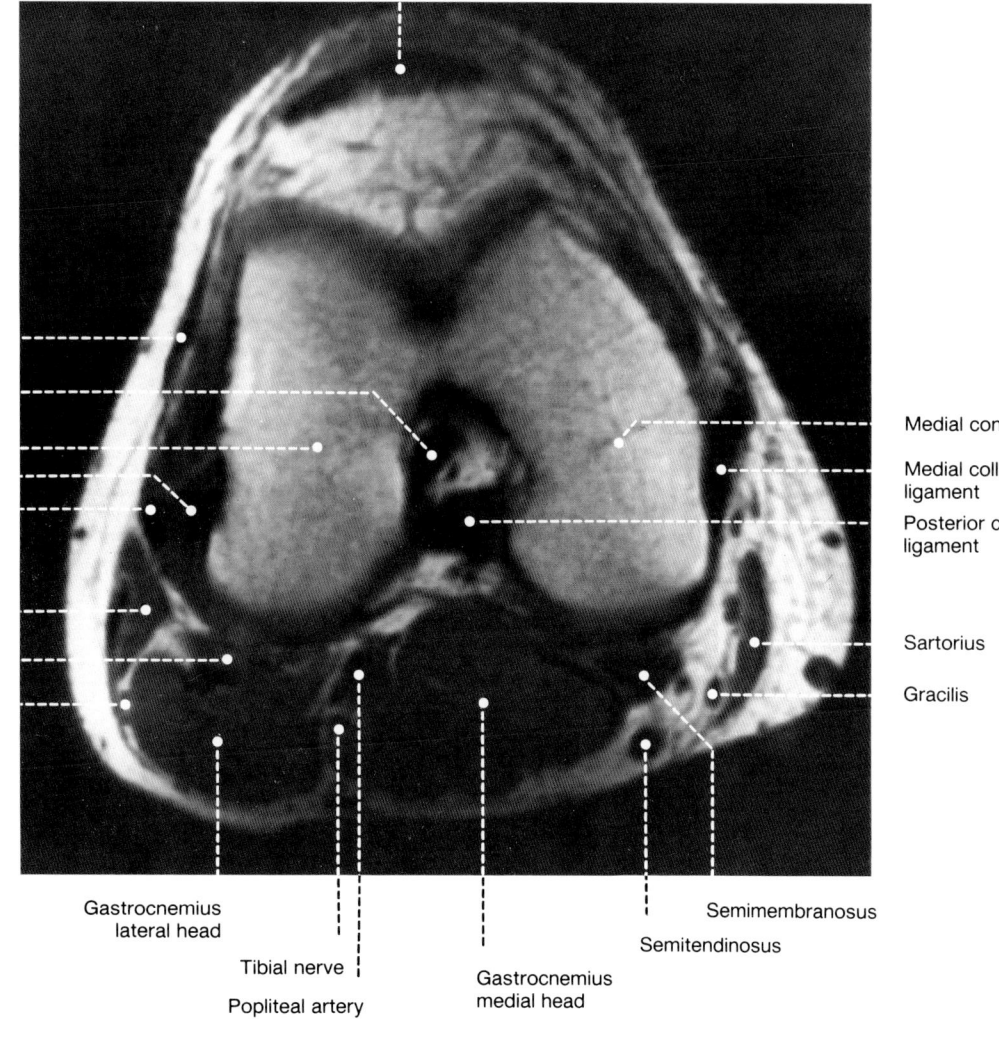

Patellar tendon

Iliotibial tract
Anterior cruciate ligament
Lateral condyle
Popliteus tendon
Lateral collateral ligament

Biceps femoris
Plantaris
Peroneal nerve

Medial condyle
Medial collateral ligament
Posterior cruciate ligament

Sartorius
Gracilis

Gastrocnemius lateral head
Tibial nerve
Popliteal artery
Gastrocnemius medial head
Semitendinosus
Semimembranosus

Anatomy and MRI of the Joints

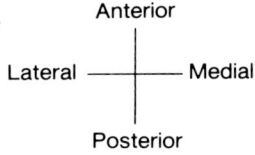

FIG. 8-15

AXIAL

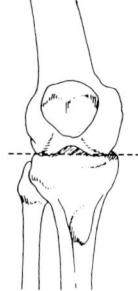

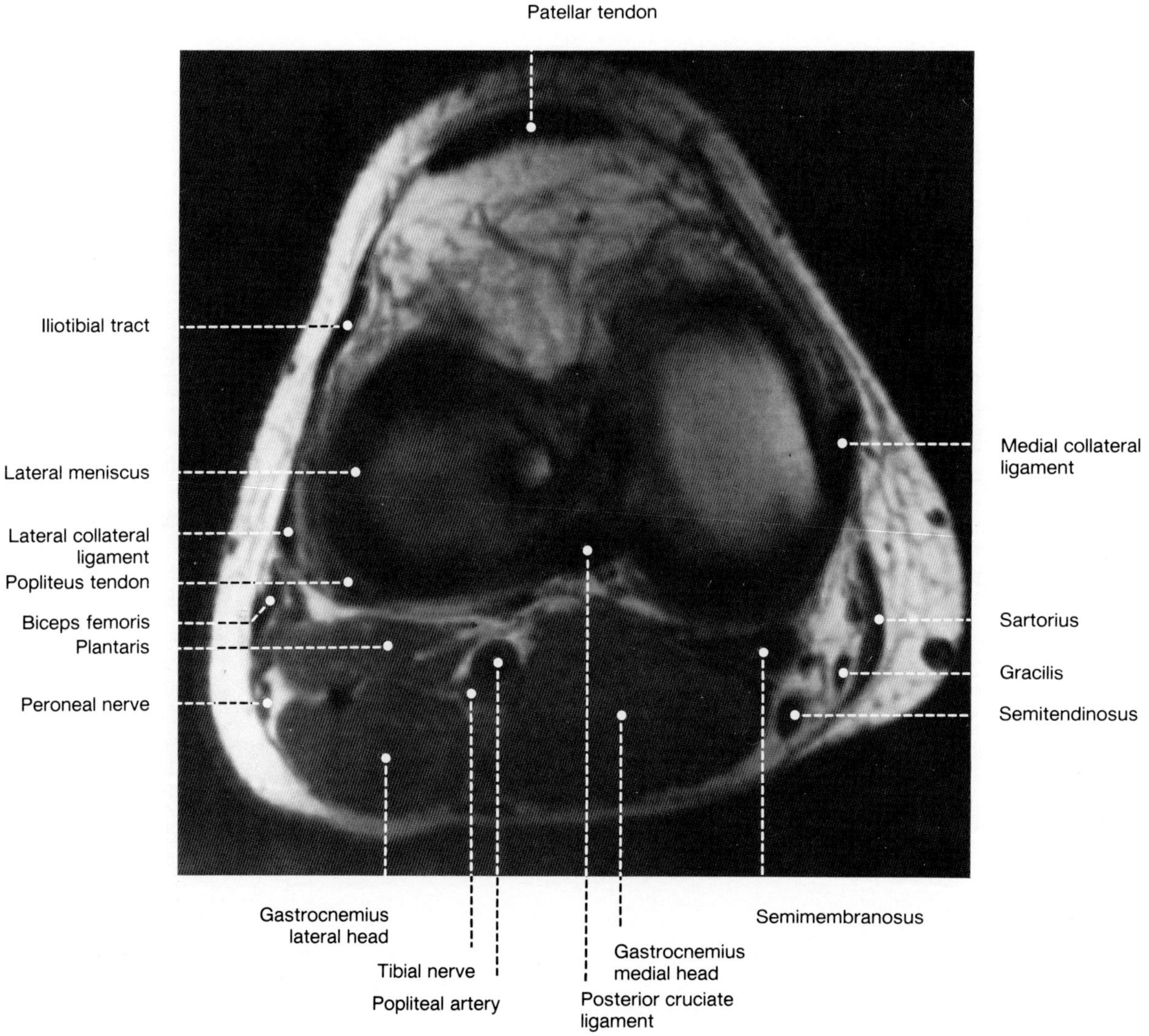

Anterior
Lateral
Medial
Posterior

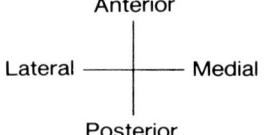

FIG. 8–16
AXIAL

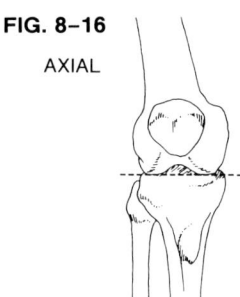

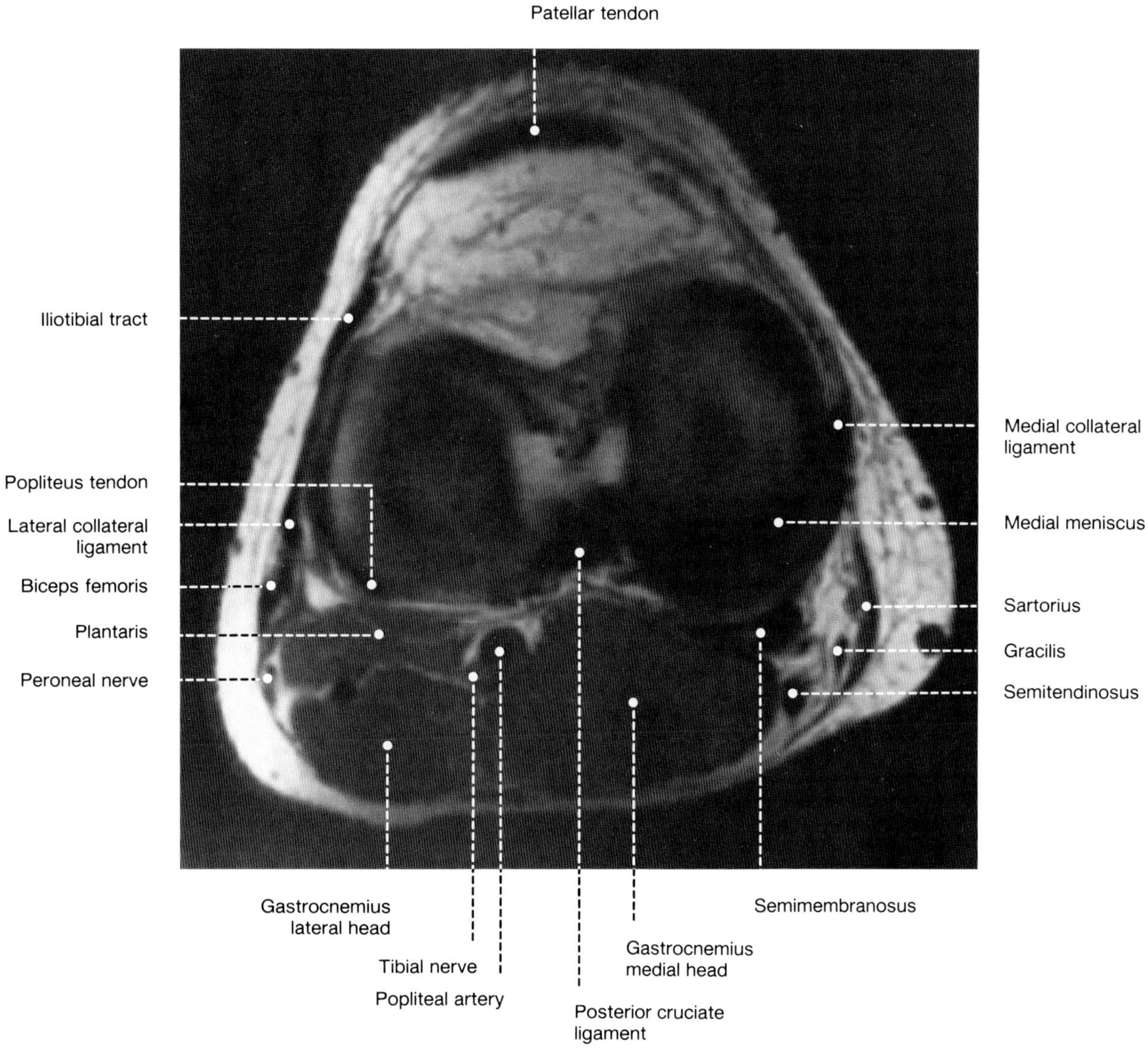

Patellar tendon
Iliotibial tract
Popliteus tendon
Lateral collateral ligament
Biceps femoris
Plantaris
Peroneal nerve
Medial collateral ligament
Medial meniscus
Sartorius
Gracilis
Semitendinosus
Gastrocnemius lateral head
Tibial nerve
Popliteal artery
Posterior cruciate ligament
Gastrocnemius medial head
Semimembranosus

Anatomy and MRI of the Joints 222

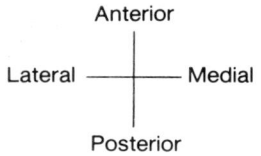

FIG. 8-17

AXIAL

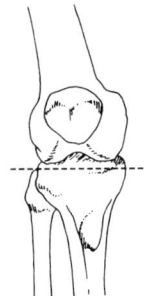

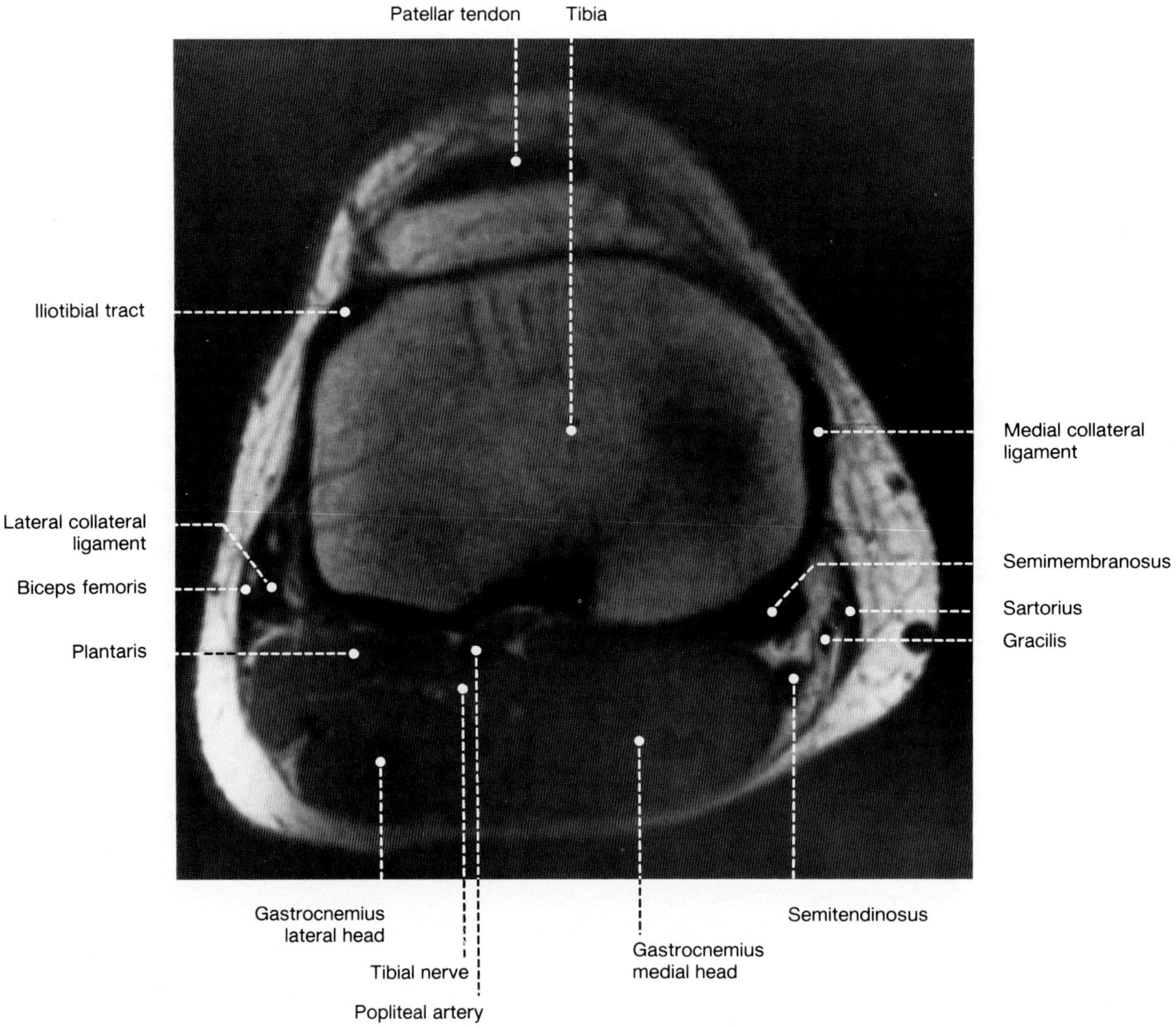

Labels: Patellar tendon, Tibia, Iliotibial tract, Medial collateral ligament, Lateral collateral ligament, Semimembranosus, Biceps femoris, Sartorius, Plantaris, Gracilis, Gastrocnemius lateral head, Semitendinosus, Tibial nerve, Gastrocnemius medial head, Popliteal artery

THE KNEE

FIG. 8-18

SAGITTAL

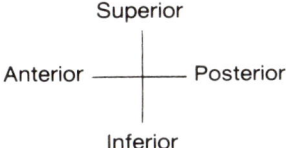
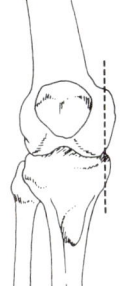
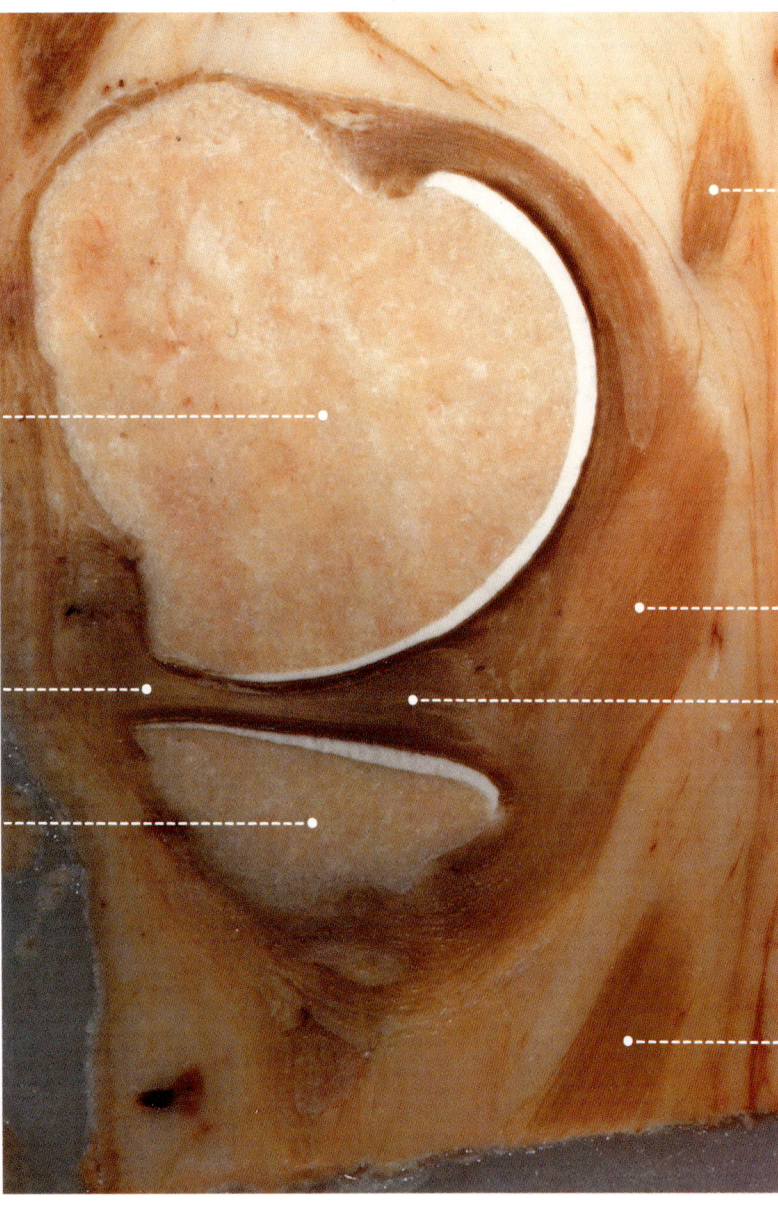

Anatomy and MRI of the Joints

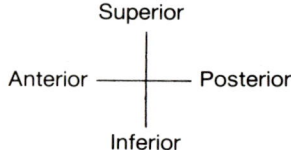

FIG. 8-19

SAGITTAL

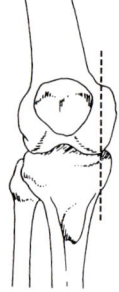

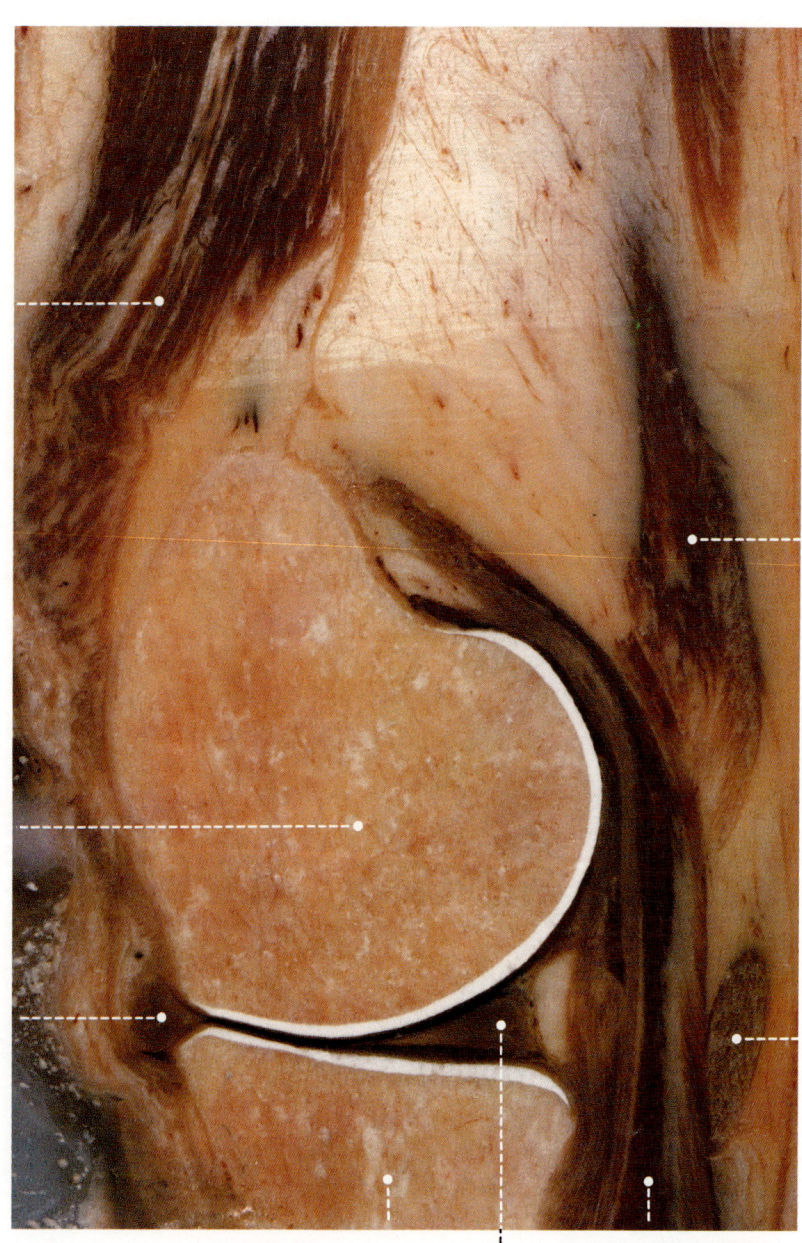

- Vastus medialis muscle
- Semimembranosus muscle
- Medial femoral condyle
- Medial meniscus anterior horn
- Semitendinosus tendon
- Medial tibial plateau
- Medial meniscus posterior horn
- Gastrocnemius medial head

Superior
Anterior — Posterior
Inferior

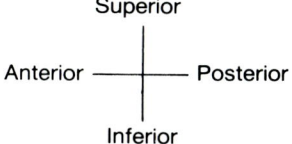

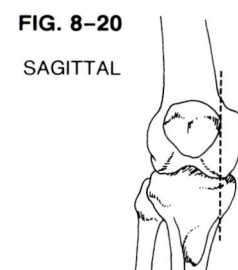

FIG. 8–20

SAGITTAL

Semimembranosus muscle
Medial femoral condyle
Semitendinosus tendon
Medial meniscus anterior horn
Medial meniscus posterior horn
Gastrocnemius muscle medial head
Medial tibial plateau

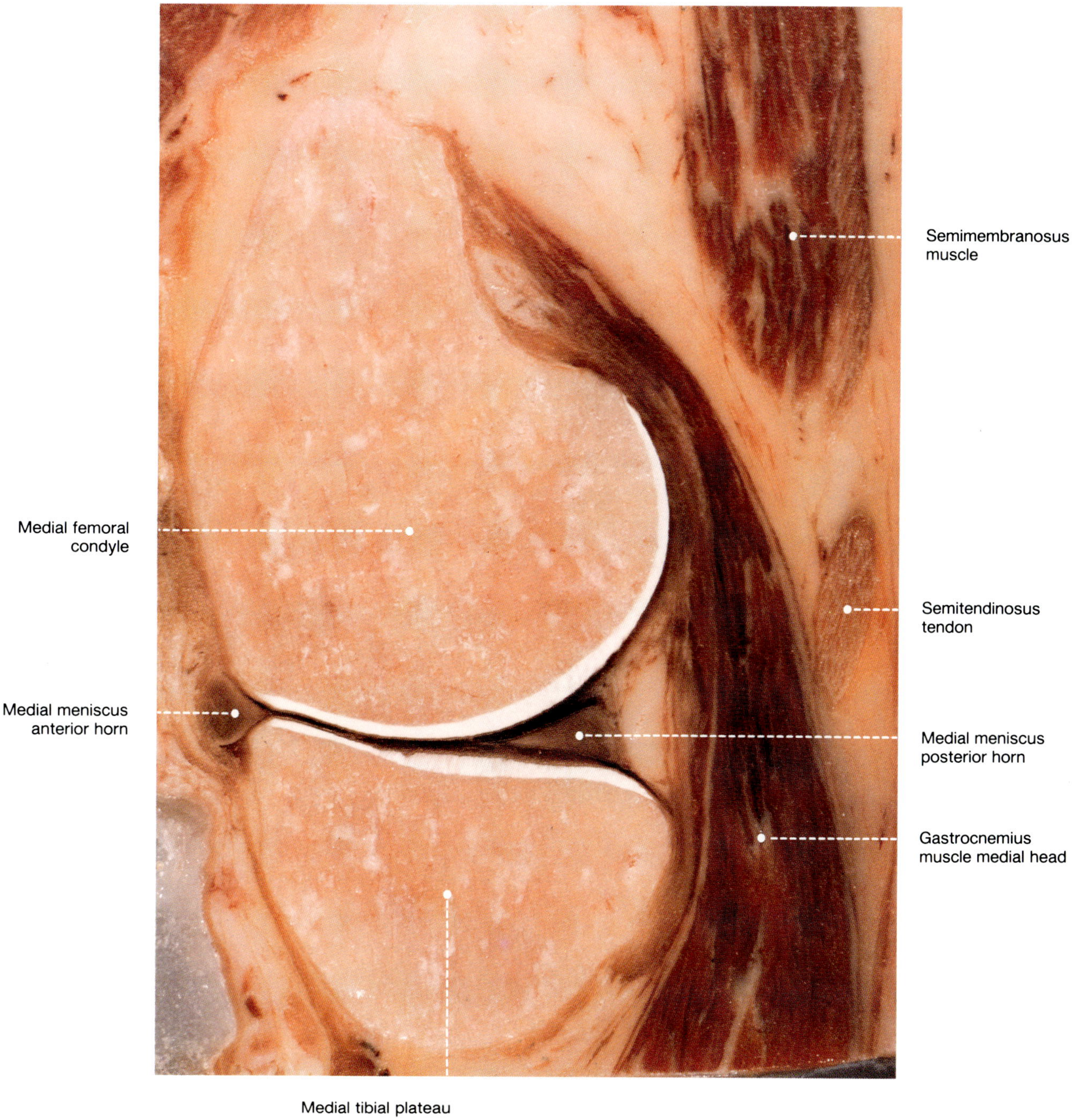

Anatomy and MRI of the Joints

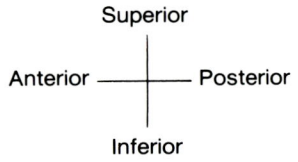

FIG. 8-21

SAGITTAL

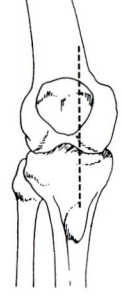

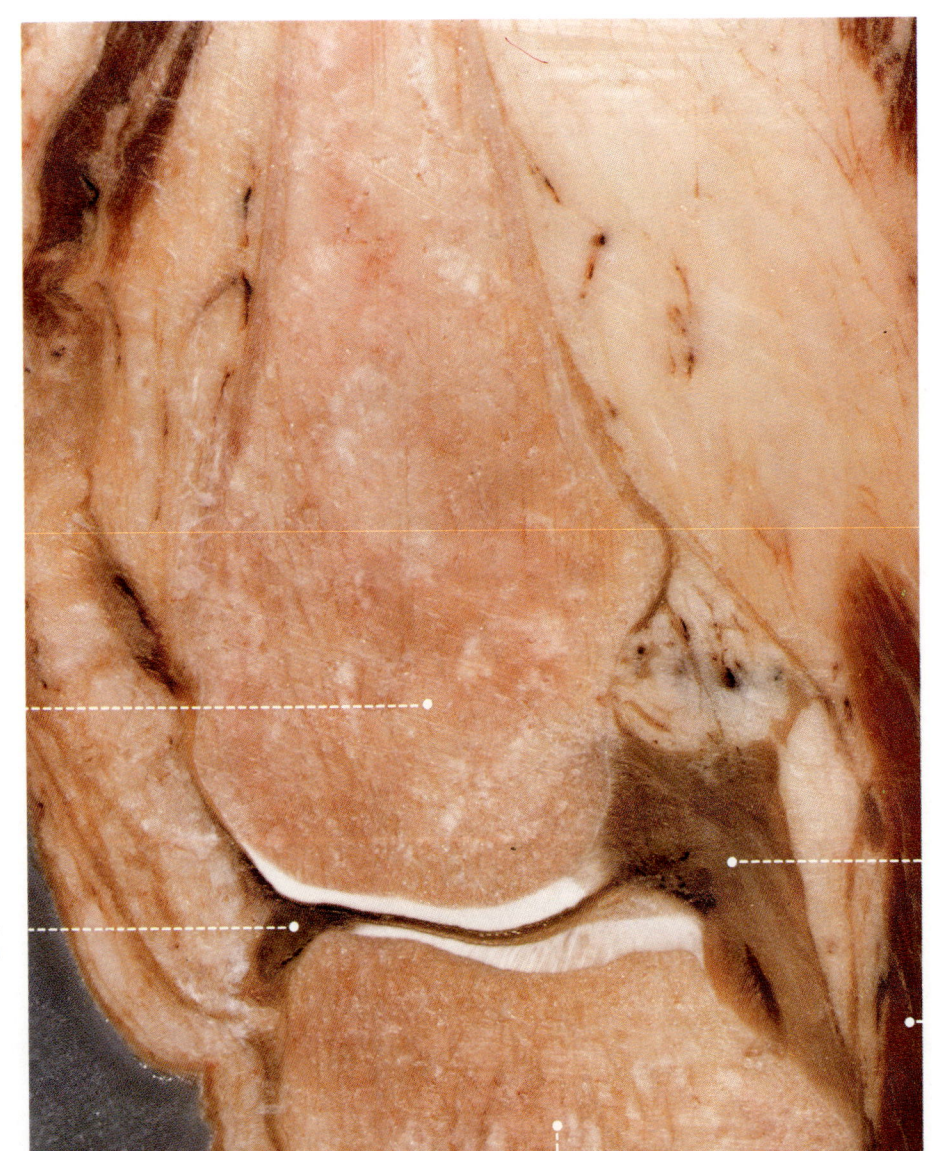

Distal femur

Medial meniscus anterior horn

Posterior cruciate ligament

Gastrocnemius medial head

Proximal tibia

227   THE KNEE

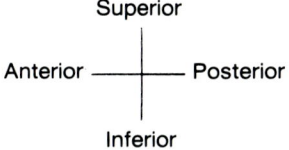

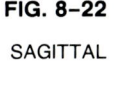
FIG. 8-22
SAGITTAL

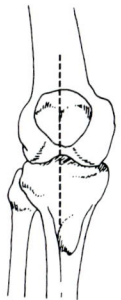

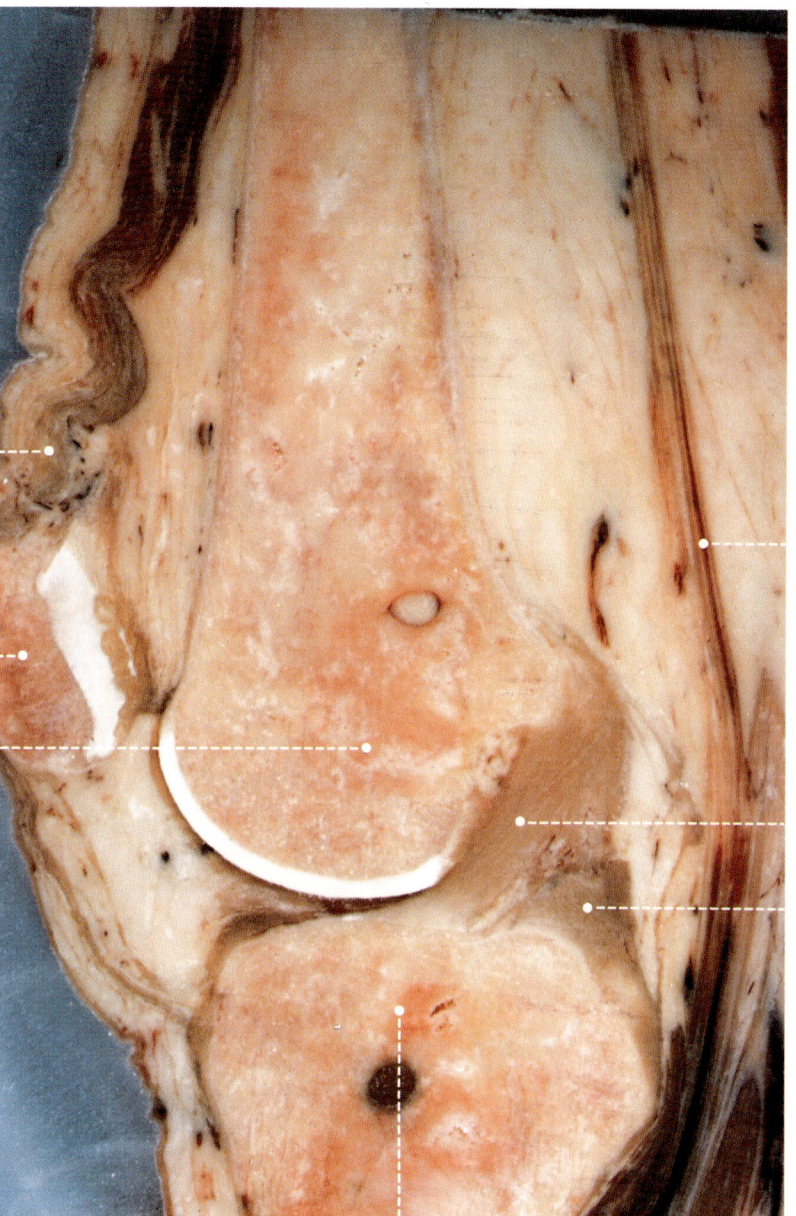

Quadriceps tendon

Patella

Distal femur

Popliteal artery

Anterior cruciate ligament

Posterior cruciate ligament

Proximal tibia

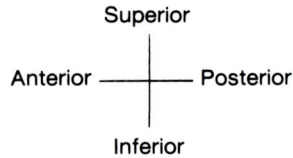

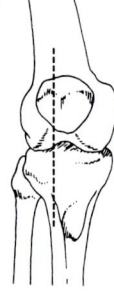

FIG. 8-23
SAGITTAL

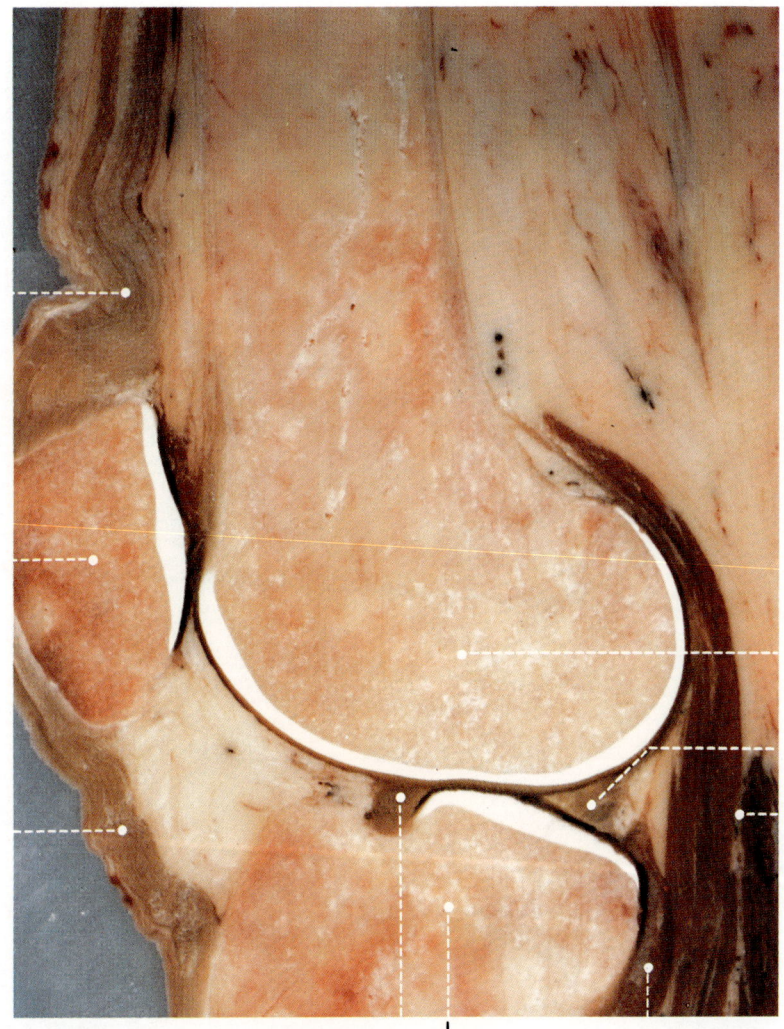

229 THE KNEE

FIG. 8-24
SAGITTAL

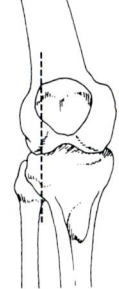

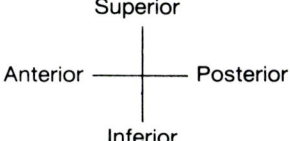

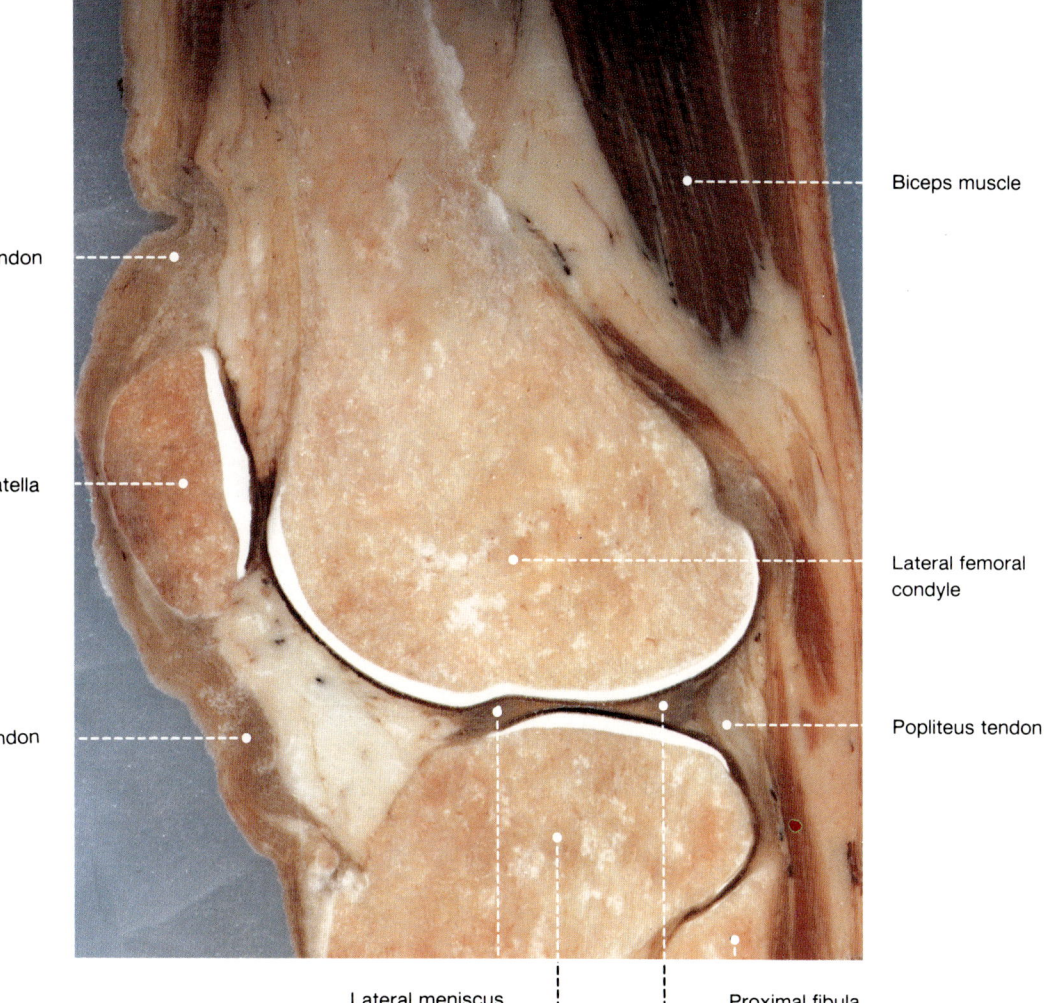

- Quadriceps tendon
- Patella
- Patellar tendon
- Biceps muscle
- Lateral femoral condyle
- Popliteus tendon
- Lateral meniscus anterior horn
- Proximal tibia
- Lateral meniscus posterior horn
- Proximal fibula

Anatomy and MRI of the Joints

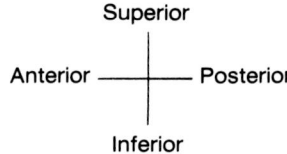

FIG. 8-25

SAGITTAL

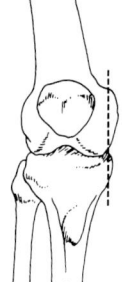

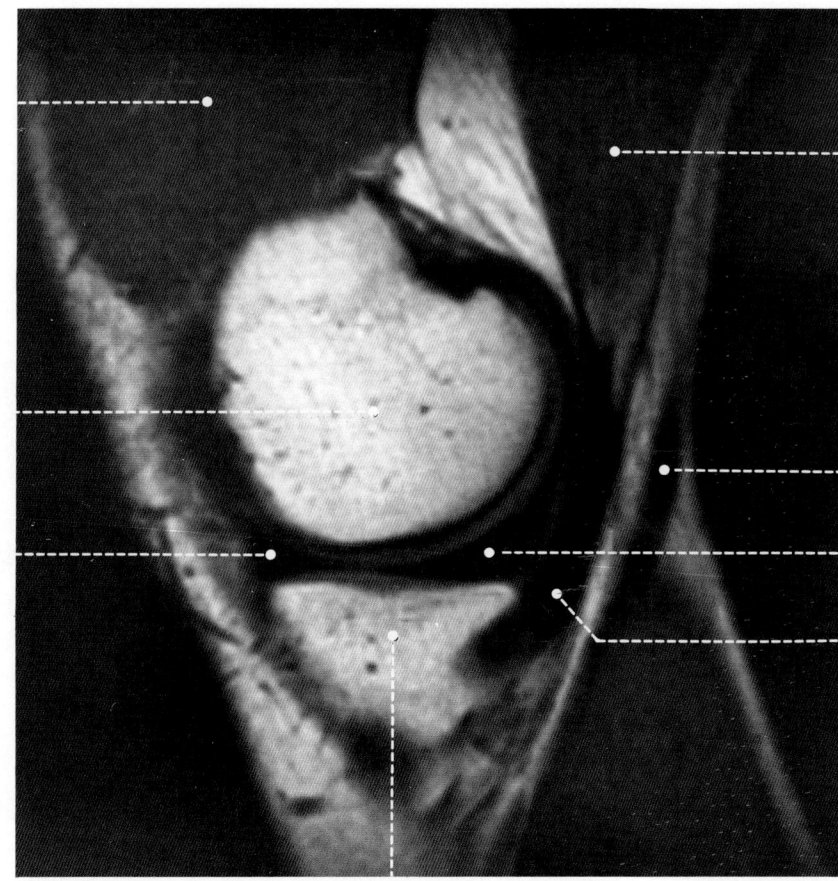

- Vastus medialis
- Medial condyle
- Medial meniscus anterior horn
- Semimembranosus muscle
- Semitendinosus tendon
- Medial meniscus posterior horn
- Semimembranosus tendon
- Tibial plateau

THE KNEE

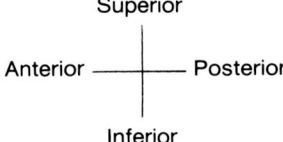

FIG. 8-26
SAGITTAL

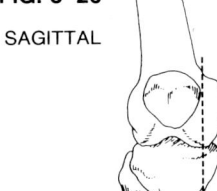

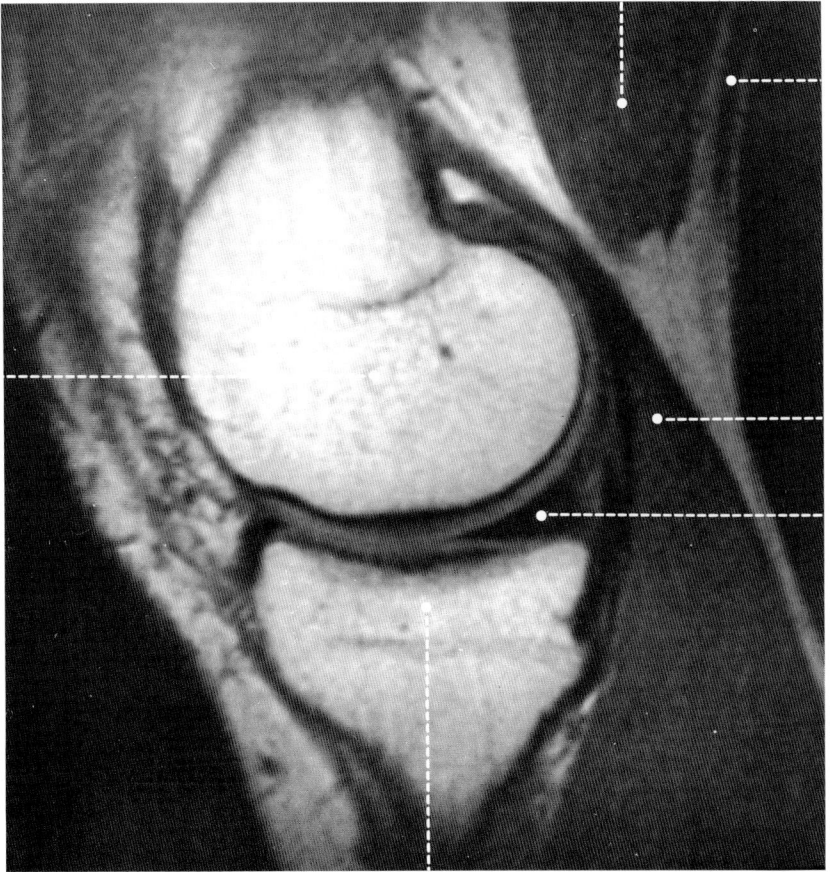

- Semimembranosus
- Semitendinosus tendon
- Medial condyle
- Gastrocnemius medial head
- Medial meniscus posterior horn
- Tibial plateau

Anatomy and MRI of the Joints 232

FIG. 8-27
SAGITTAL

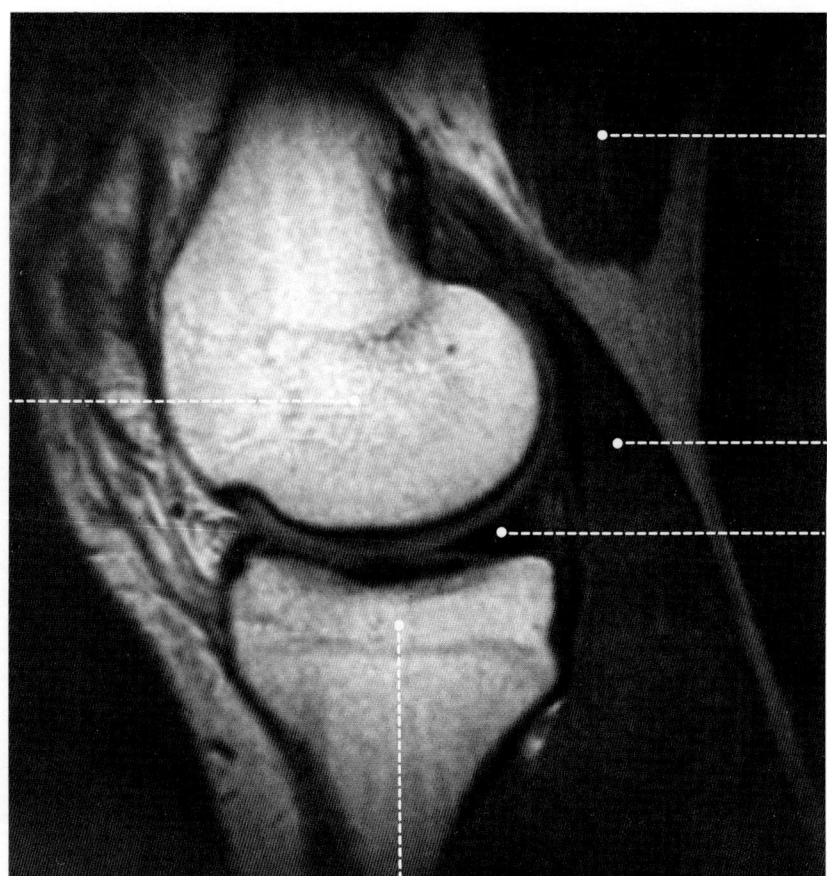

233 THE KNEE

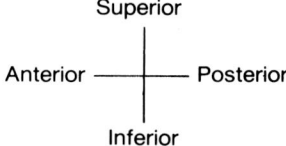

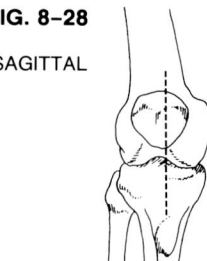

FIG. 8-28

SAGITTAL

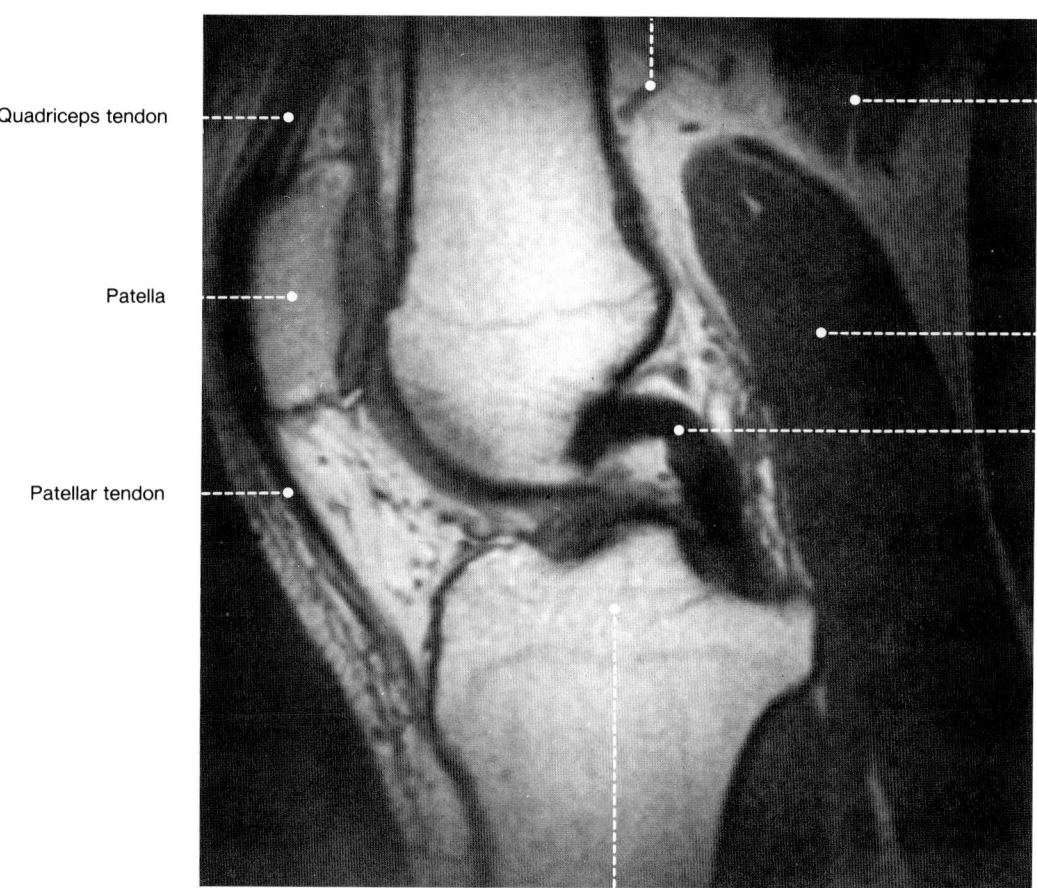

Anatomy and MRI of the Joints 234

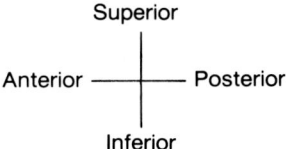

FIG. 8-29
SAGITTAL

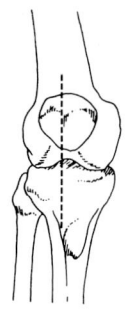

- Quadriceps tendon
- Patella
- Anterior cruciate ligament
- Patellar tendon
- Popliteal artery
- Semimembranosus
- Gastrocnemius medial head
- Posterior cruciate ligament
- Tibial plateau

THE KNEE

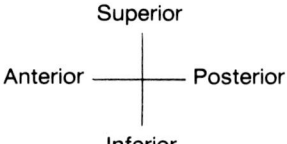

FIG. 8-30

SAGITTAL

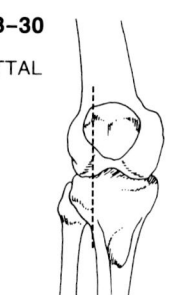

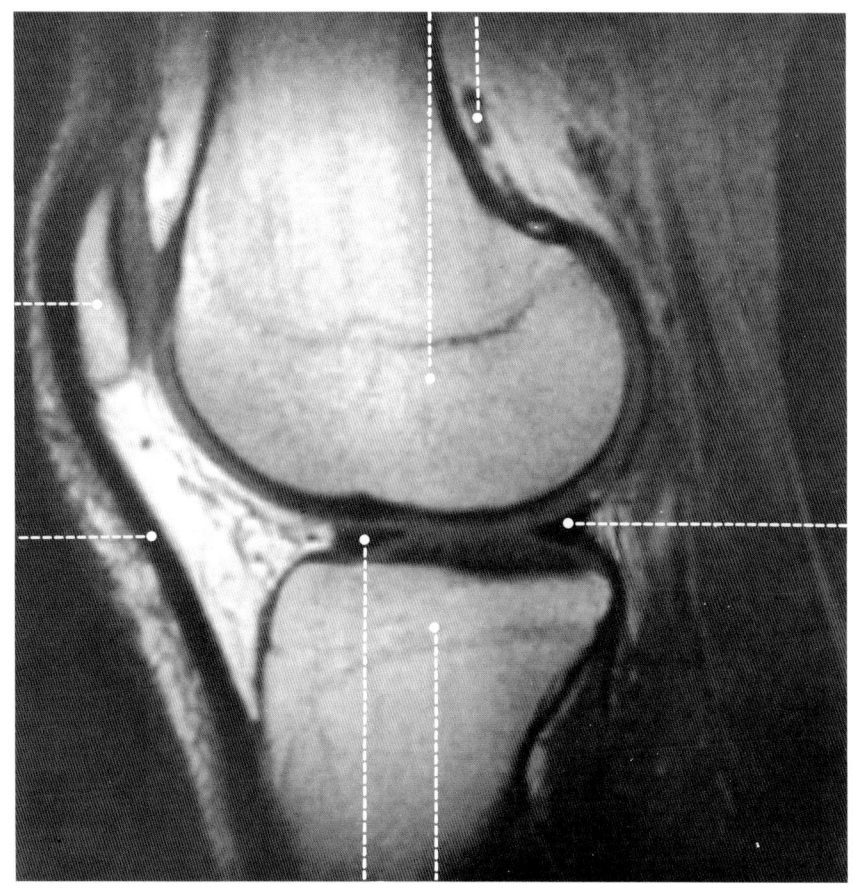

Lateral condyle
Superior lateral genicular vessels
Patella
Patellar tendon
Lateral meniscus posterior horn
Lateral meniscus anterior horn
Tibial plateau

Anatomy and MRI of the Joints 236

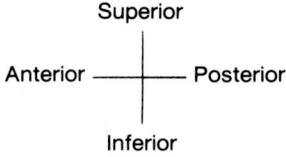

FIG. 8-31
SAGITTAL

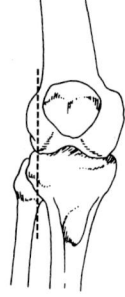

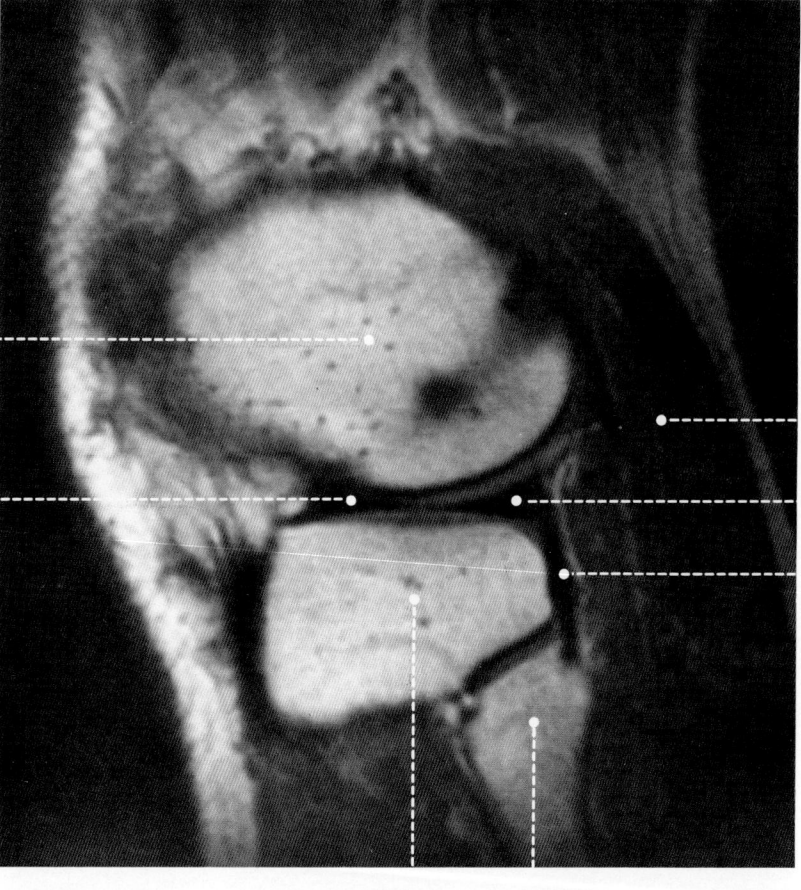

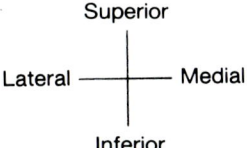
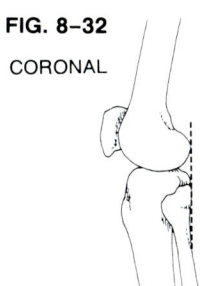

FIG. 8-32
CORONAL

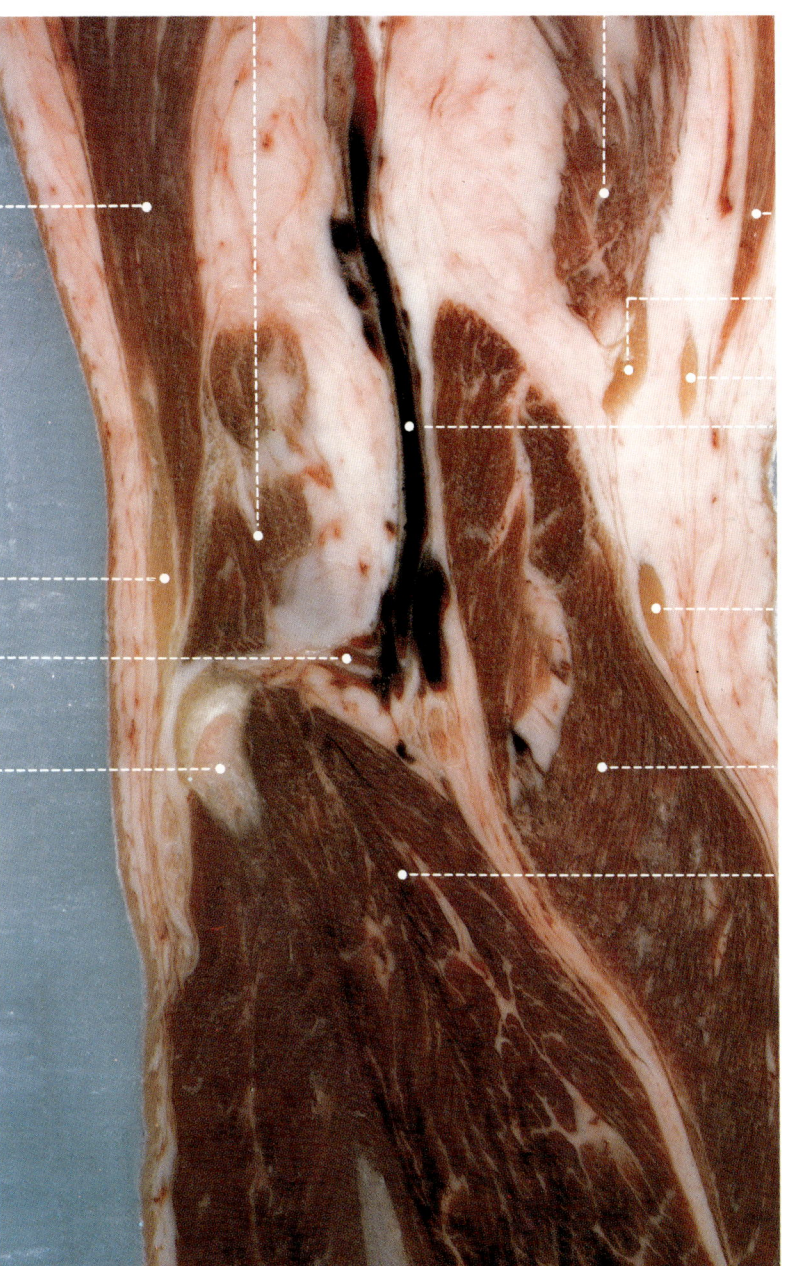

Anatomy and MRI of the Joints

FIG. 8-33
CORONAL

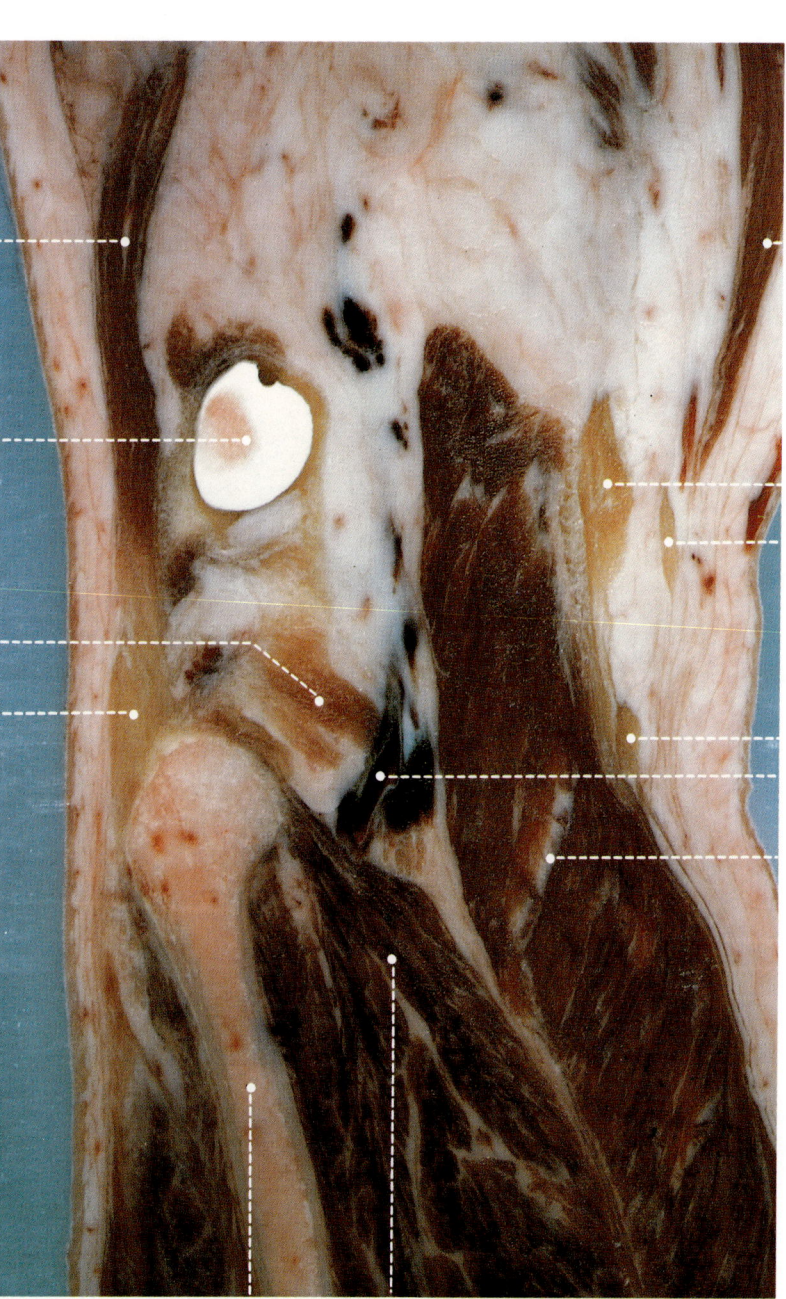

239 THE KNEE

FIG. 8–34
CORONAL

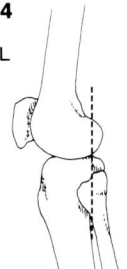

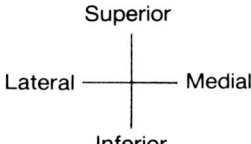

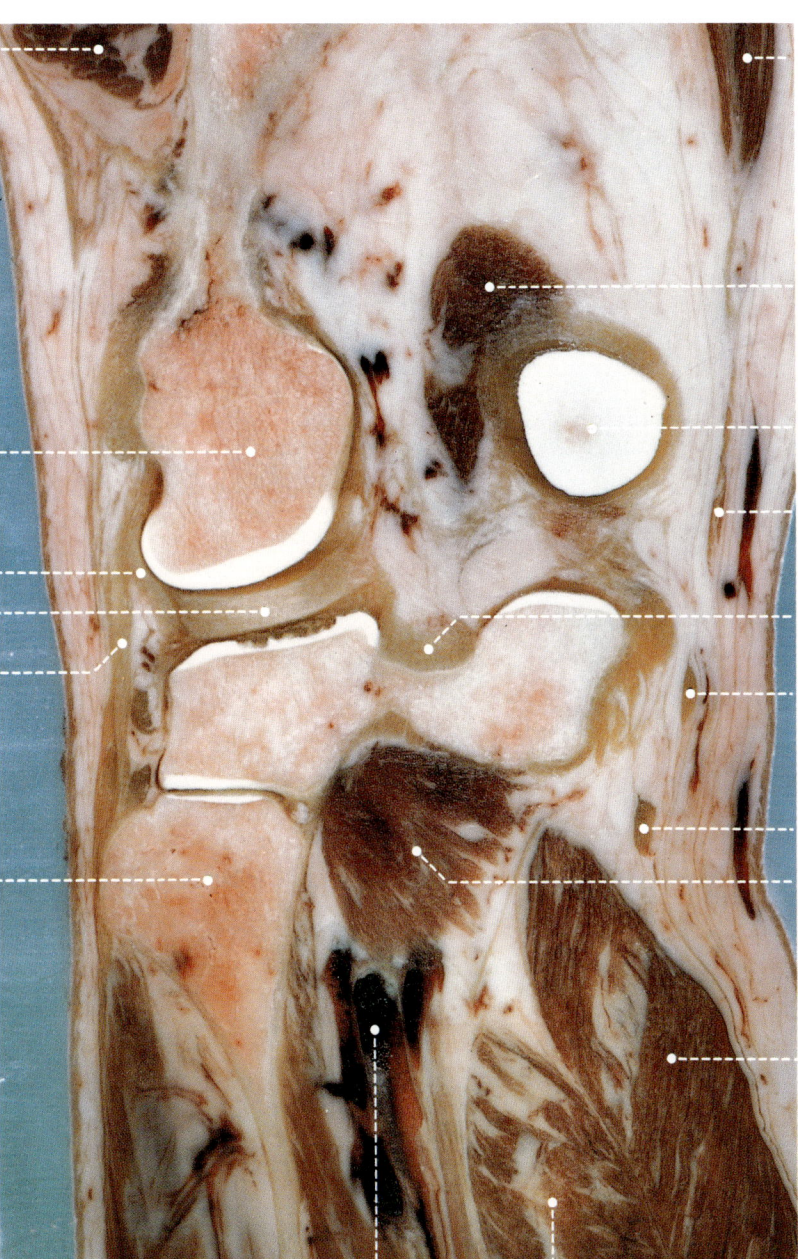

- Vastus lateralis
- Lateral condyle
- Popliteus tendon
- Lateral meniscus
- Lateral collateral ligament
- Fibula
- Popliteal artery

- Sartorius muscle
- Gastrocnemius medial head
- Medial condyle
- Sartorius tendon
- Posterior cruciate ligament
- Gracilis
- Semitendinosus
- Popliteus muscle
- Gastrocnemius medial head
- Soleus

Anatomy and MRI of the Joints   240

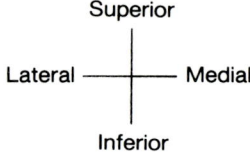

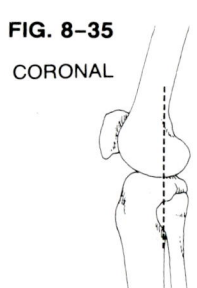

FIG. 8–35

CORONAL

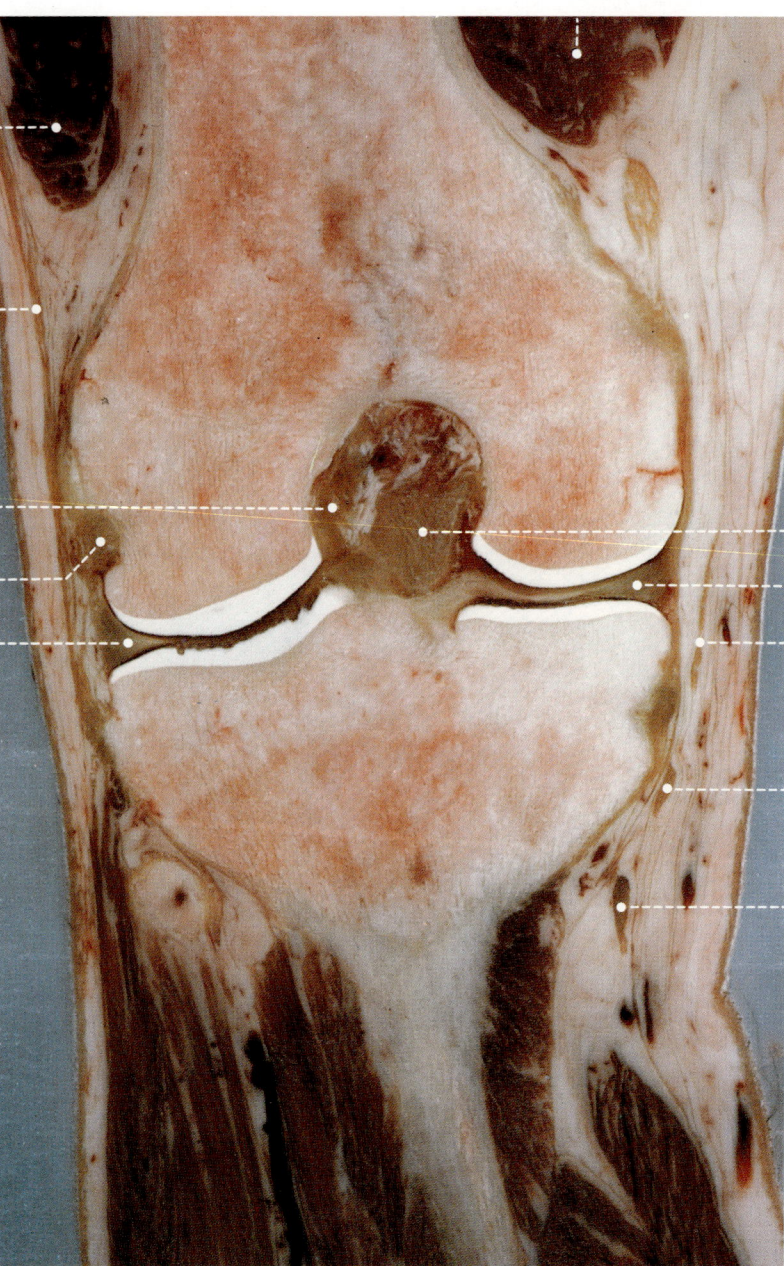

- Vastus medialis
- Vastus lateralis
- Iliotibial tract
- Anterior cruciate ligament
- Popliteus tendon
- Lateral meniscus
- Posterior cruciate ligament
- Medial meniscus
- Sartorius
- Gracilis
- Semitendinosus

THE KNEE

FIG. 8-36
CORONAL

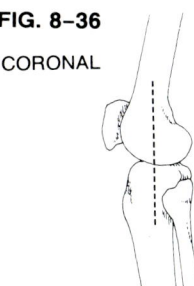

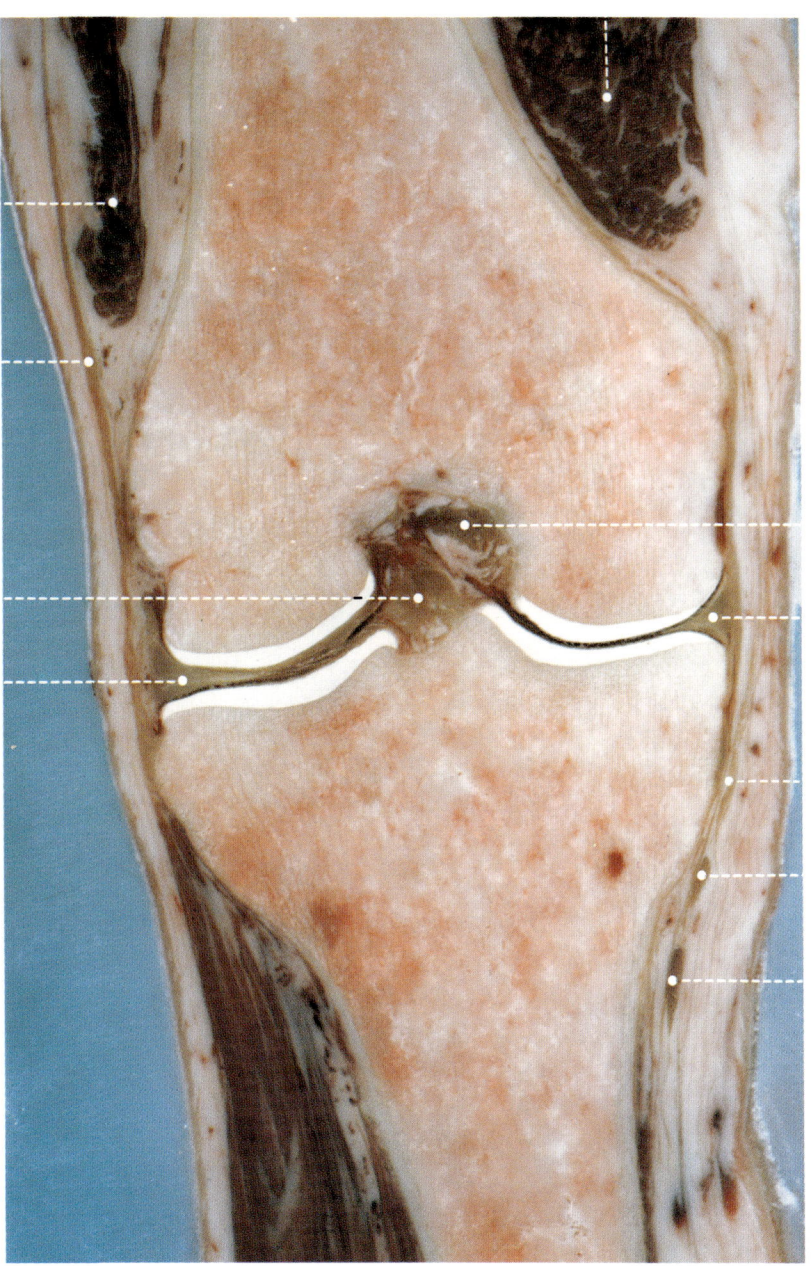

Anatomy and MRI of the Joints 242

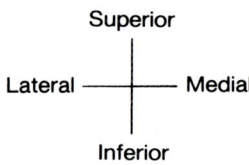

FIG. 8-37
CORONAL

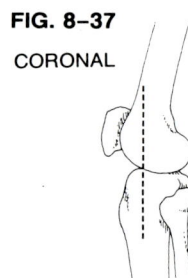

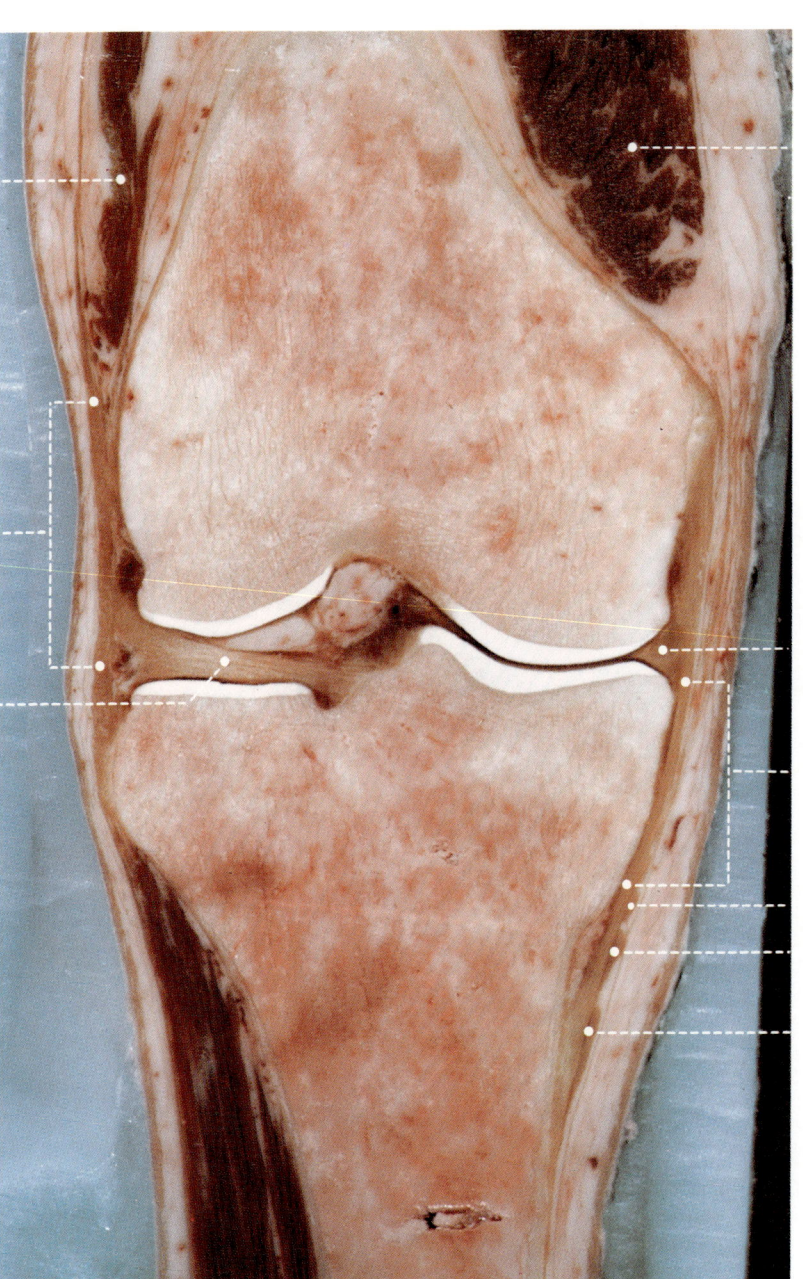

- Vastus lateralis
- Iliotibial tract
- Lateral meniscus
- Vastus medialis
- Medial meniscus
- Medial collateral ligament
- Sartorius
- Gracilis
- Semitendinosus

243 THE KNEE

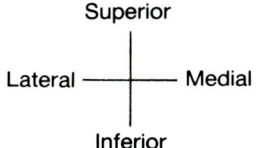

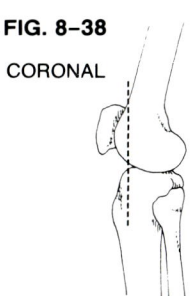

FIG. 8-38
CORONAL

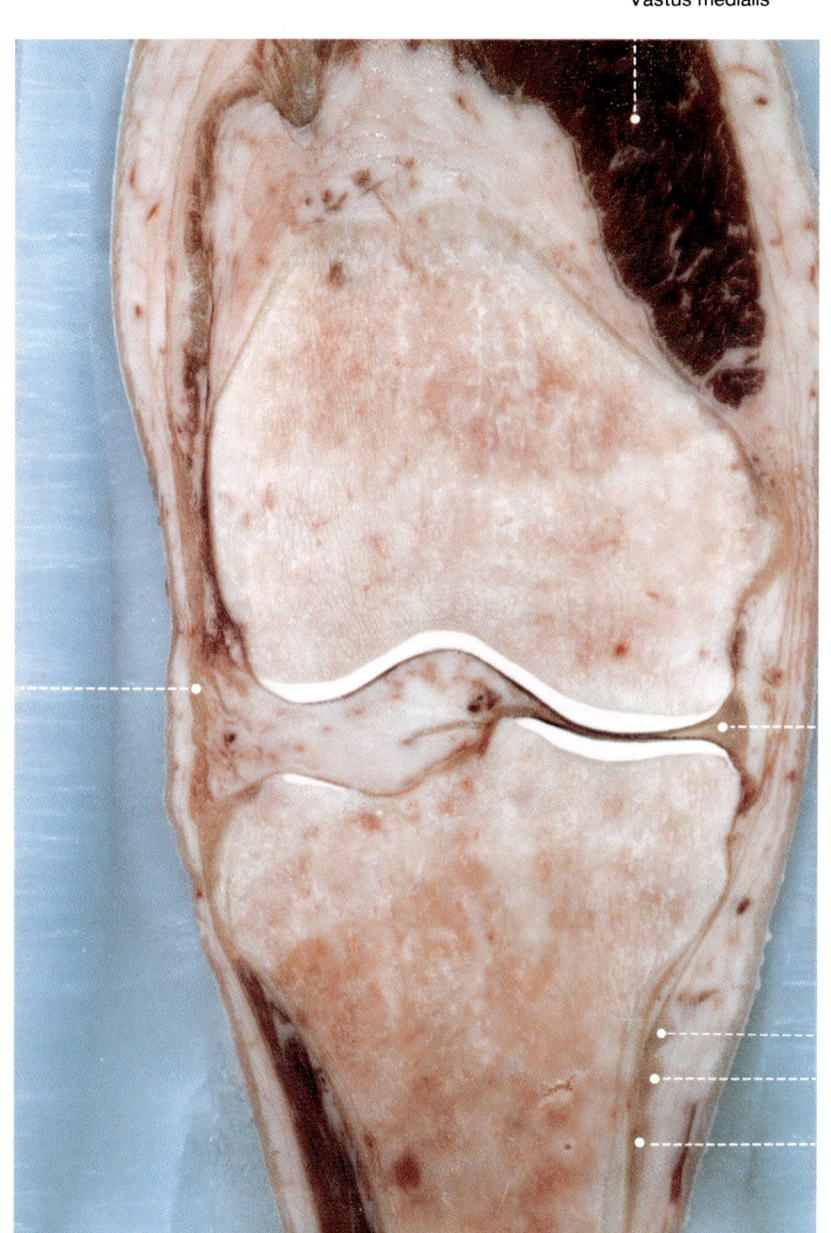

Vastus medialis

Iliotibial tract

Medial meniscus

Sartorius

Gracilis

Semitendinosus

Superior

Lateral —— Medial

Inferior

FIG. 8–39

CORONAL

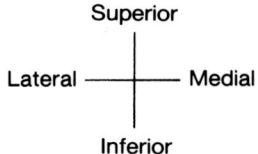

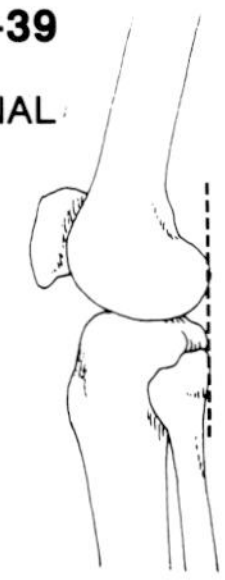

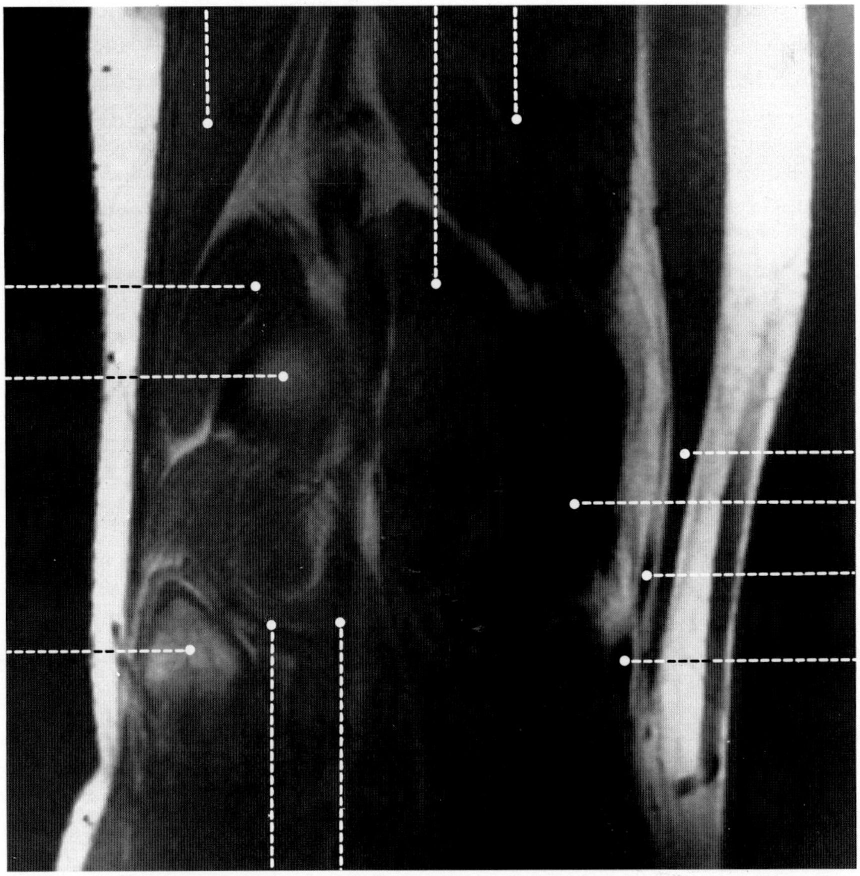

245 THE KNEE

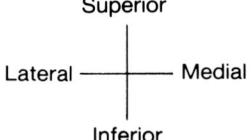

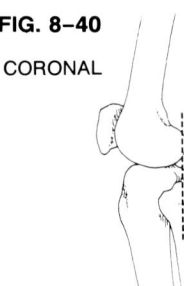

FIG. 8-40
CORONAL

Anatomy and MRI of the Joints

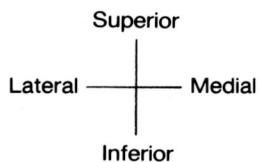

FIG. 8-41
CORONAL

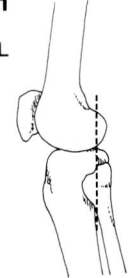

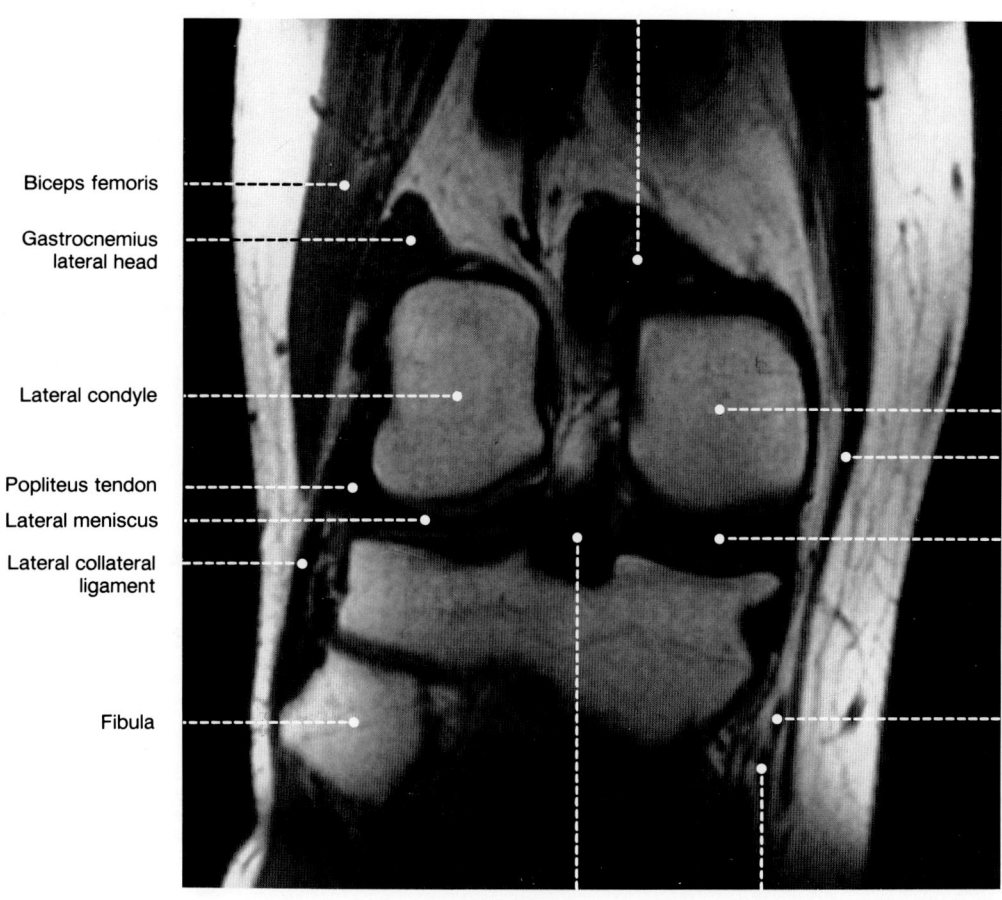

Gastrocnemius lateral head

Biceps femoris
Gastrocnemius lateral head

Lateral condyle

Popliteus tendon
Lateral meniscus
Lateral collateral ligament

Fibula

Medial condyle
Sartorius

Medial meniscus

Gracilis

Posterior cruciate ligament

Semitendinosus

THE KNEE

FIG. 8-42

CORONAL

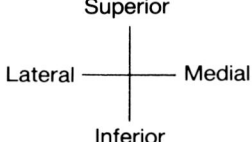
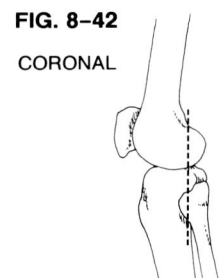
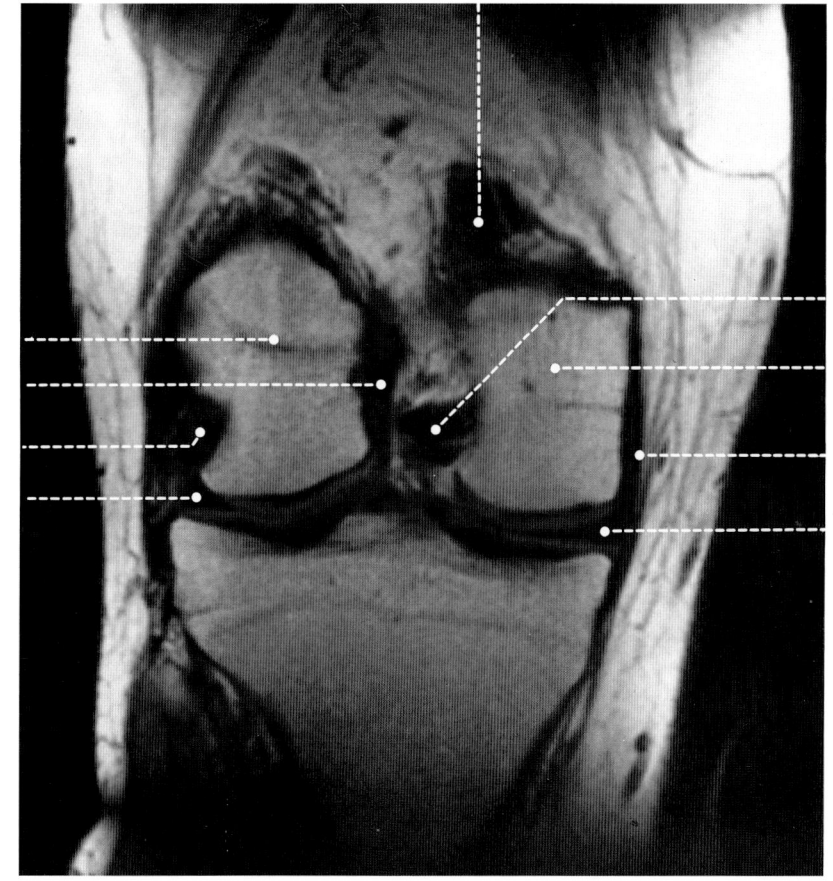

- Gastrocnemius medial head
- Lateral condyle
- Anterior cruciate ligament
- Popliteus tendon
- Lateral meniscus
- Posterior cruciate ligament
- Medial condyle
- Medial collateral ligament
- Medial meniscus

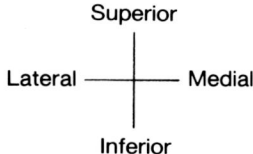

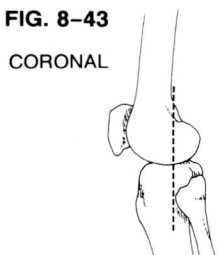

FIG. 8-43

CORONAL

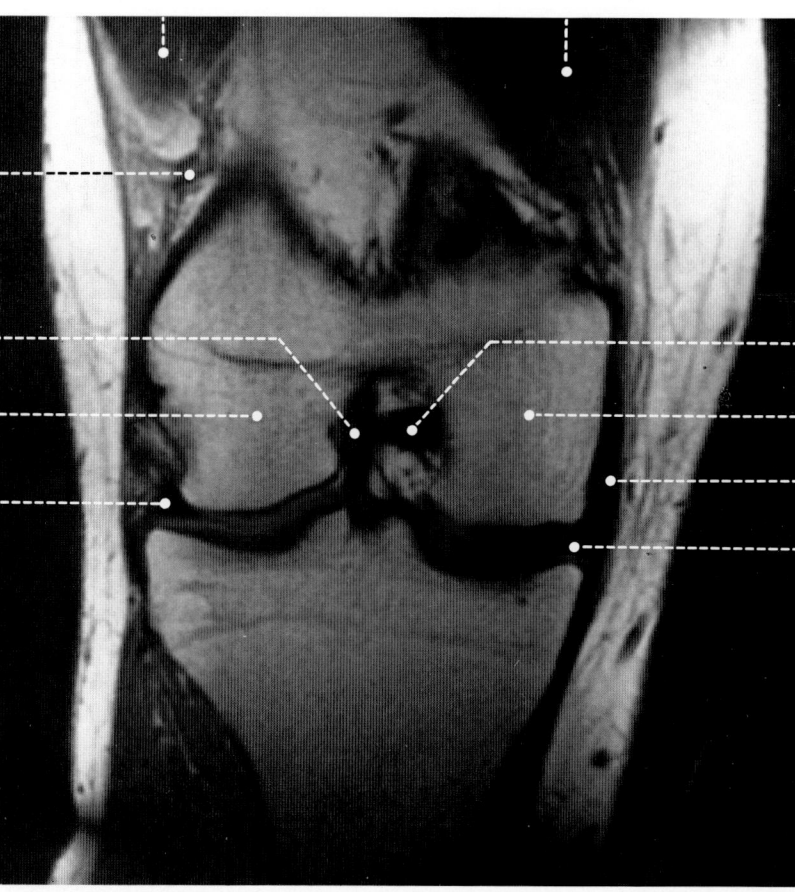

THE KNEE

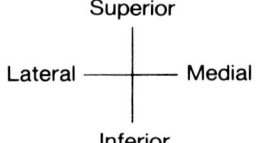

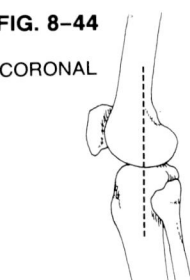

FIG. 8-44
CORONAL

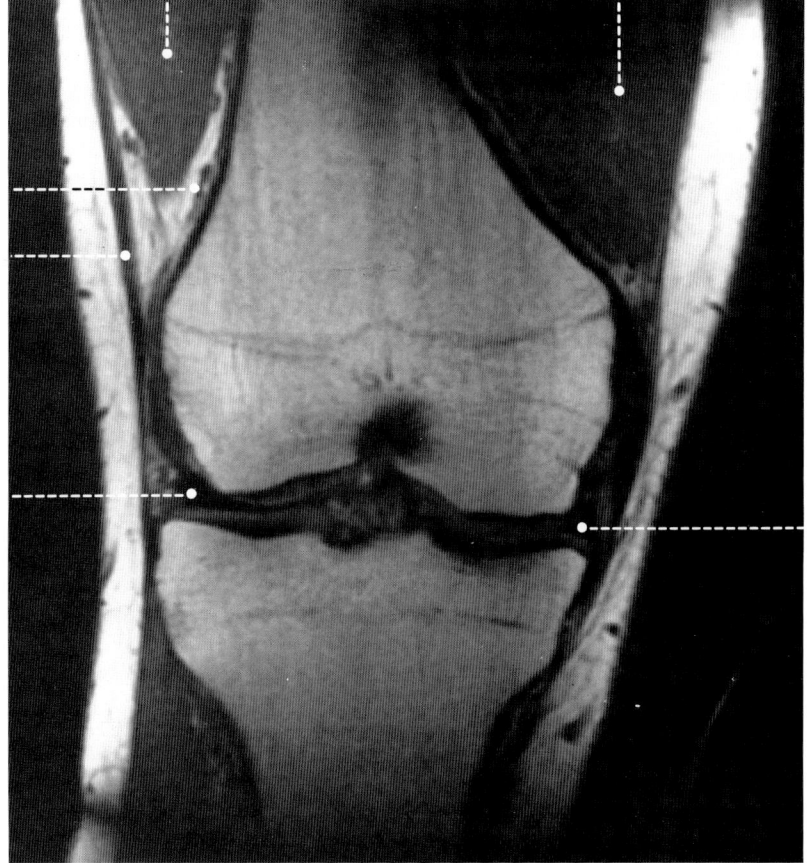

Vastus lateralis · Vastus medialis · Superior lateral genicular vessels · Iliotibial tract · Lateral meniscus · Medial meniscus

Anatomy and MRI of the Joints 250

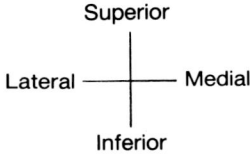

FIG. 8-45

CORONAL

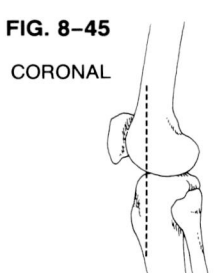

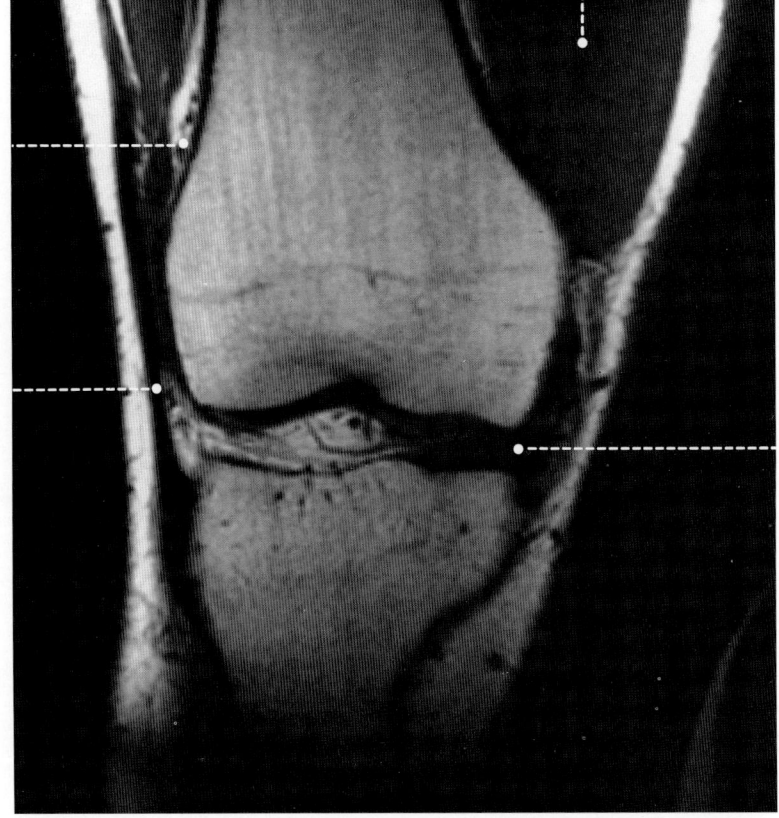

Vastus lateralis

Vastus medialis

Superior lateral genicular vessels

Iliotibial tract

Medial meniscus

Chapter 9

THE ANKLE

William D. Middleton, M.D.

Like the wrist, the ankle has a complex bony architecture with multiple ligaments, muscles, and tendons oriented in a variety of planes. Understanding the cross-sectional relationships of these various anatomic structures can be difficult if the ankle is described in isolation. Therefore, this chapter will also include discussion of the subtalar region as well as portions of the mid-foot.

The ankle joint itself is composed of the articulation between the tibia and fibula and the talus. The convex talar dome rests in the concave surface of the distal tibia and is secured medially and laterally by the medial and lateral malleoli. This arrangement allows for dorsiflexion and plantarflexion in the sagittal plane while restricting motion in the coronal and axial planes.

The subtalar joint between the talus and calcaneus consists of three separate facets. The largest is the posterior facet. The middle and anterior facets are smaller, variable in shape, and may be fused into a single unit with a continuous cartilaginous covering. The mid-subtalar facet is formed below by a ledge of bone projecting off the medial surface of the calcaneus called the sustentaculum tali. The sustentaculum tali is necessary for bony support of the talus because the talus projects medially at approximately a 15-degree angle from the long axis of the calcaneus.

Anteriorly the head of the talus articulates with the navicular and the calcaneus articulates with the cuboid. The talonavicular and calcaneocuboid joints together are known as the transverse tarsal joint. The navicular articulates anteriorly with the three cuneiforms and the cuboid articulates anteriorly with the base of the fourth and fifth metatarsals.

A number of important ligaments support the ankle. The strongest is the deltoid ligament which arises from the medial malleolus. Its strength is necessary since the medial malleolus is short and provides relatively little bony support to the medial aspect of the ankle. The deltoid ligament has many fibers. The deepest run between the medial malleolus and the talus. These fibers fan out to reach both anterior and posterior aspect of the talus. Superficial fibers also extend to the sustentaculum tali and the navicular. These superficial fibers also attach to and blend with the plantar calcaneonavicular (spring) ligament. Figure 9–1 illustrates the fibers of the deltoid ligament.

Laterally the ankle is supported by several separate ligaments. The calcaneofibular ligament extends posteriorly from the lateral malleolus to the calcaneus. The anterior talofibular ligament runs from the anterior aspect of the lateral malleolus to the neck of the talus while the posterior talofibular ligament connects these bones posteriorly. These ligaments are shown in Fig. 9–2.

The subtalar joint is supported by the interosseous ligament running between the posterior and mid-subtalar joints from the superior aspect of the calcaneus to the inferior aspect of the talus (Fig. 9–2). The space in which the interosseous ligament runs is called the tarsal sinus.

Another important ligament arising from the calcaneus is the spring ligament (also known as the plantar calcaneonavicular ligament). The spring ligament extends from the sustentaculum tali to the inferior aspect of the navicular and provides important support for the head of the talus which is lacking in significant bony support. The spring ligament blends superiorly with the tibionavicular fibers of the deltoid ligament and inferiorly with the plantar calcaneocuboid (short plantar) ligament.

The musculotendinous structures in the ankle can be divided into medial, lateral, anterior, and posterior groups. The posterior group consists of a single tendon—the Achilles tendon. This tendon arises from the soleus and gastrocnemius muscles and is the largest in the body. It attaches to the posterior surface of the calcaneus.

The medial group includes the flexor hallucis longus, flexor digitorum longus, and the tibialis posterior. The relationships of these three tendons to each other and adjacent structures is shown in Figs. 9–1 and 9–3. The flexor hallucis longus is the most posterior of the three,

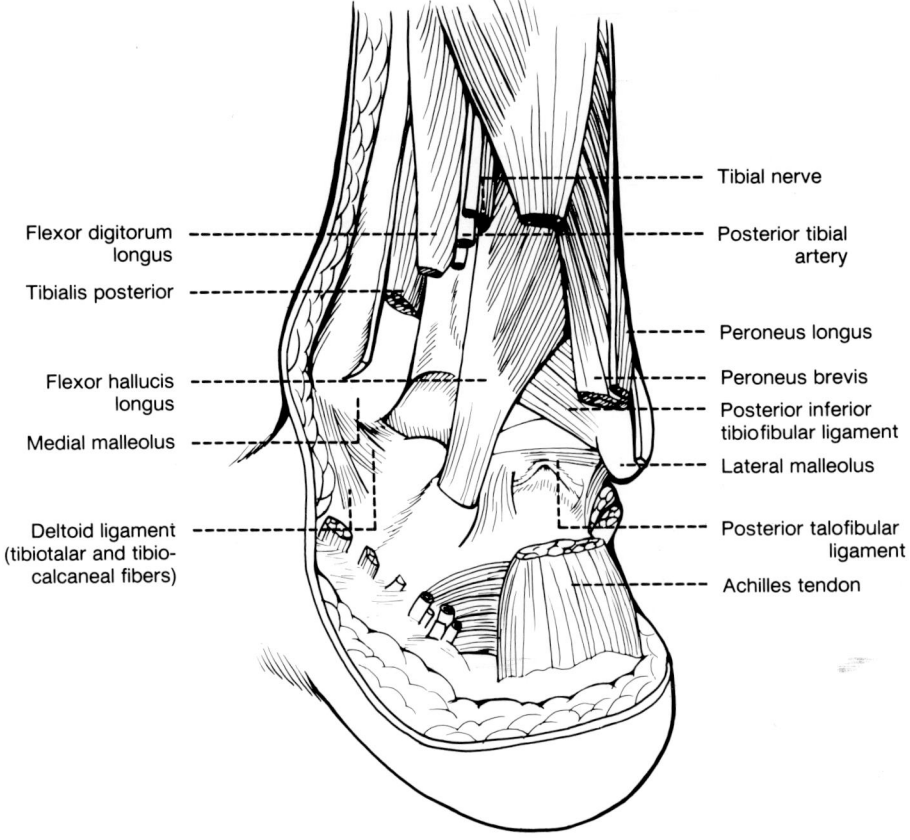

FIG. 9-1

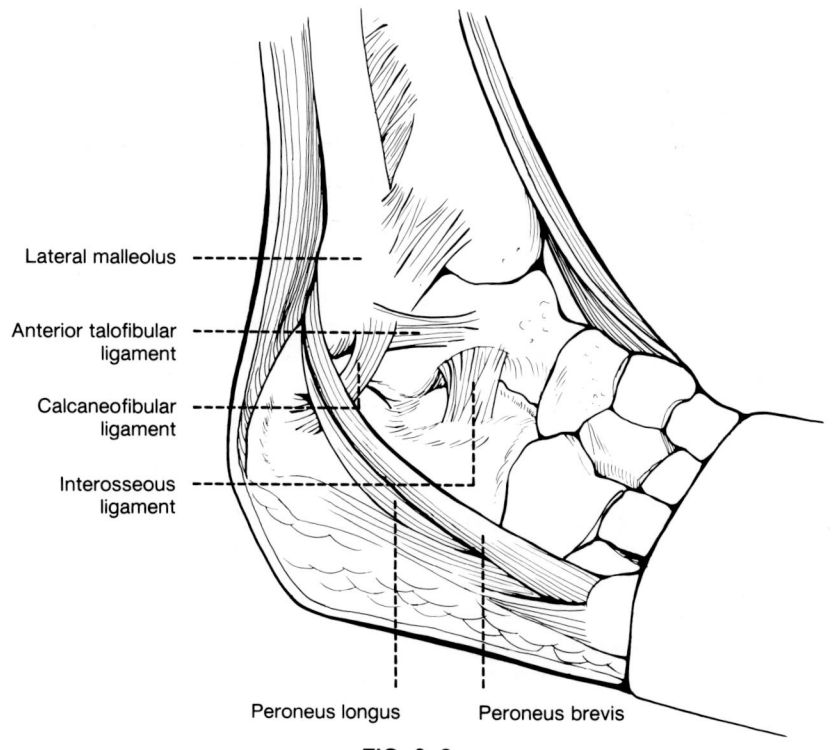

FIG. 9-2

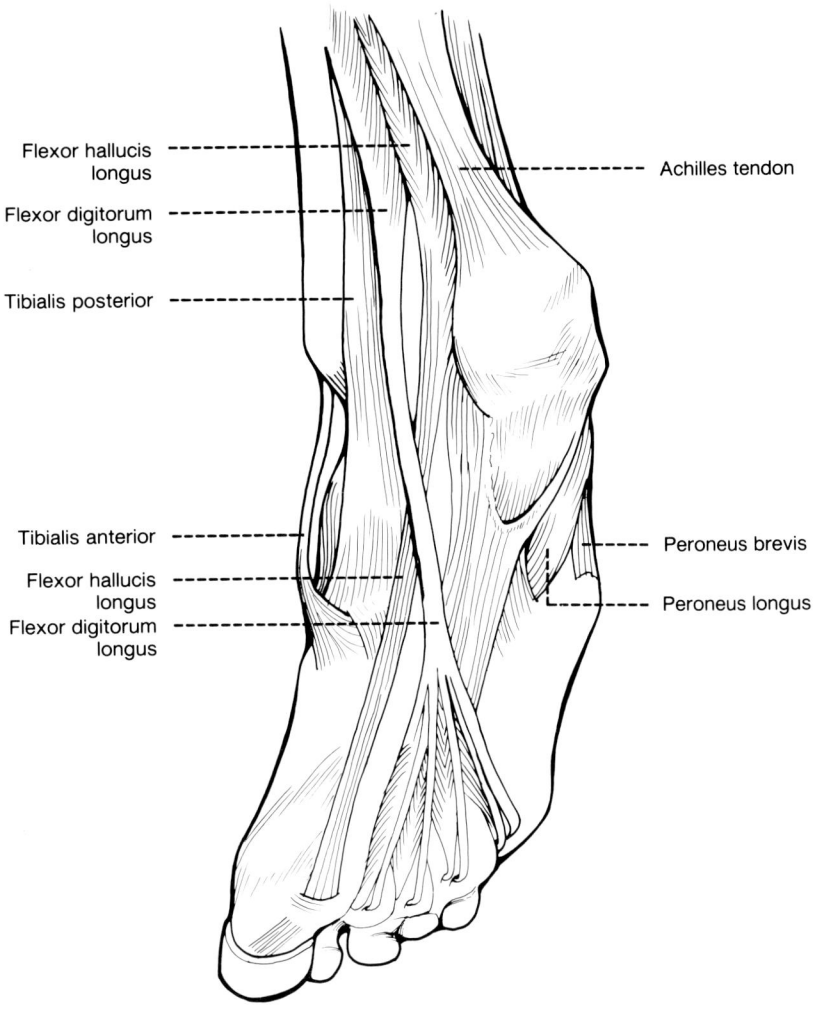

FIG. 9-3

and at the level of the ankle, both muscle and tendon are visible. The tendon of the flexor hallucis longus runs in a groove in the posterior aspect of the tibia then extends inferiorly and anteriorly below the medial tubercle of the talus and beneath the sustentaculum tali. The flexor digitorum longus tendon runs behind the medial malleolus between the flexor hallucis longus and the tibialis posterior. In the plantar aspect of the foot, the flexor digitorum longus crosses over the flexor hallucis longus. Both tendons are located deep to the abductor hallucis muscle and the flexor digitorum brevis. The tibialis posterior tendon is the most anterior of the medial group. It passes behind the medial malleolus then courses anteriorly and divides into two separate tendons. The largest of these insert on the tuberosity of the navicular and extends to insert on the inferior aspect of the medial cuneiform. The smaller division passes laterally and inserts variably onto the middle three metatarsals and the intermediate cuneiform.

The two peroneus tendons make up the lateral group. Both tendons travel in a groove on the posterior aspect of the lateral malleolus and then extend anteriorly beneath the malleolus (Figs. 9-1 and 9-2). The peroneus brevis is positioned anterior to the peroneus longus at the level of the lateral malleolus and superior to the peroneus longus beyond the malleolus. The peroneus brevis inserts on the lateral aspect of the base of the fifth metatarsal. The peroneus longus passes around the lateral malleolus and along the lateral aspect of the calcaneus inferior to the peroneal trochlea. It then changes course and extends medially in a groove on the inferior surface of the cuboid. It continues medially to insert on the base of the first metatarsal and the medial cuneiform.

The anterior group is composed of the tibialis anterior, the extensor hallucis longus, extensor digitorum longus, and peroneus tertius. The tibialis anterior is the most prominent of this group and is positioned medially. It inserts at the medial and inferior aspect of the medial cuneiform and at the base of the first metatarsal. The extensor hallucis longus runs lateral to the tibialis anterior and eventually inserts on the base of the first distal phalanx. The extensor digitorum longus and peroneus tertius are positioned most laterally and are difficult to separate

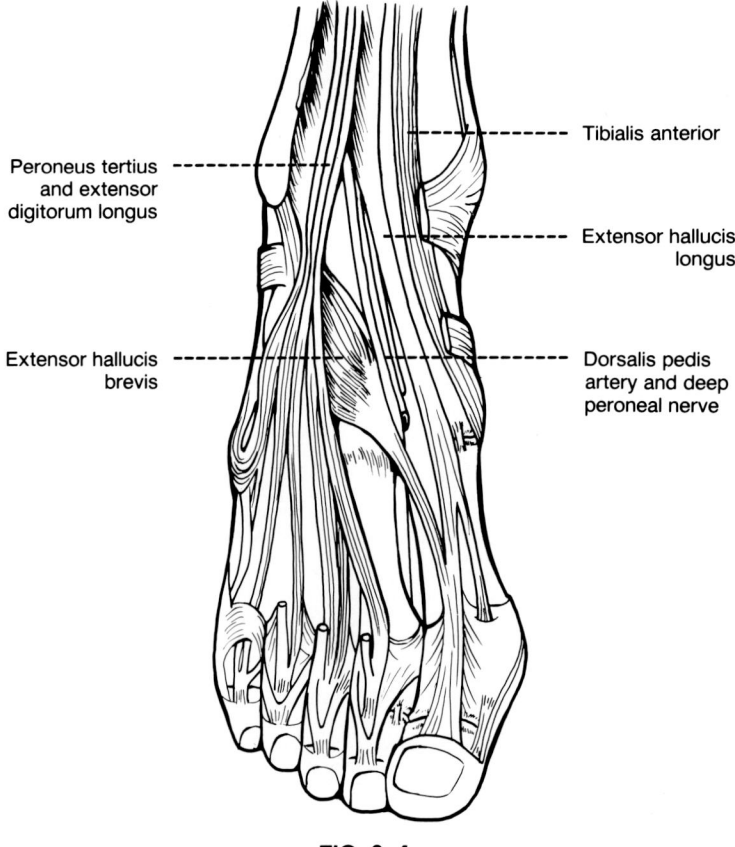

FIG. 9–4

on cross-sectional images and anatomic specimens. The peroneus tertius muscle extends inferiorly to the level of the ankle and then becomes tendinous and attaches to the base and a portion of the shaft of the fifth metatarsal. In the region of the ankle, the extensor digitorum longus divides into four separate tendons which ultimately separate from each other and extend to the second through fifth digits. Figure 9–4 shows the orientation of these anterior tendons.

A number of muscles are present on the plantar aspect of the foot. The abductor hallucis is most medial and arises from the posterior medial surface of the calcaneus. As it extends anteriorly it covers the plantar arteries and nerves. The flexor digitorum brevis is located lateral to the abductor hallucis and also covers the lateral plantar artery and nerve. The abductor digit minimi is the most lateral of the plantar muscles. Deep to these three superficial muscles is the quadratus plantae.

Several neurovascular structures are visible in cross section and deserve attention. The posterior tibial artery and tibial nerve roughly run superficial to the flexor hallucis longus and flexor digitorum longus with the artery positioned medial to the nerve (Fig. 9–1). Both course anteriorly at the level of the medial malleolus and extend to the plantar surface of the foot. Prior to entering the foot the nerve and artery divide into medial and lateral plantar branches. Both branches course between the abductor hallucis and the quadratus plantae. In the region of the ankle the medial branch is anterior and superior to the lateral branch.

The anterior tibial artery runs deep to the extensor hallucis longus in the ankle, then extends into the foot as the dorsalis pedis artery between the extensor hallucis longus and extensor digitorum longus (Fig. 9–4). The anterior tibial artery is accompanied by the deep peroneal nerve.

The peroneal artery is positioned posteriorly near the inferior tibiofibular joint. It is variably seen in cross-sectional images and anatomic specimens.

THE ANKLE

AXIAL
    Cryomicrotomes . . . . FIGS. 9–5 to 9–9
    MR Images . . . . FIGS. 9–10 to 9–15

SAGITTAL
    Cryomicrotomes . . . . FIGS. 9–16 to 9–21
    MR Images . . . . FIGS. 9–22 to 9–29

CORONAL
    Cryomicrotomes . . . . FIGS. 9–30 to 9–35
    MR Images . . . . FIGS. 9–36 to 9–41

Anatomy and MRI of the Joints

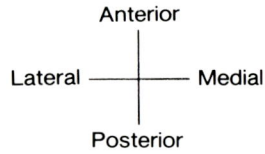

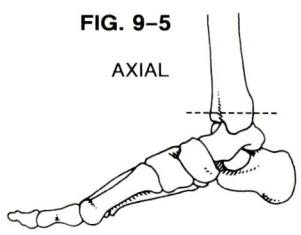

FIG. 9-5

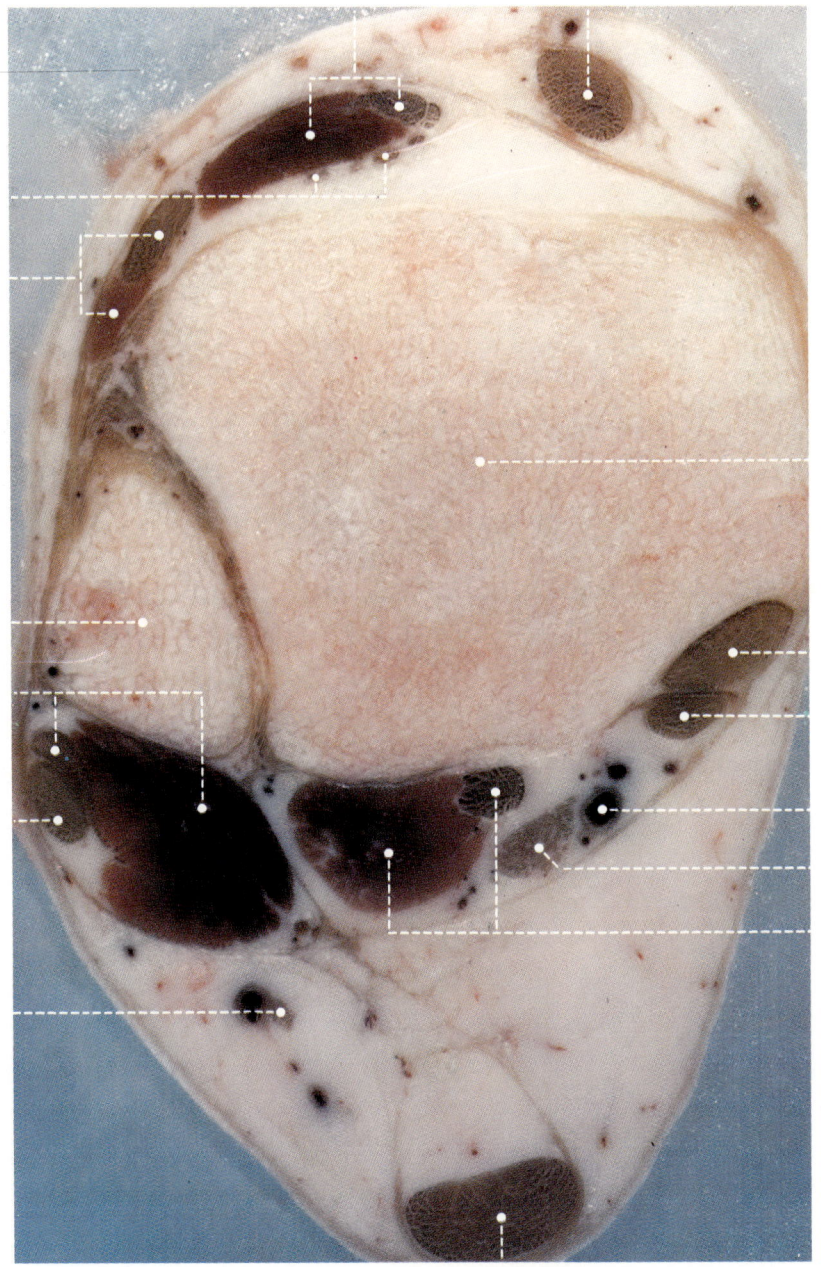

257 THE ANKLE

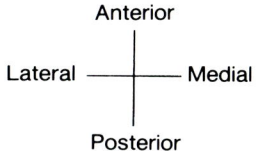

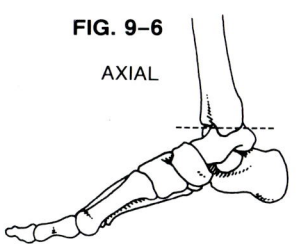

FIG. 9-6
AXIAL

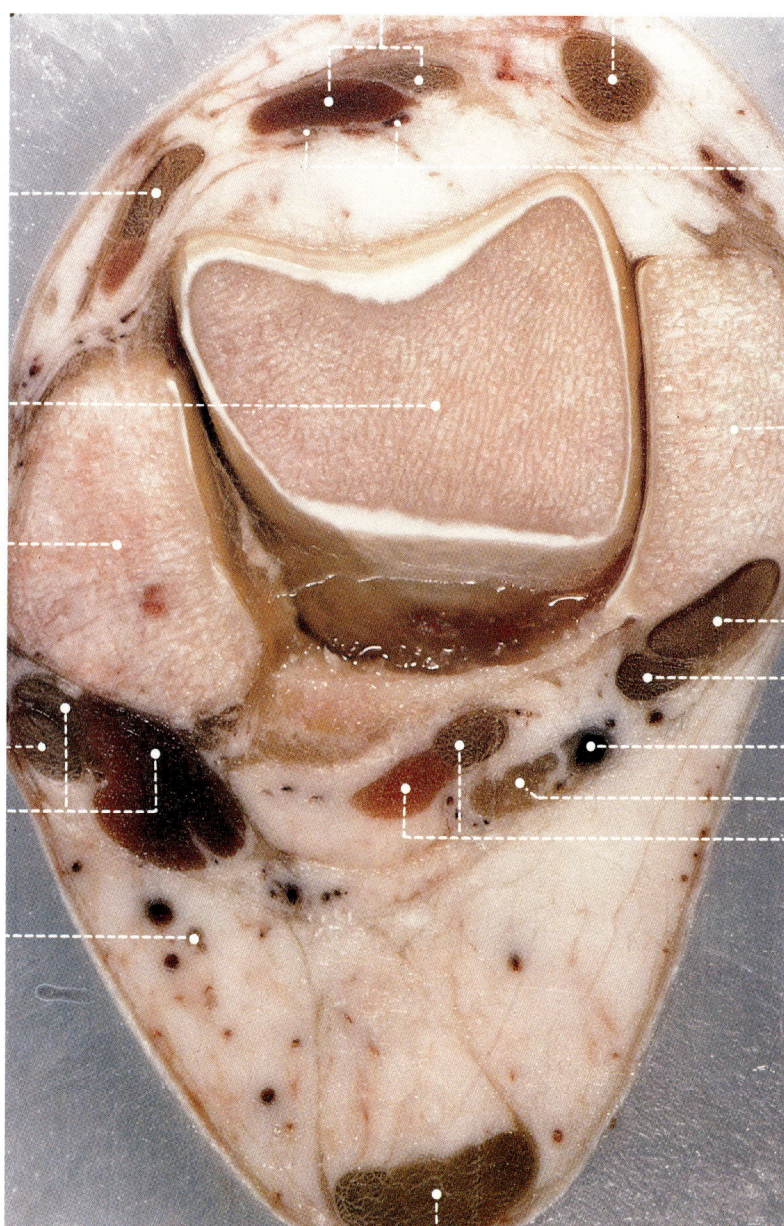

Anatomy and MRI of the Joints 258

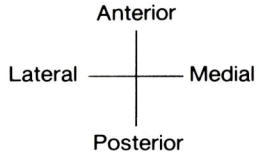

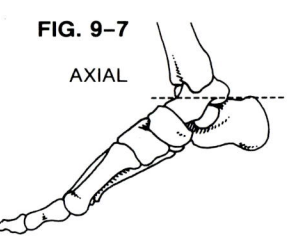

FIG. 9-7
AXIAL

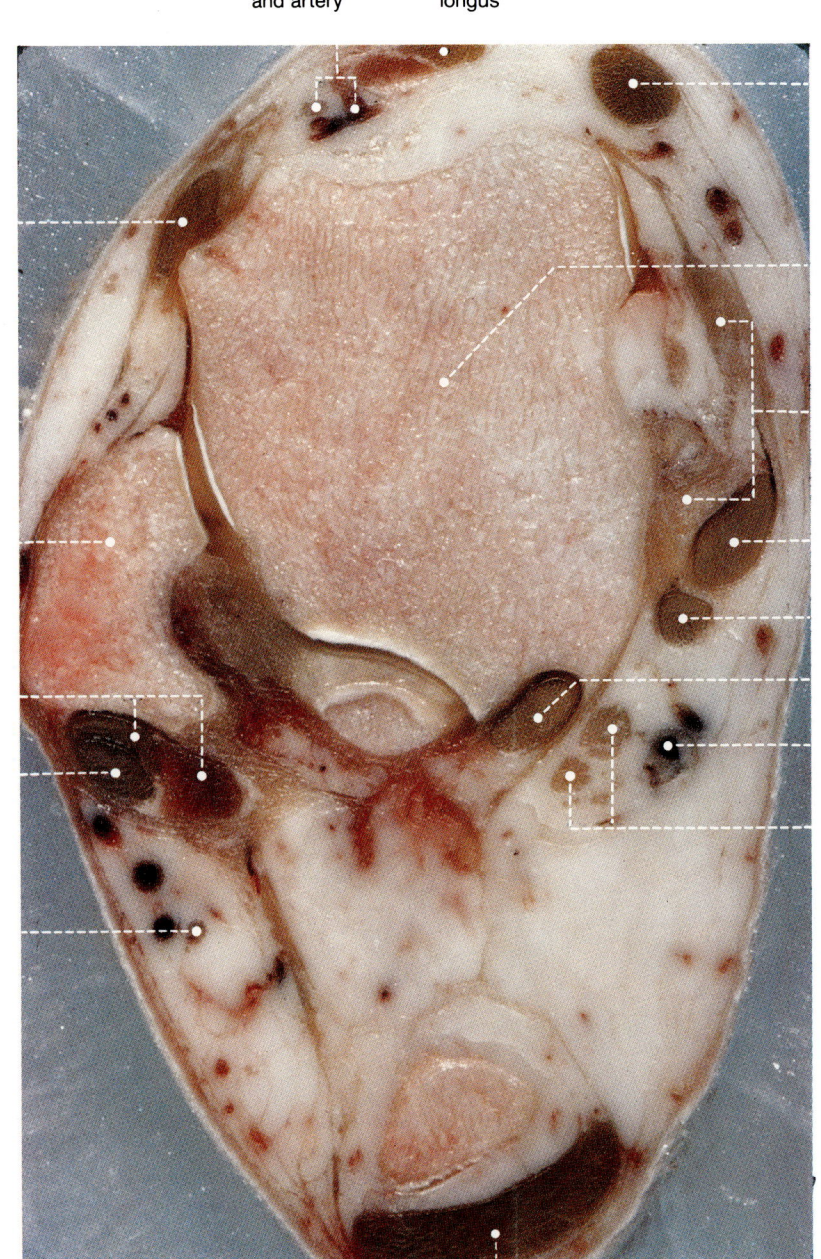

Achilles tendon

259 THE ANKLE

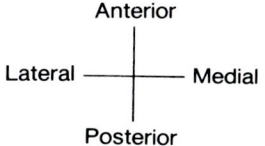

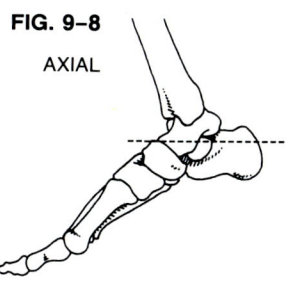

FIG. 9-8
AXIAL

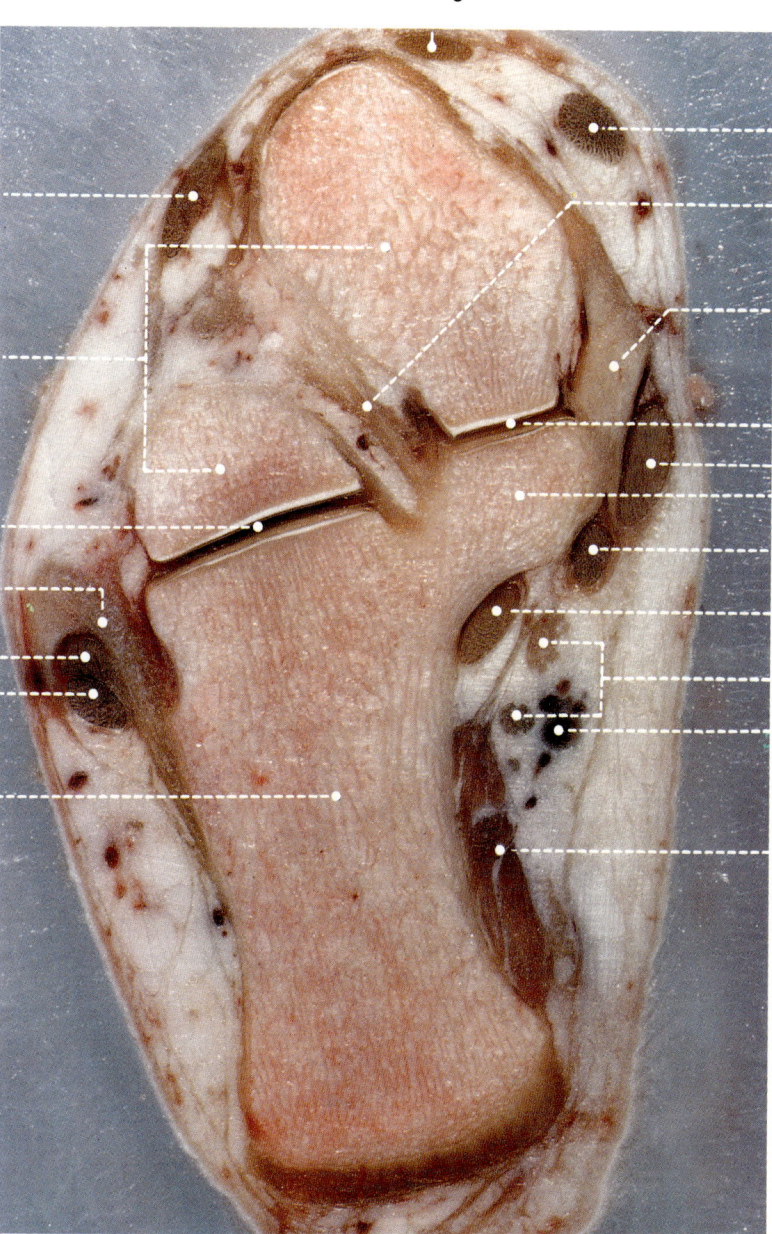

- Extensor hallucis longus
- Extensor digitorum longus and peroneus tertius
- Talus
- Posterior subtalar joint
- Calcaneofibular ligament
- Peroneus brevis
- Peroneus longus
- Calcaneus
- Tibialis anterior
- Interosseous ligament
- Deltoid ligament (tibiocalcaneal fibers) and spring ligament
- Middle subtalar joint
- Tibialis posterior
- Sustentaculum tali
- Flexor digitorum longus
- Flexor hallucis longus
- Medial and lateral plantar nerves
- Posterior tibial artery
- Quadratus plantae

Anatomy and MRI of the Joints

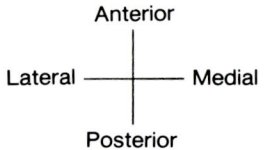

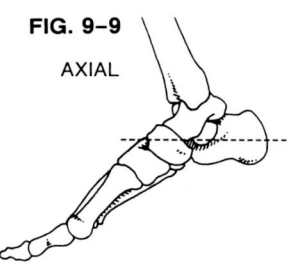

FIG. 9-9
AXIAL

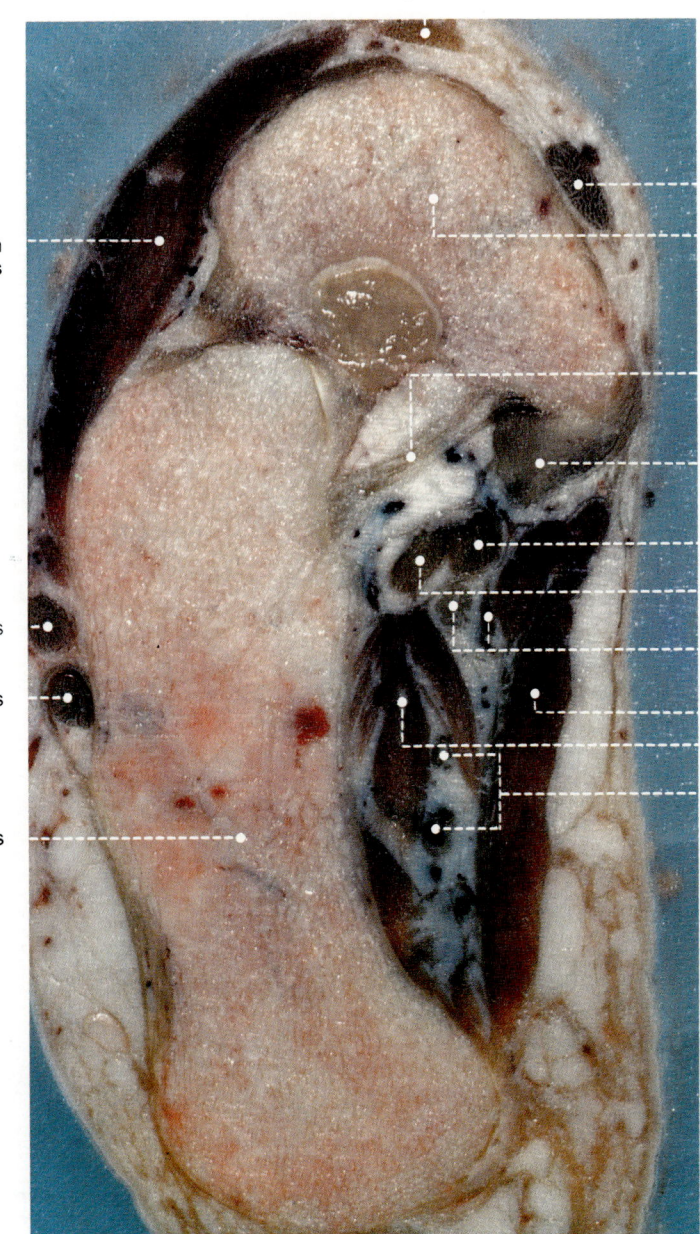

- Extensor hallucis longus
- Extensor digitorum brevis
- Peroneus brevis
- Peroneus longus
- Calcaneus
- Tibialis anterior
- Navicular
- Plantar calcaneo-navicular (spring) ligament
- Tibialis posterior
- Flexor digitorum longus
- Flexor hallucis longus
- Medial plantar nerve and artery
- Abductor hallucis
- Quadratus plantae
- Lateral plantar nerve and artery

THE ANKLE

FIG. 9-10
AXIAL

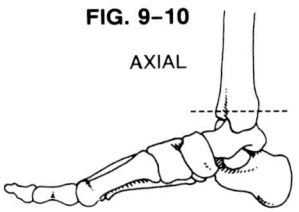

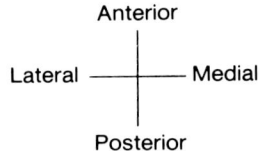

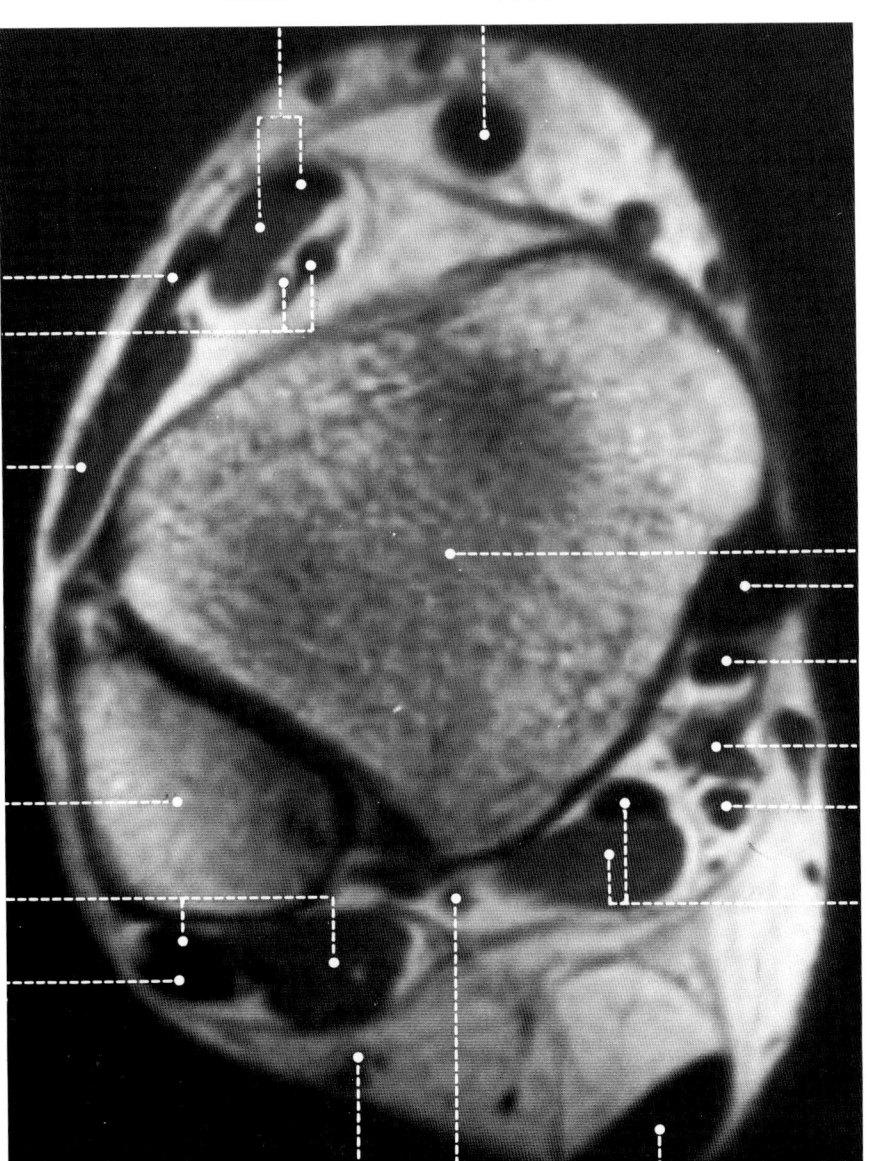

Anatomy and MRI of the Joints 262

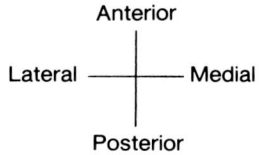

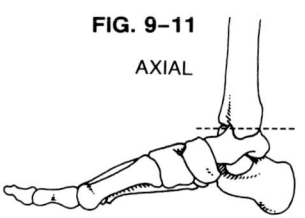

FIG. 9–11
AXIAL

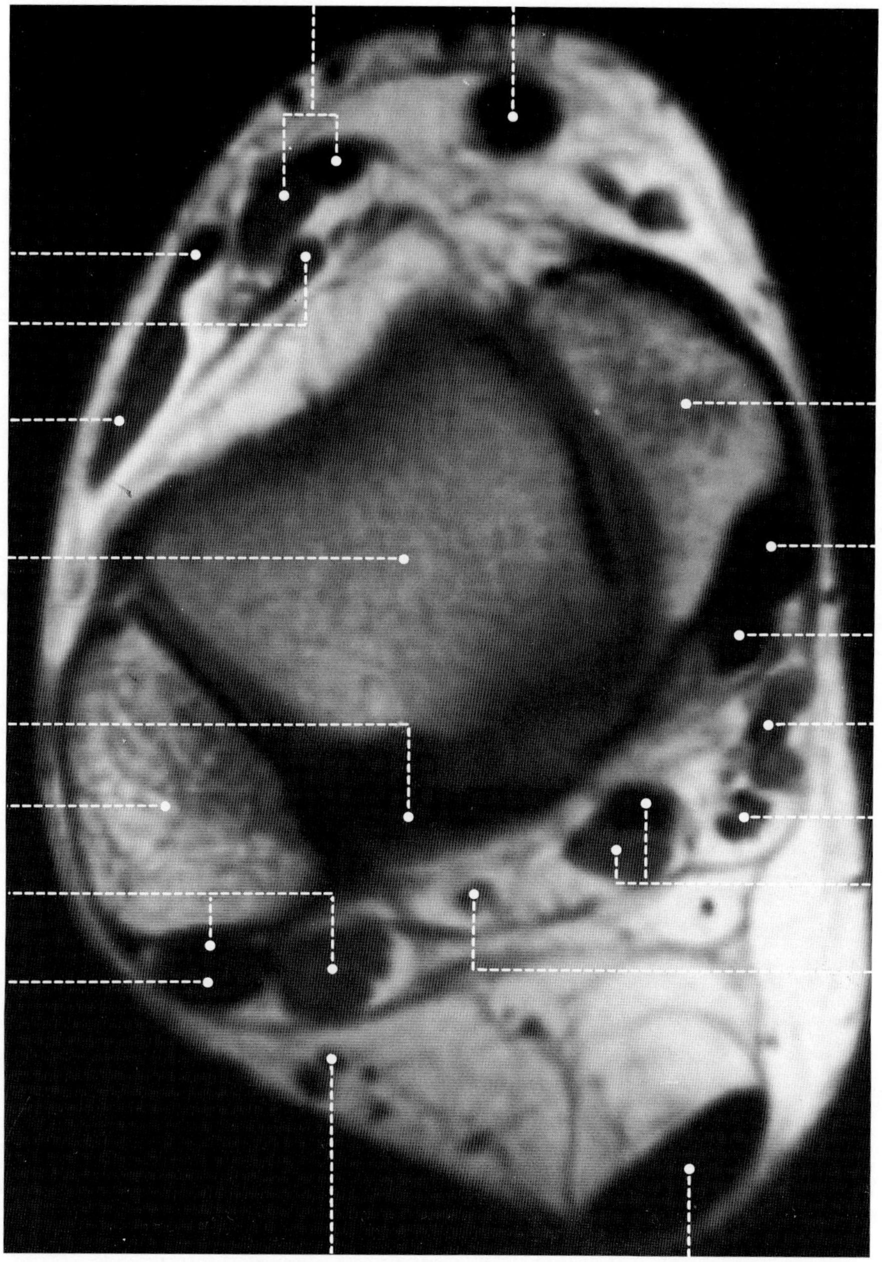

263 THE ANKLE

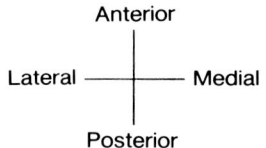

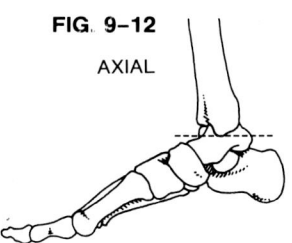

FIG. 9-12
AXIAL

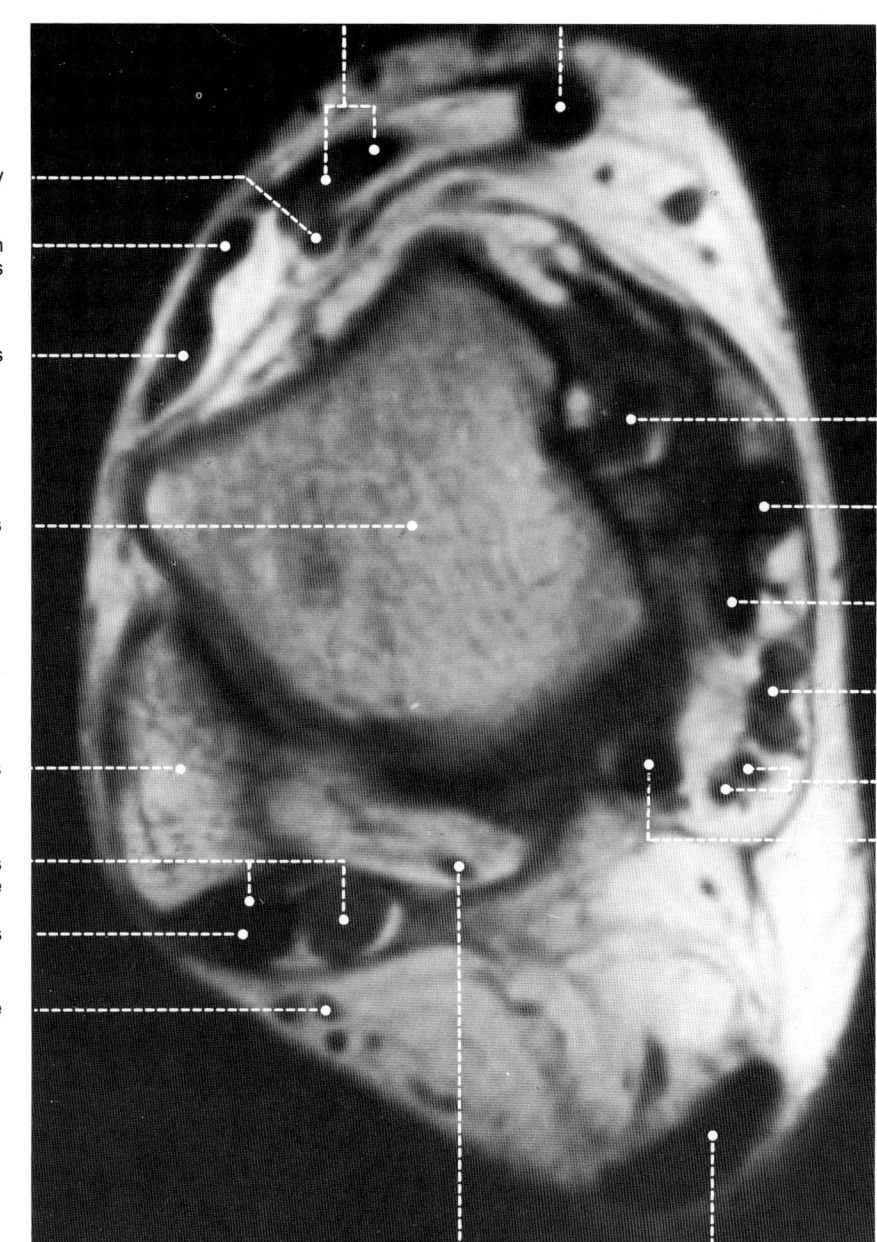

Anatomy and MRI of the Joints 264

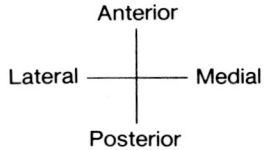

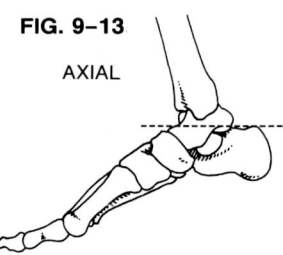

FIG. 9-13
AXIAL

- Extensor hallucis longus
- Tibialis anterior
- Anterior tibial artery
- Extensor digitorum longus
- Peroneus tertius
- Talus
- Peroneus brevis tendon and muscle
- Peroneus longus
- Sural nerve
- Deltoid ligament (tibiocalcaneal fibers)
- Tibialis posterior
- Flexor digitorum longus
- Posterior tibial artery
- Medial and lateral plantar nerves
- Flexor hallucis longus
- Achilles tendon

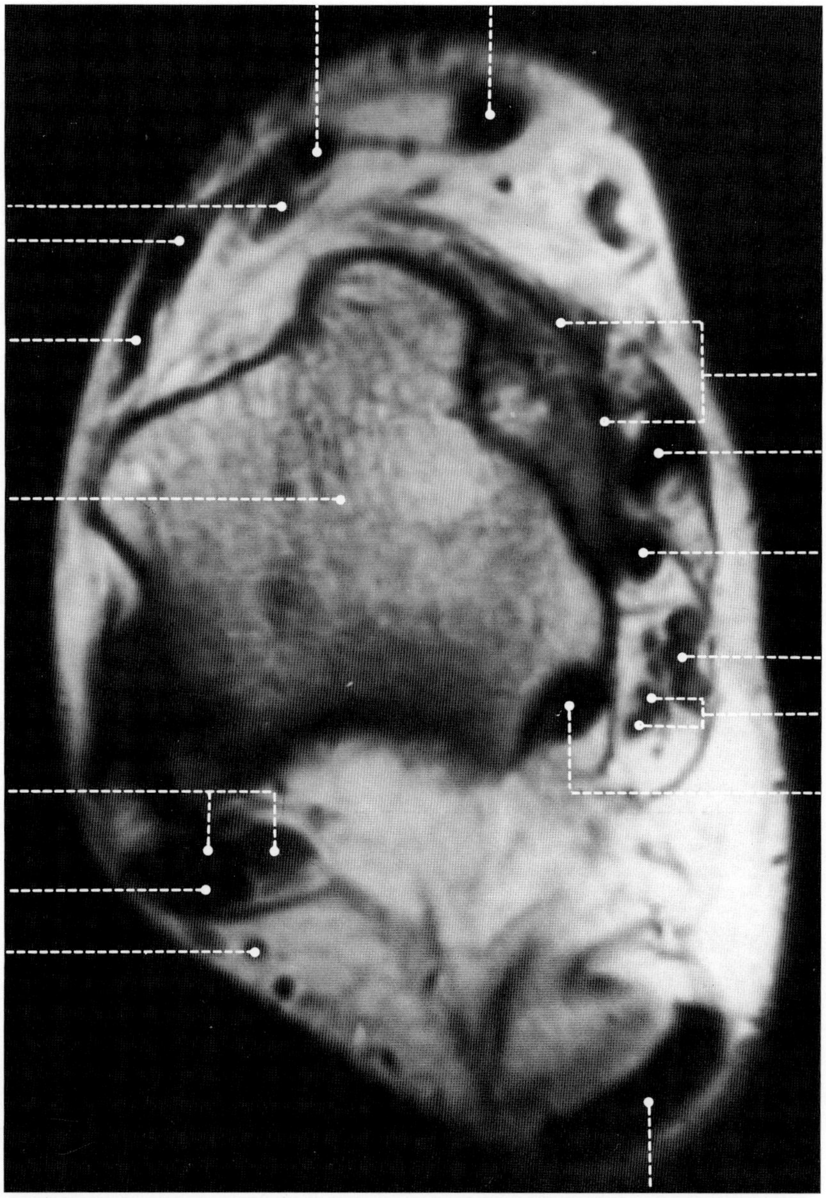

THE ANKLE

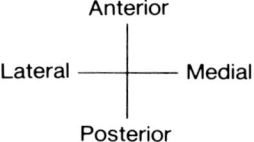

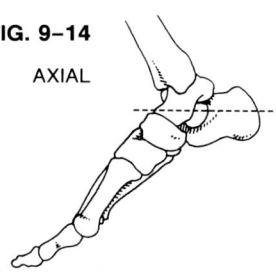

FIG. 9-14
AXIAL

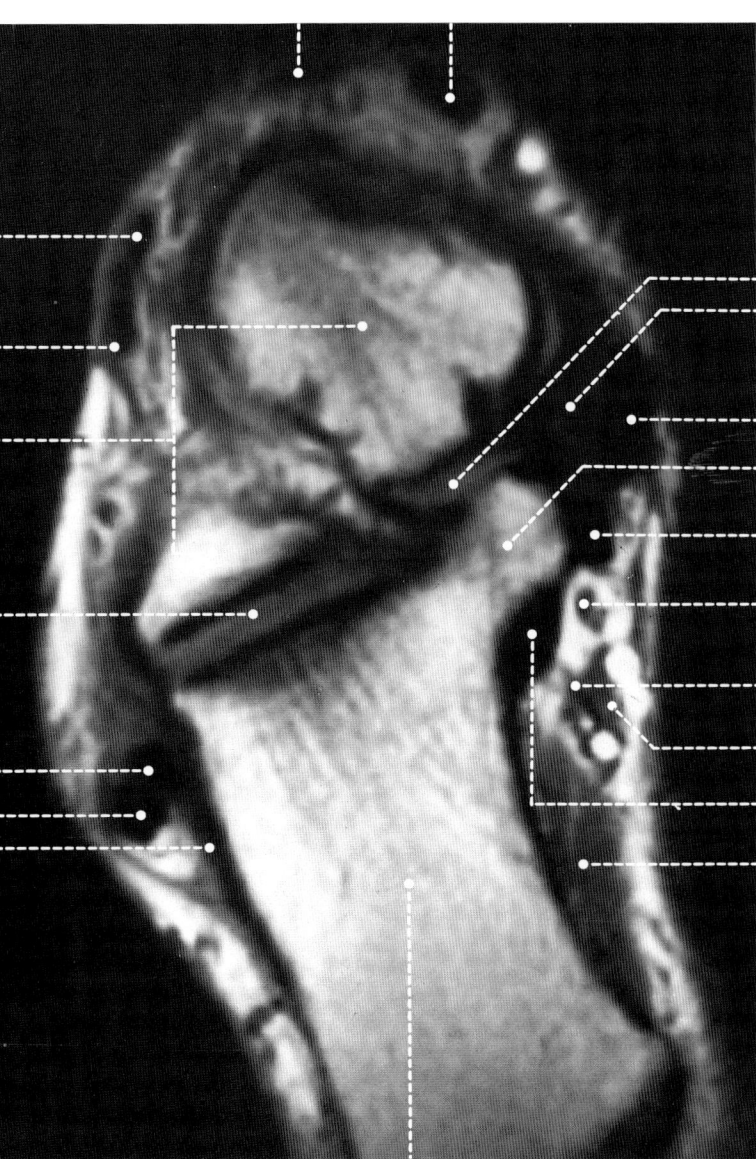

Extensor hallucis longus — Tibialis anterior

Extensor digitorum longus
Peroneus tertius
Talus
Posterior facet subtalar joint
Peroneus brevis
Peroneus longus
Calcaneofibular ligament

Middle subtalar joint
Deltoid ligament and plantar calcaneo-navicular (spring) ligament
Tibialis posterior
Sustentaculum tali
Flexor digitorum longus
Medial plantar nerve
Lateral plantar nerve
Posterior tibial artery
Flexor hallucis longus
Quadratus plantae

Calcaneus

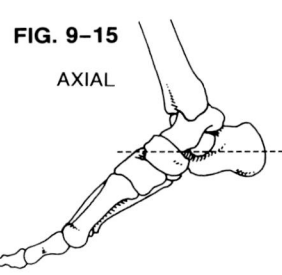

FIG. 9-15
AXIAL

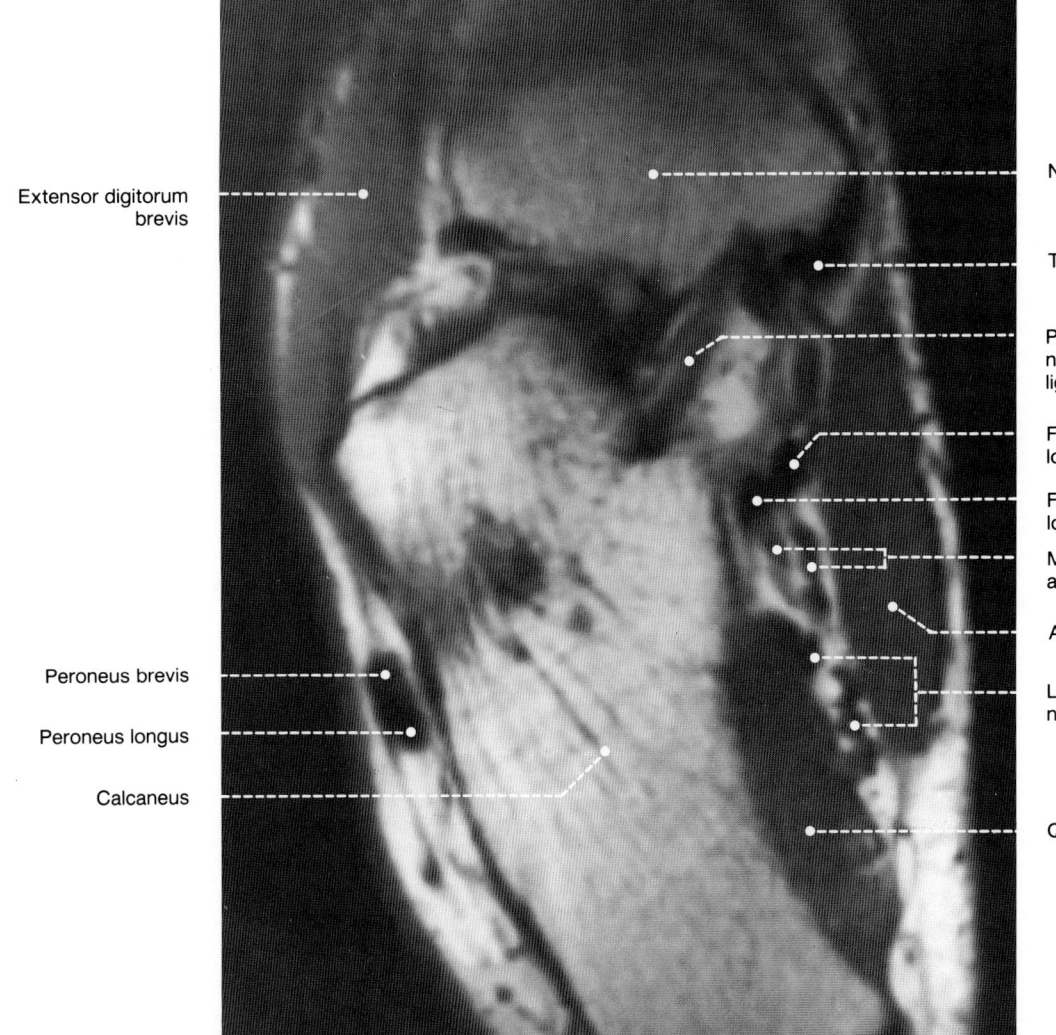

- Extensor digitorum brevis
- Peroneus brevis
- Peroneus longus
- Calcaneus
- Navicular
- Tibialis posterior
- Plantar calcaneo-navicular (spring) ligament
- Flexor digitorum longus
- Flexor hallucis longus
- Medial plantar nerve and artery
- Abductor hallucis
- Lateral plantar nerve and artery
- Quadratus plantae

267 THE ANKLE

FIG. 9-16

SAGITTAL

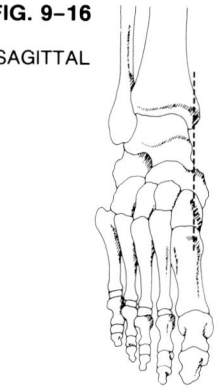

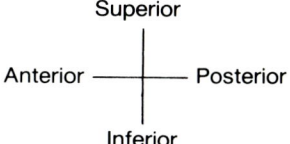

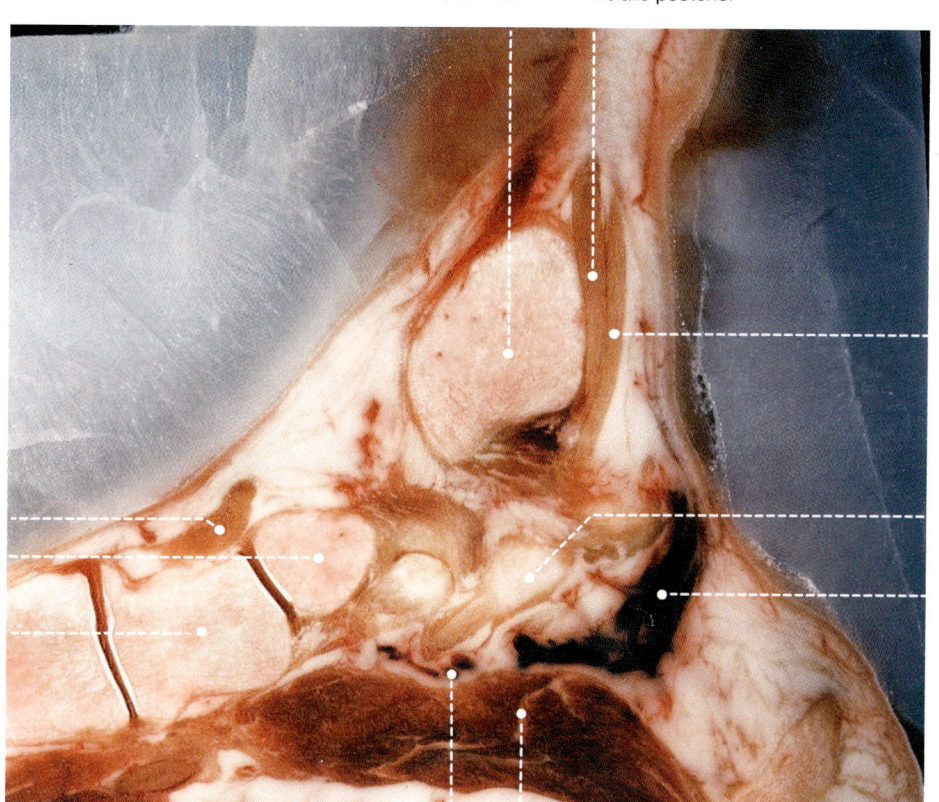

Labels: Distal tibia, Tibialis posterior, Flexor digitorum longus, Tibialis anterior, Navicular, Medial cuneiform, Sustentaculum tali, Posterior tibial artery, Medial plantar neurovascular bundle, Abductor hallucis

Anatomy and MRI of the Joints 268

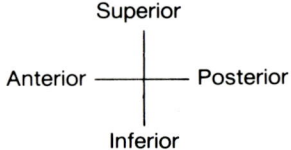

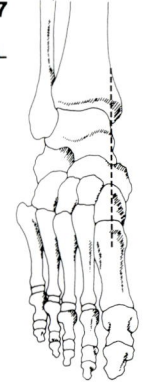

FIG. 9-17
SAGITTAL

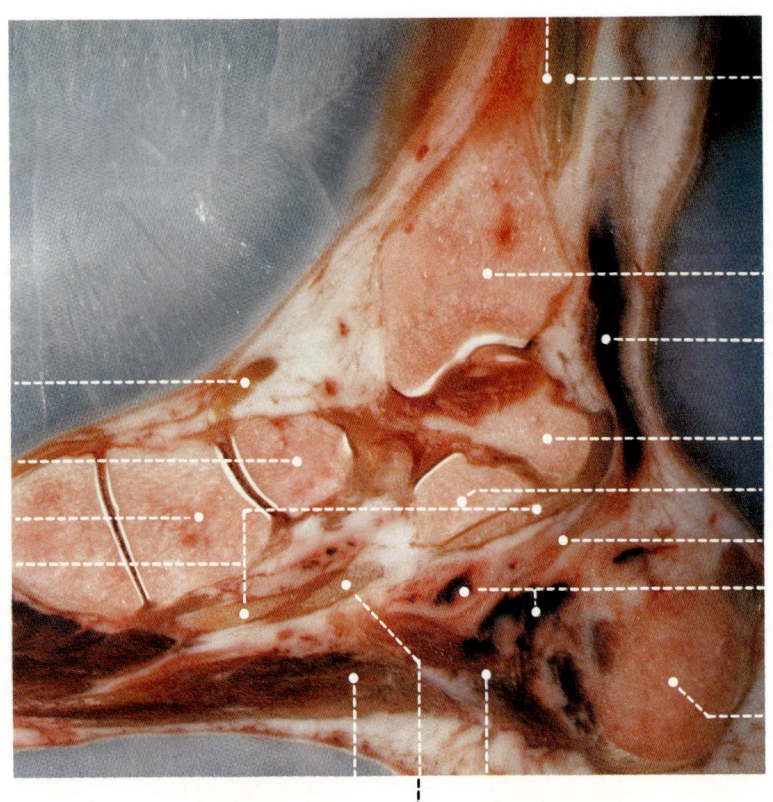

Labels:
- Tibialis posterior
- Flexor digitorum longus
- Distal tibia
- Posterior tibial artery
- Medial tubercle talus
- Sustentaculum tali
- Medial plantar nerve
- Medial and lateral plantar neurovascular bundles
- Calcaneus
- Tibialis anterior
- Navicular
- Medial cuneiform
- Flexor hallucis longus
- Flexor digitorum brevis
- Flexor digitorum longus
- Abductor hallucis

THE ANKLE

FIG. 9-18

SAGITTAL

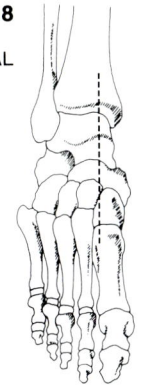

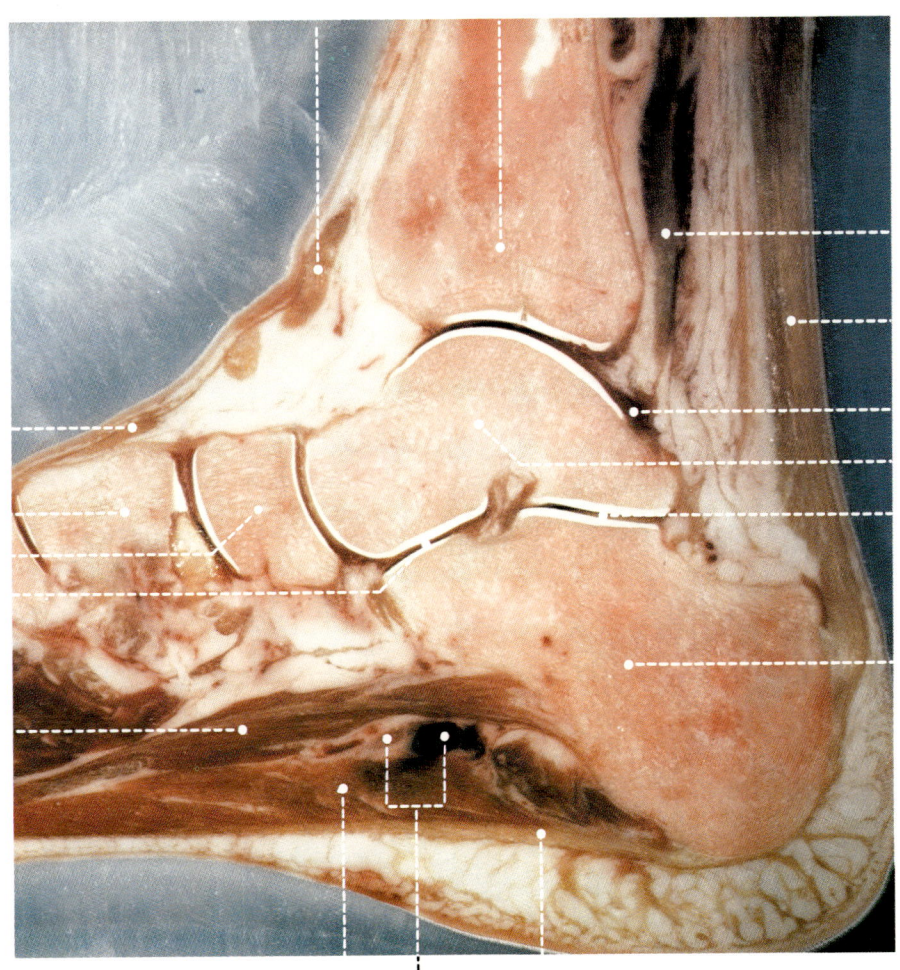

Figure labels:
- Tibialis anterior
- Distal tibia
- Flexor hallucis longus
- Achilles tendon
- Posterior talofibular ligament
- Talus
- Posterior subtalar joint
- Extensor hallucis longus
- Medial cuneiform
- Navicular
- Middle subtalar joint
- Calcaneus
- Quadratus plantae
- Flexor digitorum brevis
- Lateral plantar nerve and artery
- Plantar aponeurosis

Orientation: Superior / Inferior / Anterior / Posterior

Anatomy and MRI of the Joints 270

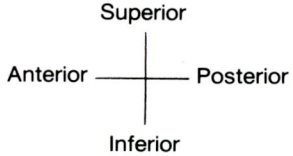

FIG. 9-19
SAGITTAL

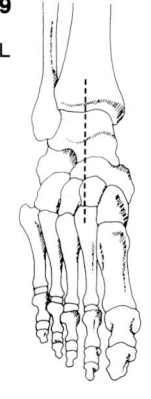

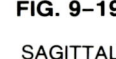

Labels:
- Tibialis anterior
- Distal tibia
- Flexor hallucis longus muscle
- Extensor hallucis longus
- Anterior subtalar joint
- Navicular
- Intermediate cuneiform
- Sustentaculum tali
- Lateral cuneiform
- Cuboid
- Peroneus longus
- Posterior inferior tibiofibular ligament
- Posterior talofibular ligament
- Talus
- Posterior subtalar joint
- Calcaneus
- Quadratus plantae
- Lateral plantar artery
- Short plantar (calcaneocuboid) ligament
- Flexor digitorum brevis

THE ANKLE

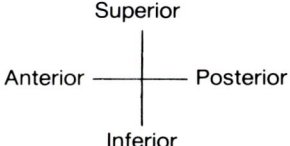

FIG. 9-20
SAGITTAL

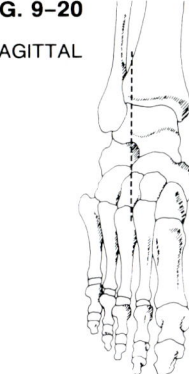

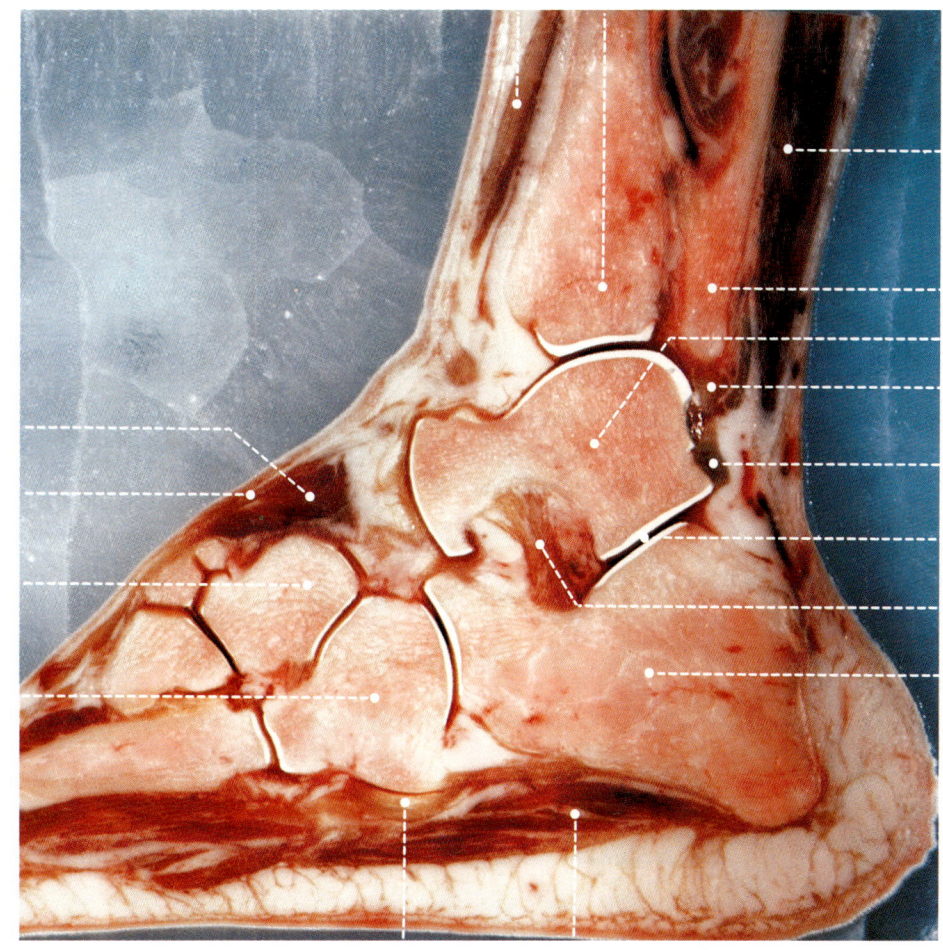

- Extensor hallucis longus
- Distal tibia
- Peroneus brevis muscle
- Distal fibula
- Talus
- Posterior inferior tibiofibular ligament
- Extensor digitorum brevis
- Extensor digitorum longus
- Lateral cuneiform
- Posterior talofibular ligament
- Posterior subtalar joint
- Interosseous ligament
- Calcaneus
- Cuboid
- Peroneus longus
- Abductor digiti minimi

Anatomy and MRI of the Joints

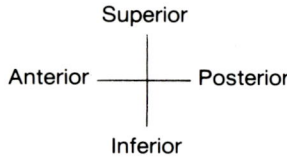

FIG. 9–21

SAGITTAL

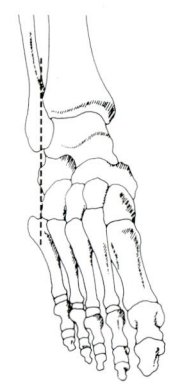

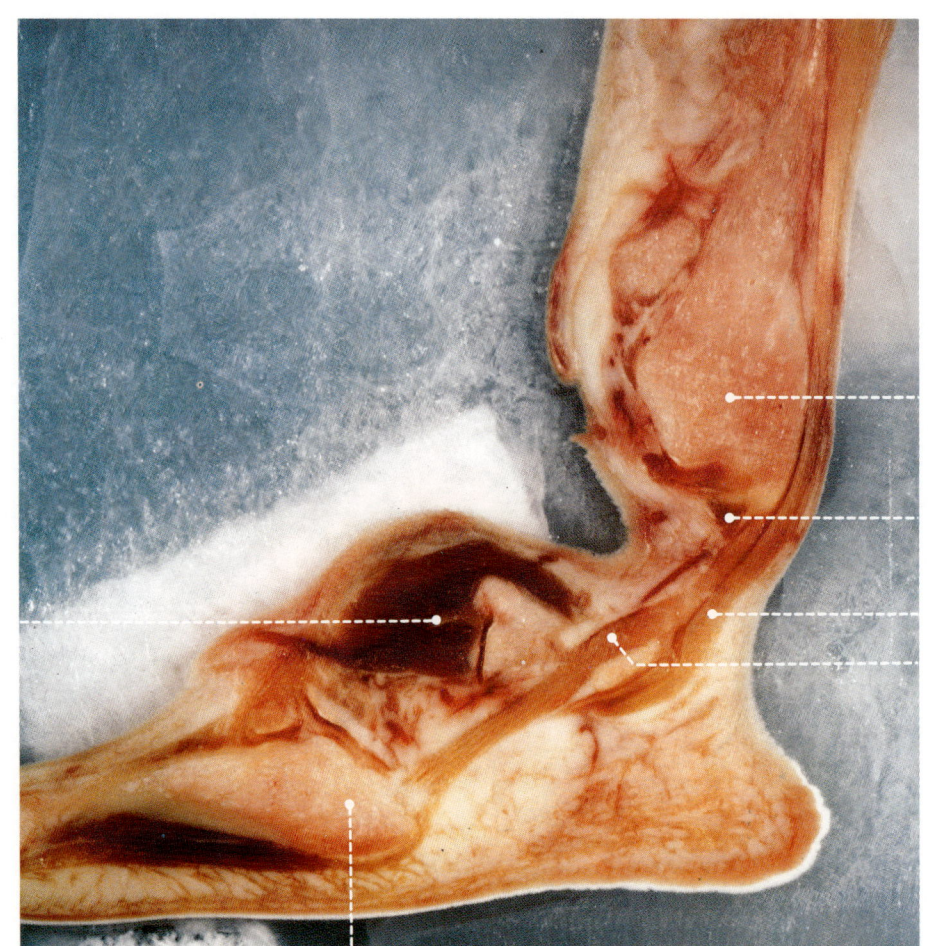

- Distal fibula
- Posterior talofibular ligament
- Peroneus longus
- Peroneus brevis
- Extensor digitorum brevis
- Fifth metatarsal

THE ANKLE

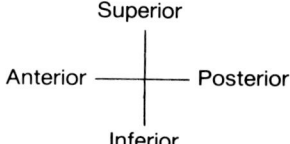

FIG. 9-22
SAGITTAL

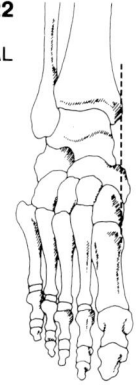

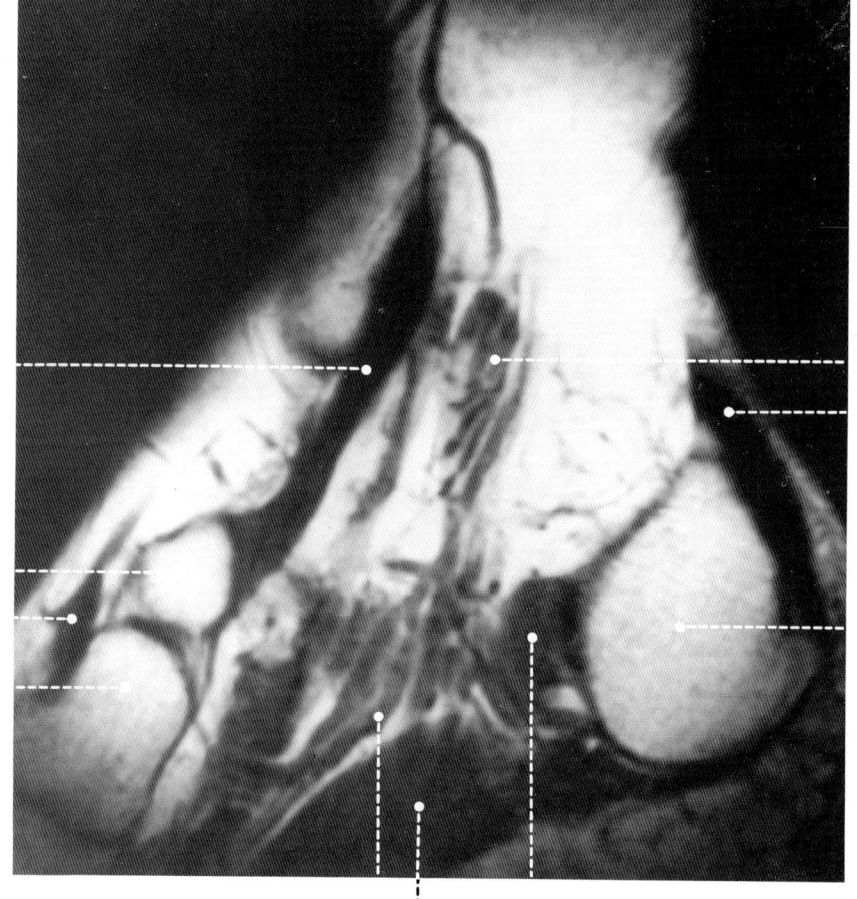

- Tibialis posterior
- Navicular
- Tibialis anterior
- Medial cuneiform
- Medial plantar artery
- Abductor hallucis
- Quadratus plantae
- Posterior tibial artery and veins
- Achilles tendon
- Calcaneus

Anatomy and MRI of the Joints

Superior | Anterior — Posterior | Inferior

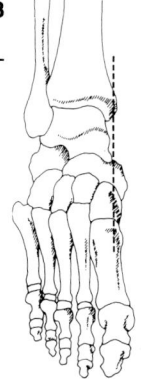

FIG. 9-23
SAGITTAL

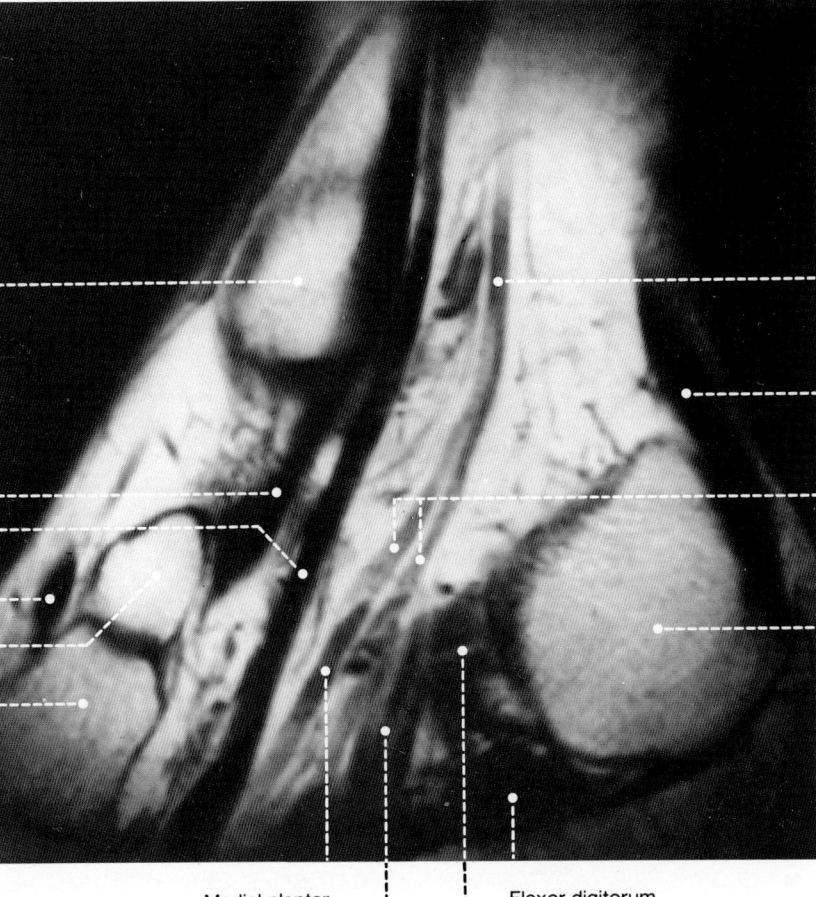

- Distal tibia
- Tibialis posterior
- Flexor digitorum longus
- Tibialis posterior
- Navicular
- Medial cuneiform
- Medial plantar artery
- Lateral plantar artery
- Flexor digitorum brevis
- Quadratus plantae
- Tibial nerve
- Achilles tendon
- Medial and lateral plantar nerves
- Calcaneus

Superior
Anterior — Posterior
Inferior

FIG. 9–24

SAGITTAL

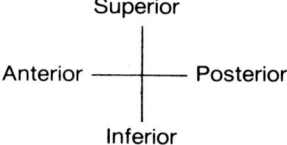

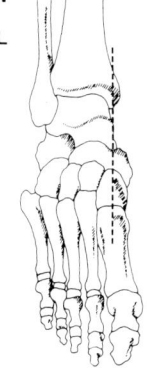

Tibialis posterior
Flexor digitorum longus
Distal tibia
Achilles tendon
Medial tubercle talus
Tibialis anterior
Navicular
Calcaneus
Medial cuneiform
Sustentaculum tali
Flexor hallucis longus
Lateral plantar neurovascular bundle
Quadratus plantae
Flexor digitorum brevis

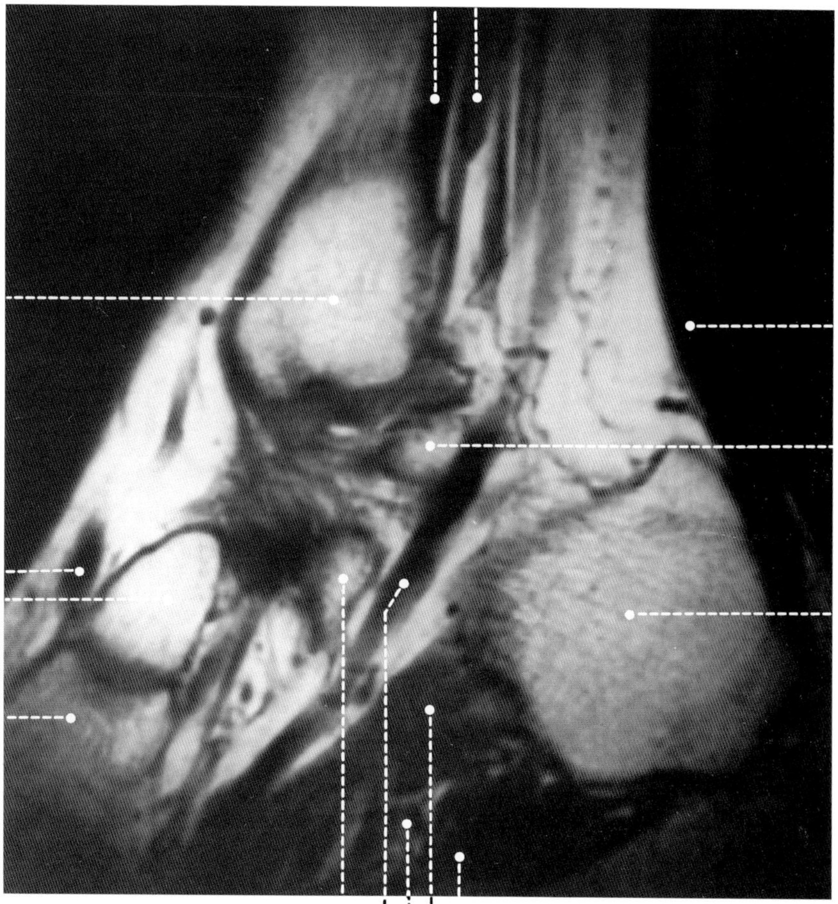

Anatomy and MRI of the Joints

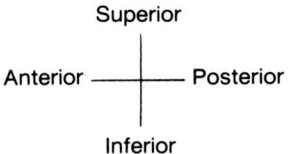

FIG. 9–25
SAGITTAL

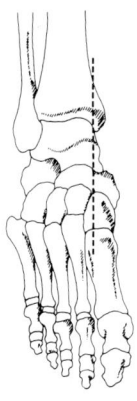

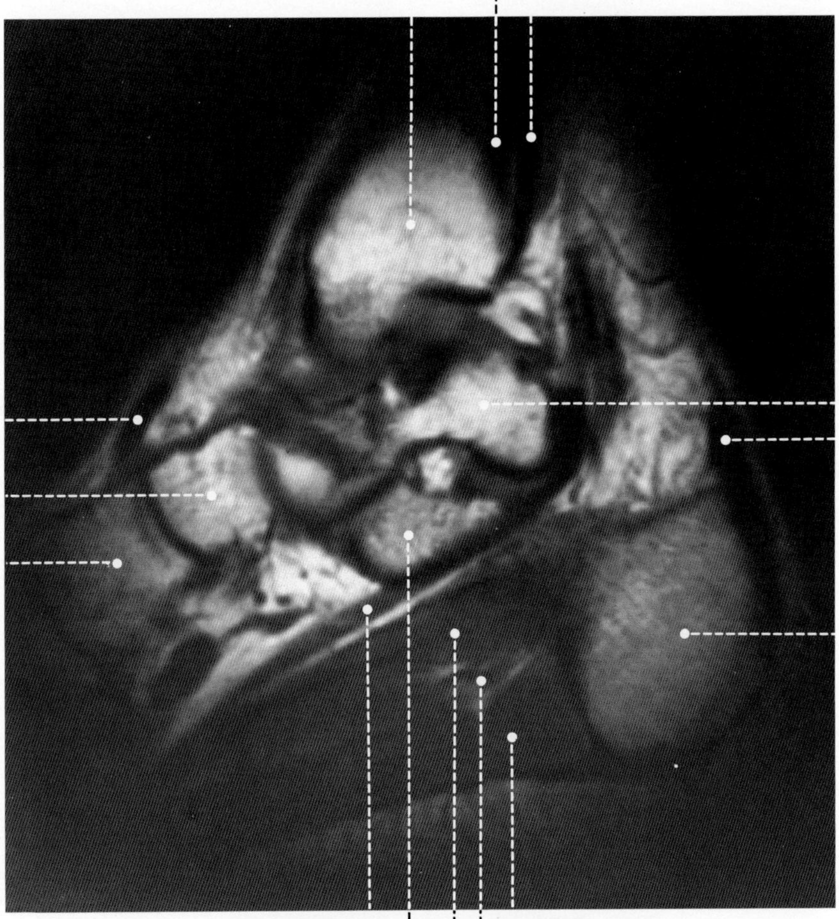

Labels:
- Distal tibia
- Tibialis posterior
- Flexor digitorum longus
- Tibialis anterior
- Navicular
- Medial cuneiform
- Talus
- Achilles tendon
- Calcaneus
- Flexor hallucis longus
- Sustentaculum tali
- Flexor digitorum brevis
- Lateral plantar neurovascular bundle
- Quadratus plantae

THE ANKLE

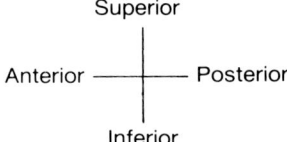

FIG. 9-26
SAGITTAL

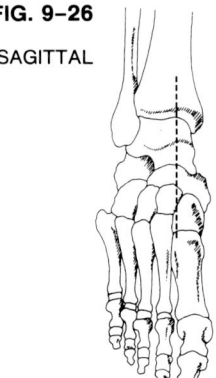

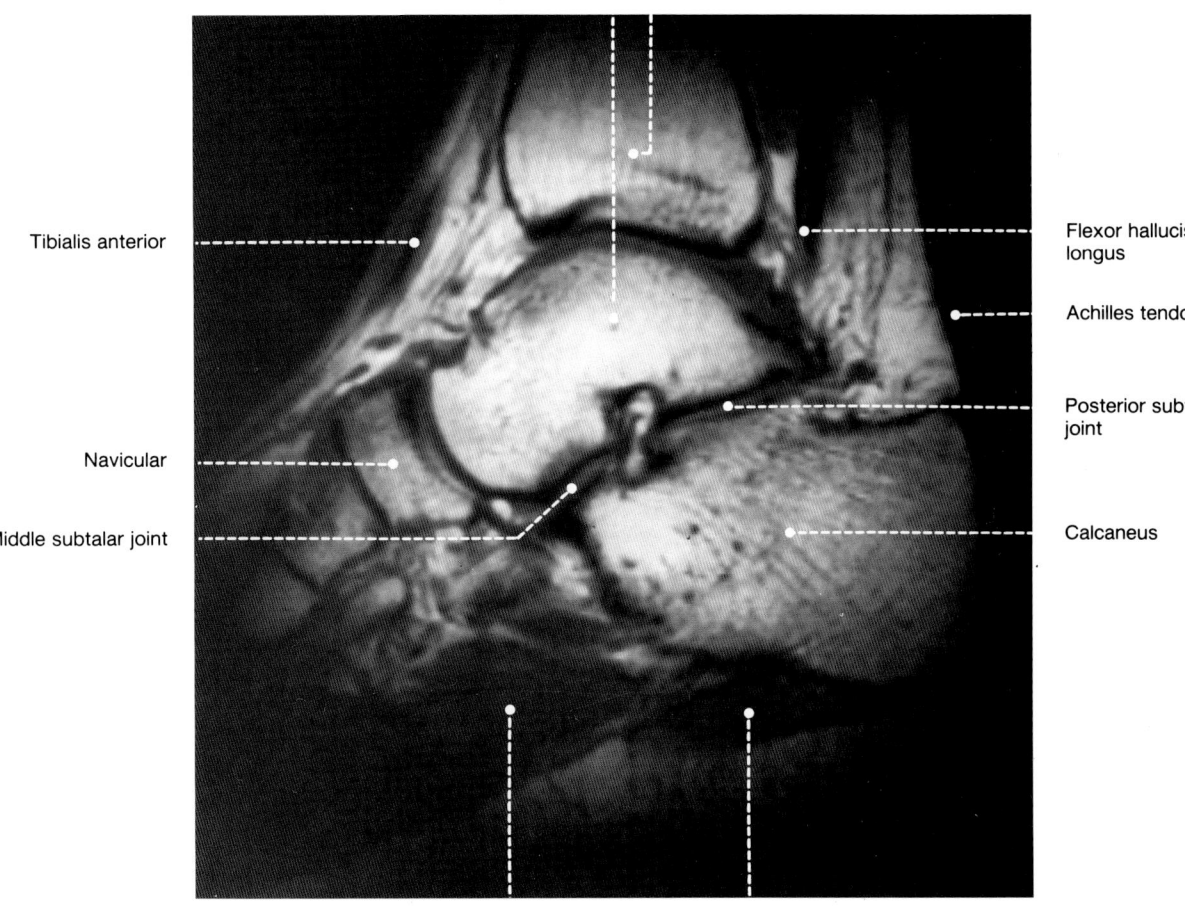

Talus   Distal tibia

Tibialis anterior — Flexor hallucis longus

Achilles tendon

Posterior subtalar joint

Navicular

Middle subtalar joint — Calcaneus

Flexor digitorum brevis   Abductor digiti minimi

Anatomy and MRI of the Joints

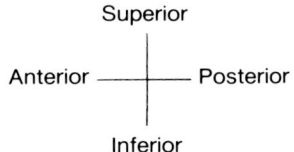

FIG. 9-27
SAGITTAL

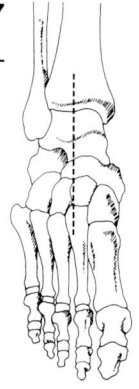

Tibialis anterior — Talus — Distal tibia — Flexor hallucis longus

Achilles tendon
Posterior inferior tibiofibular ligament
Posterior talofibular ligament
Posterior subtalar joint
Calcaneus

Extensor hallucis longus
Anterior subtalar joint
Navicular
Intermediate cuneiform
Lateral cuneiform
Cuboid

Plantar calcaneo-cuboid ligament — Abductor digiti minimi

279 THE ANKLE

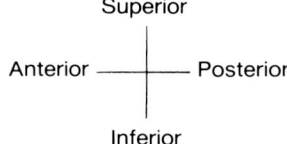

FIG. 9-28
SAGITTAL

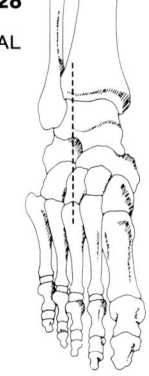

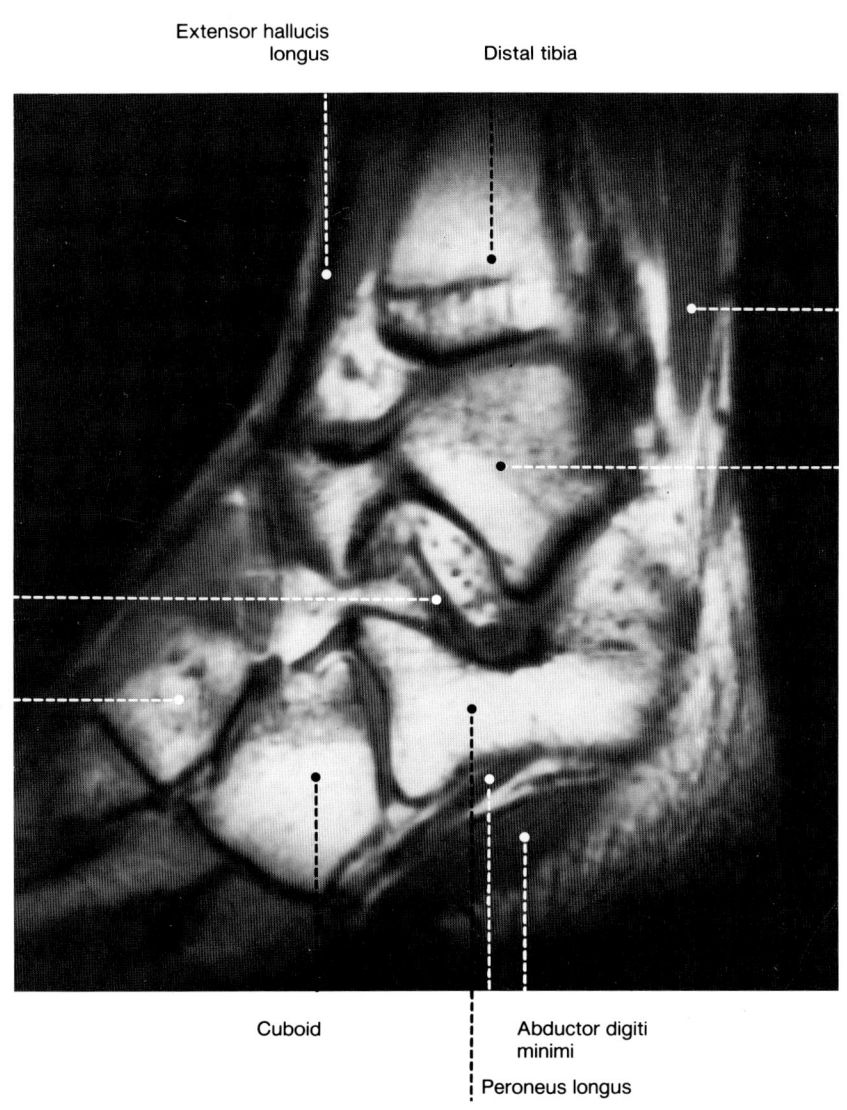

Extensor hallucis longus
Distal tibia
Peroneus brevis muscle
Talus
Interosseous ligament
Lateral cuneiform
Cuboid
Abductor digiti minimi
Peroneus longus
Calcaneus

Anatomy and MRI of the Joints   280

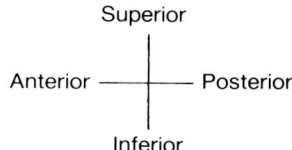

FIG. 9-29

SAGITTAL

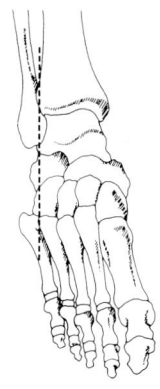

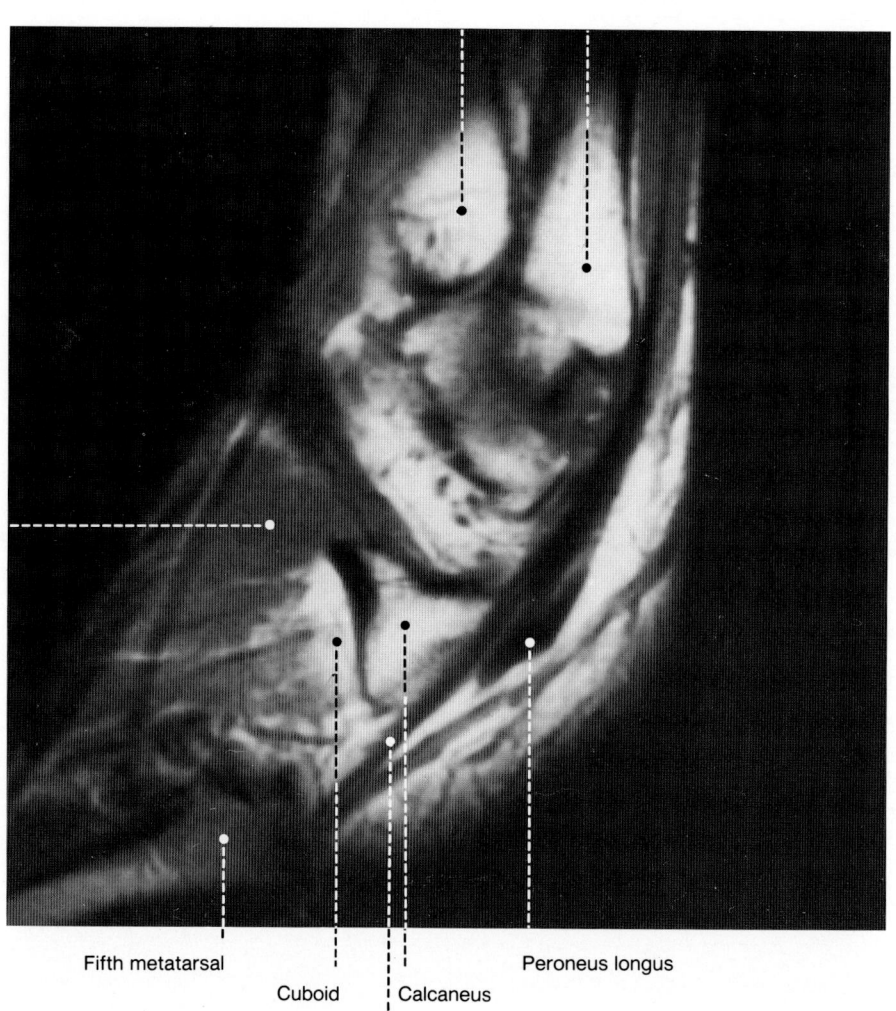

Distal tibia   Distal fibula

Extensor digitorum brevis

Fifth metatarsal   Cuboid   Calcaneus   Peroneus longus

Peroneus brevis

281 THE ANKLE

FIG. 9-30
CORONAL

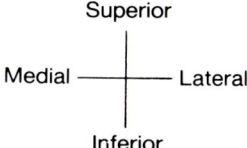
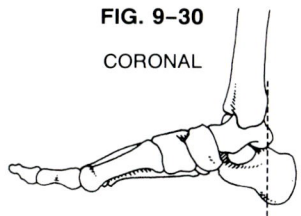
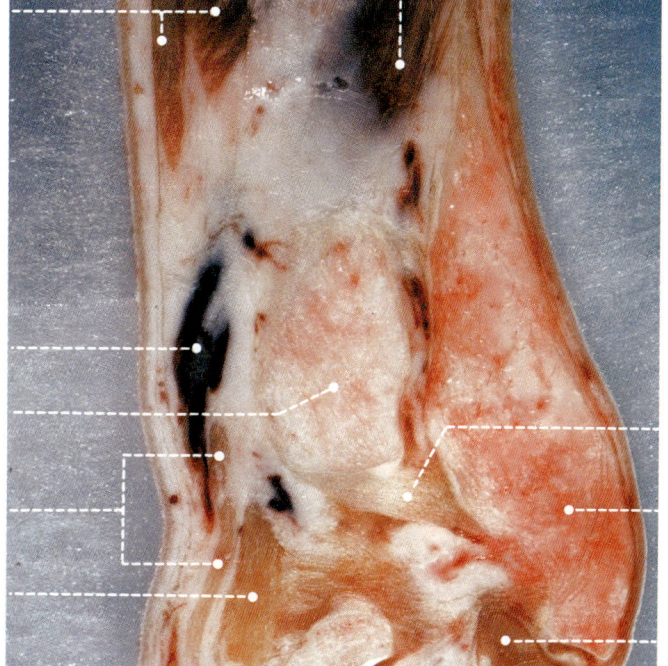

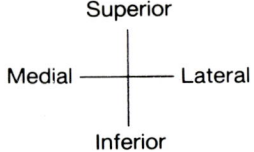
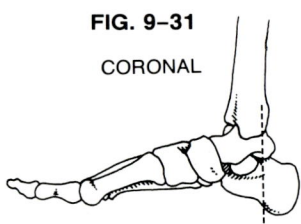

FIG. 9-31
CORONAL

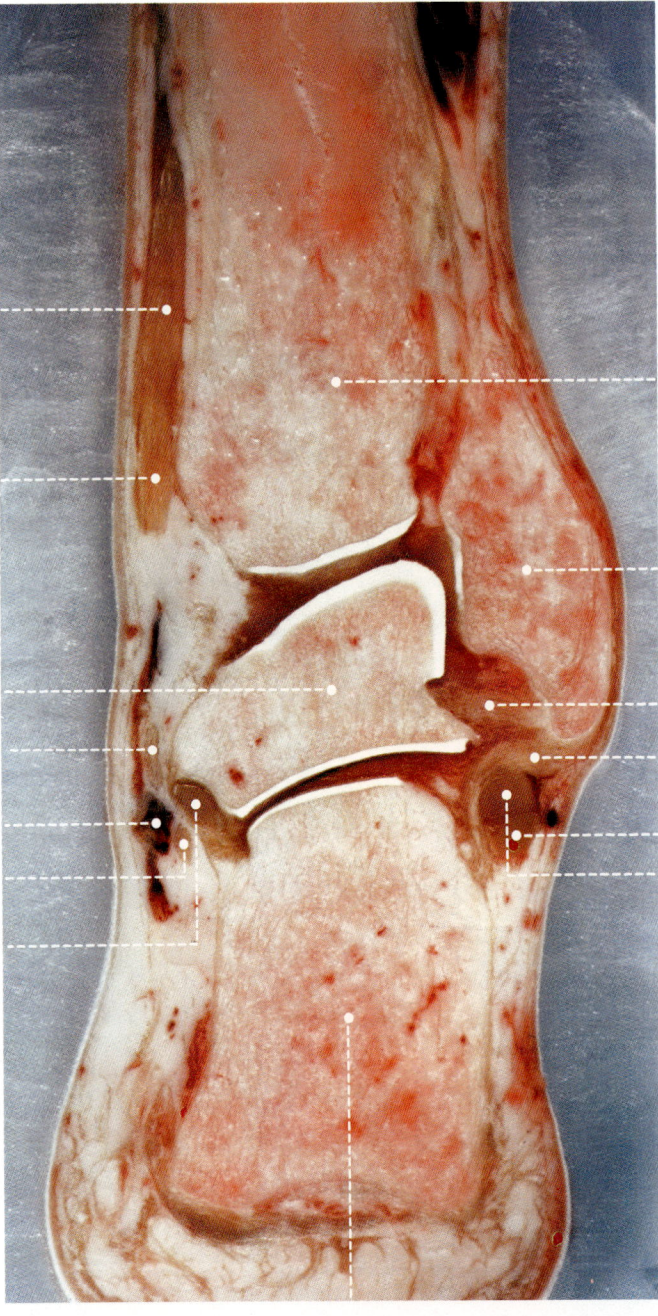

- Tibialis posterior
- Flexor digitorum longus
- Talus
- Medial plantar nerve
- Posterior tibial artery
- Lateral plantar nerve
- Flexor hallucis longus
- Distal tibia
- Lateral malleolus
- Posterior talofibular ligament
- Calcaneofibular ligament
- Peroneus longus
- Peroneus brevis
- Calcaneus

283 THE ANKLE

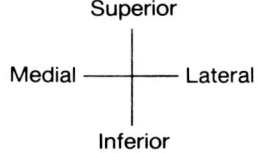

FIG. 9-32

CORONAL

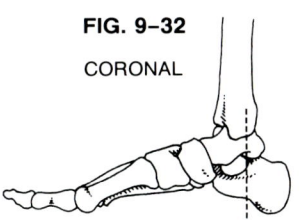

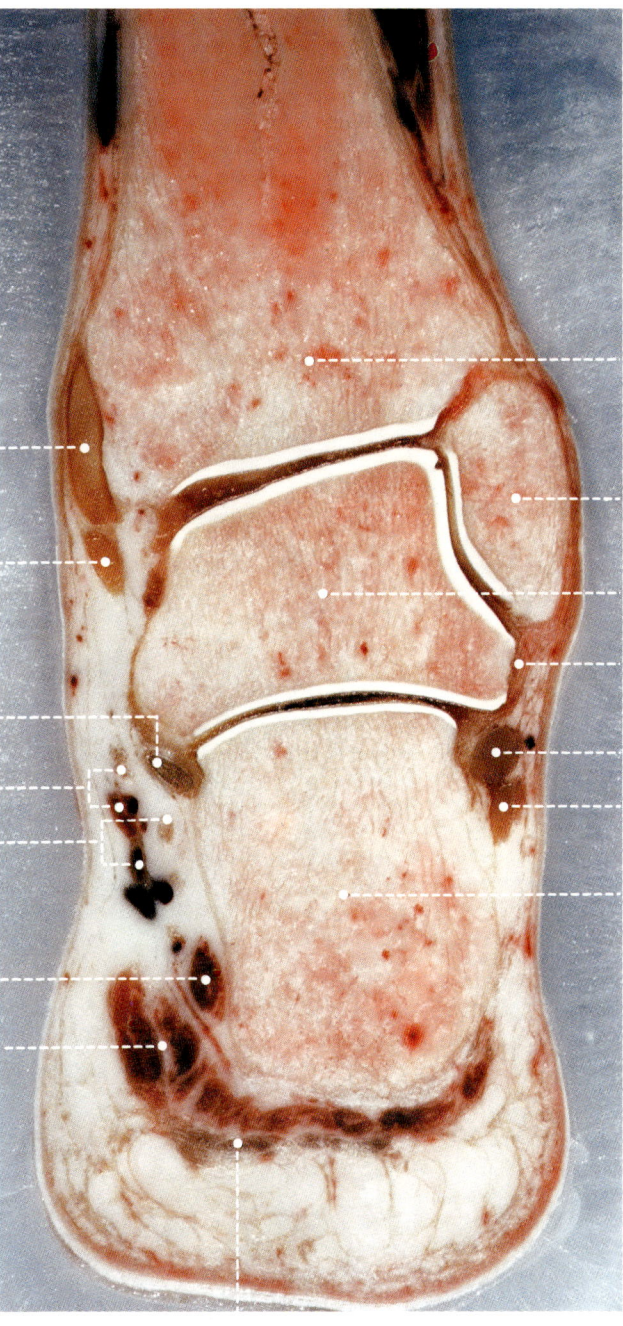

- Tibialis posterior
- Flexor digitorum longus
- Flexor hallucis longus
- Medial plantar nerve and artery
- Lateral plantar nerve and artery
- Quadratus plantae
- Abductor hallucis longus

- Distal tibia
- Lateral malleolus
- Talus
- Anterior talofibular ligament
- Peroneus brevis
- Peroneus longus
- Calcaneus

Plantar aponeurosis

Anatomy and MRI of the Joints

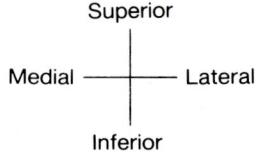

FIG. 9-33
CORONAL

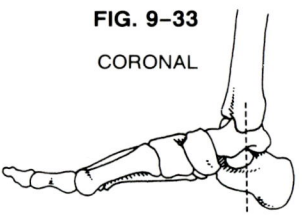

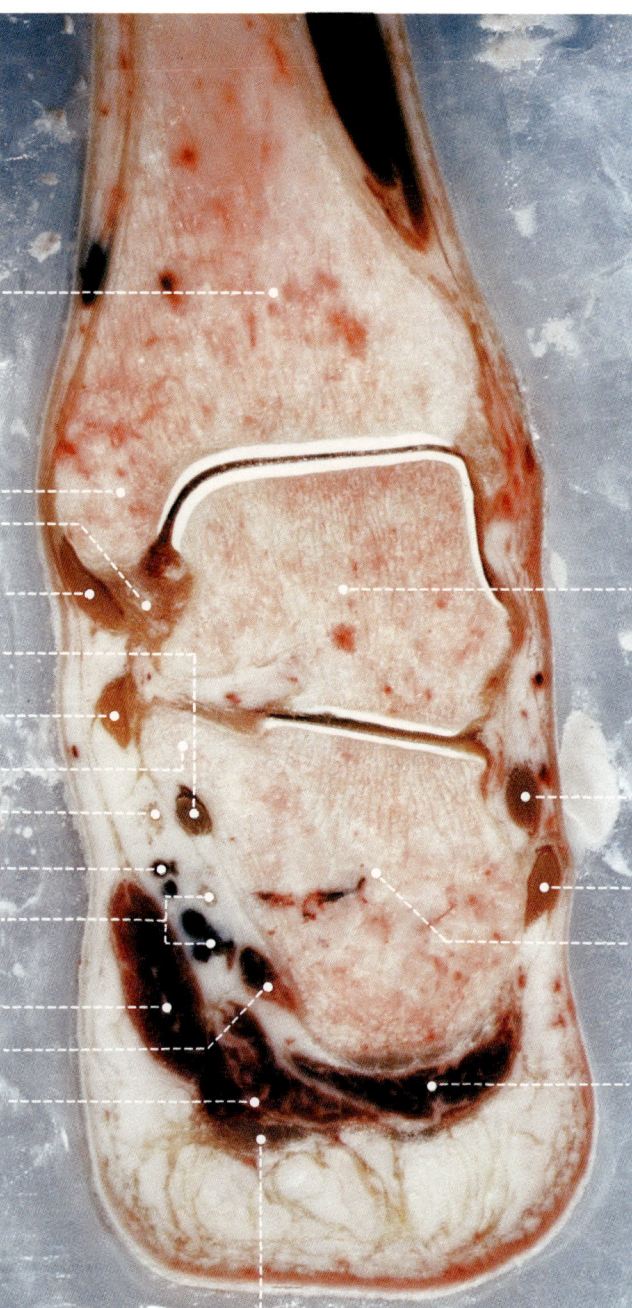

Distal tibia

Medial malleolus
Deltoid ligament (tibiotalar fiber)
Tibialis posterior
Flexor hallucis longus
Flexor digitorum longus
Sustentaculum tali
Medial plantar nerve
Medial plantar artery
Lateral plantar nerve and artery
Abductor hallucis
Quadratus plantae
Flexor digitorum brevis

Talus

Peroneus brevis

Peroneus longus
Calcaneus

Abductor digiti minimi

Plantar aponeurosis

285 THE ANKLE

FIG. 9-34
CORONAL

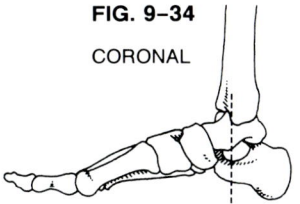

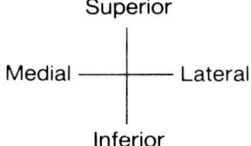

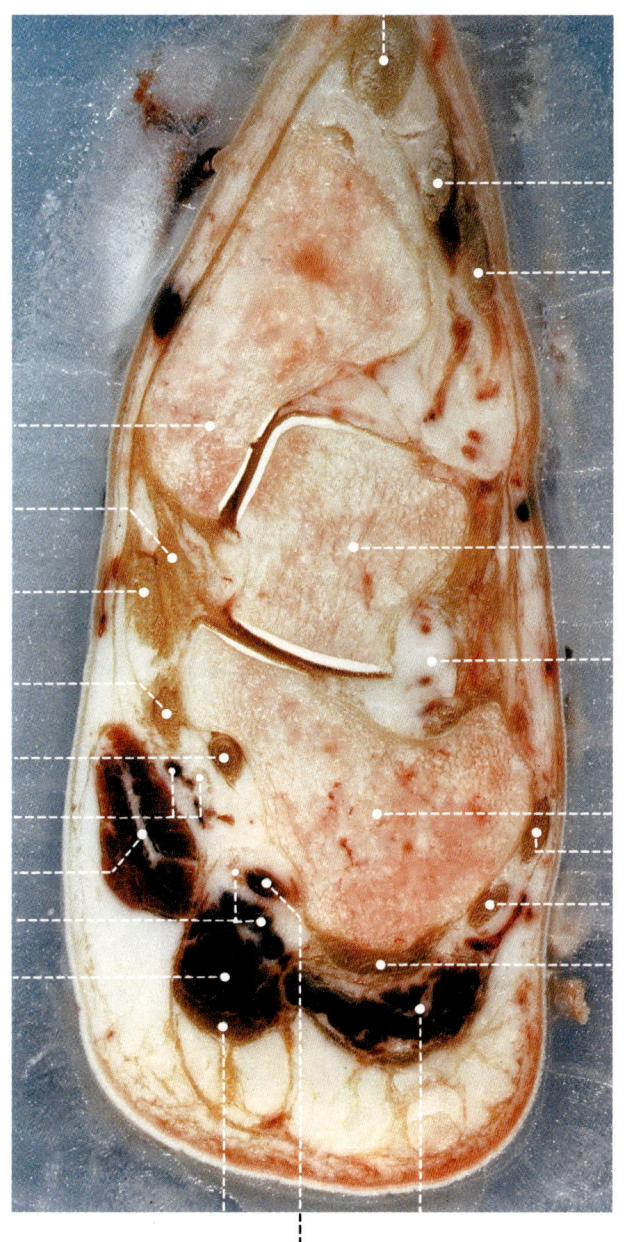

Tibialis anterior — Extensor hallucis longus — Extensor digiti minimi and peroneus tertius — Medial malleolus — Talus — Deltoid ligament (tibiocalcaneal fibers) — Tibialis posterior — Tarsal sinus — Flexor digitorum longus — Flexor hallucis longus — Medial plantar artery and nerve — Abductor hallucis — Calcaneus — Peroneus brevis — Lateral plantar nerve and artery — Peroneus longus — Flexor digitorum brevis — Long plantar ligament — Plantar aponeurosis — Quadratus plantae — Abductor digiti minimi

Anatomy and MRI of the Joints 286

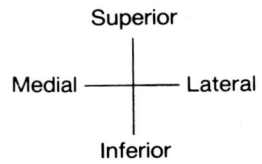

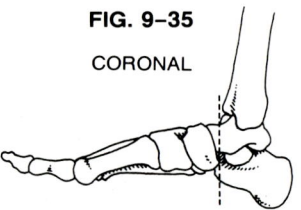
FIG. 9-35
CORONAL

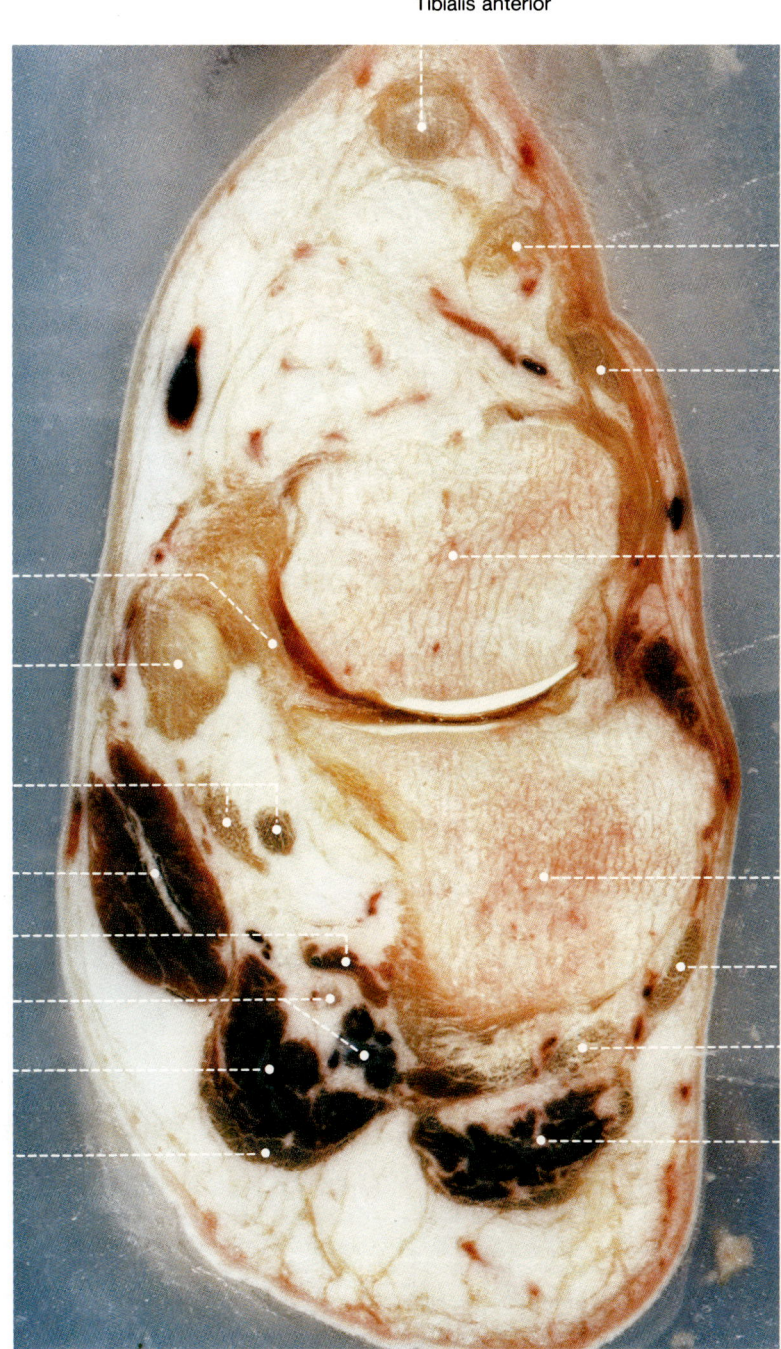

Tibialis anterior

Extensor hallucis longus

Extensor digitorum longus and peroneus tertius

Talus

Plantar calcaneo-navicular (spring) ligament

Tibialis posterior

Flexor digitorum longus and flexor hallucis longus

Abductor hallucis longus

Quadratus plantae

Calcaneus

Peroneus brevis

Lateral plantar nerve and artery

Peroneus longus

Extensor digitorum brevis

Plantar aponeurosis

Abductor digiti minimi

287 THE ANKLE

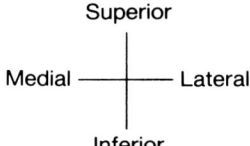

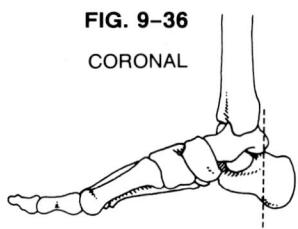
FIG. 9-36
CORONAL

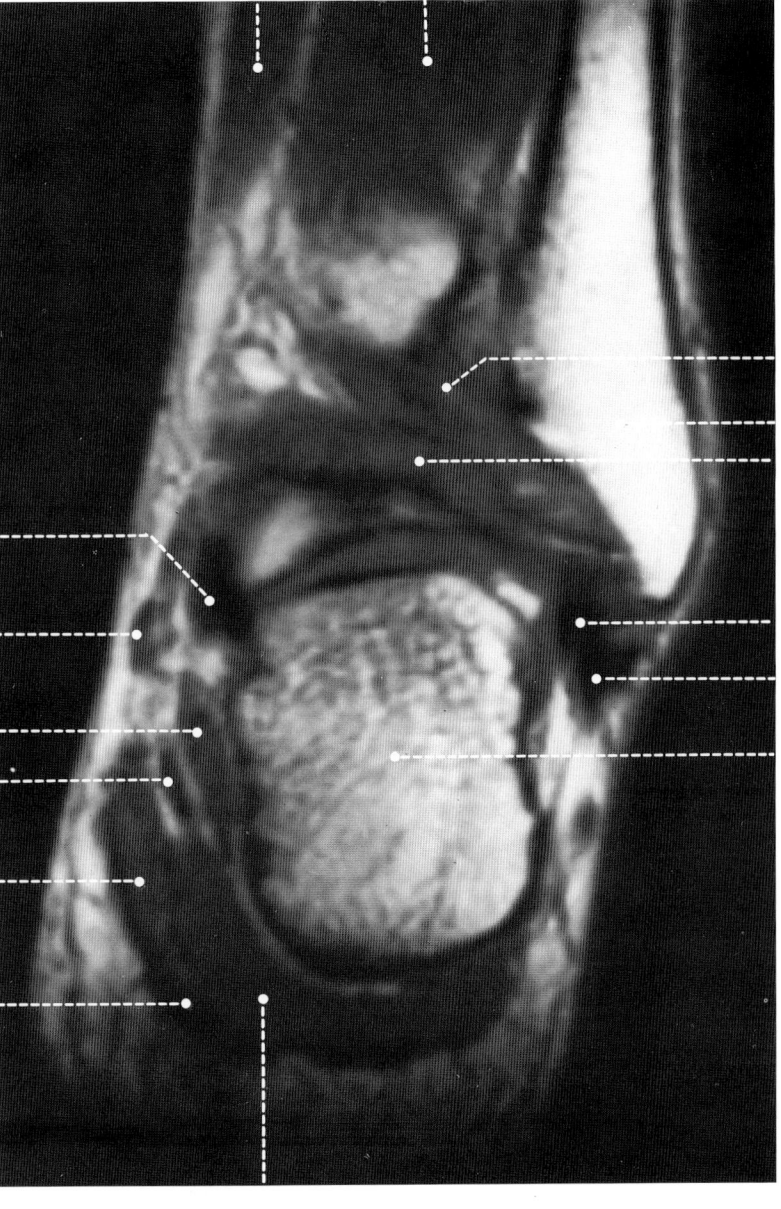

Flexor digitorum longus muscle
Flexor hallucis longus muscle
Posterior inferior tibiofibular ligament
Distal fibula
Posterior talofibular ligament
Flexor hallucis longus tendon
Medial plantar neurovascular bundle
Peroneus brevis
Peroneus longus
Quadratus plantae
Lateral plantar neurovascular bundle
Calcaneus
Abductor hallucis
Plantar aponeurosis
Flexor digitorum brevis

Anatomy and MRI of the Joints 288

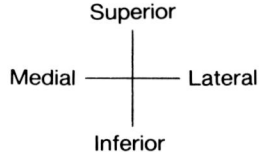

FIG. 9–37
CORONAL

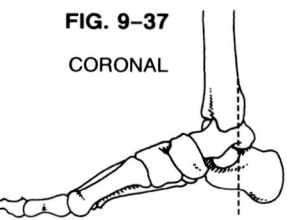

- Tibialis posterior
- Distal tibia
- Flexor digitorum longus
- Lateral malleolus
- Talus
- Posterior talofibular ligament
- Flexor hallucis longus
- Calcaneofibular ligament
- Medial plantar neurovascular bundle
- Peroneus brevis
- Quadratus plantae
- Peroneus longus
- Abductor hallucis
- Calcaneus
- Lateral plantar neurovascular bundle
- Flexor digitorum brevis
- Plantar aponeurosis
- Abductor digiti minimi

Superior
Medial — Lateral
Inferior

FIG. 9-38
CORONAL

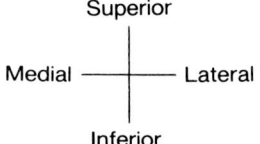

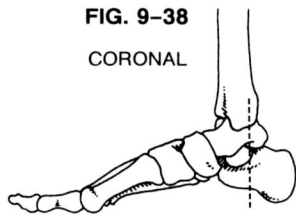

Distal tibia
Tibialis posterior
Flexor digitorum longus
Flexor hallucis longus
Medial plantar neurovascular bundle
Abductor hallucis
Quadratus plantae
Flexor digitorum brevis
Lateral malleolus
Talus
Anterior talofibular ligament
Peroneus brevis
Peroneus longus
Plantar aponeurosis
Lateral plantar neurovascular bundle
Abductor digiti minimi
Calcaneus

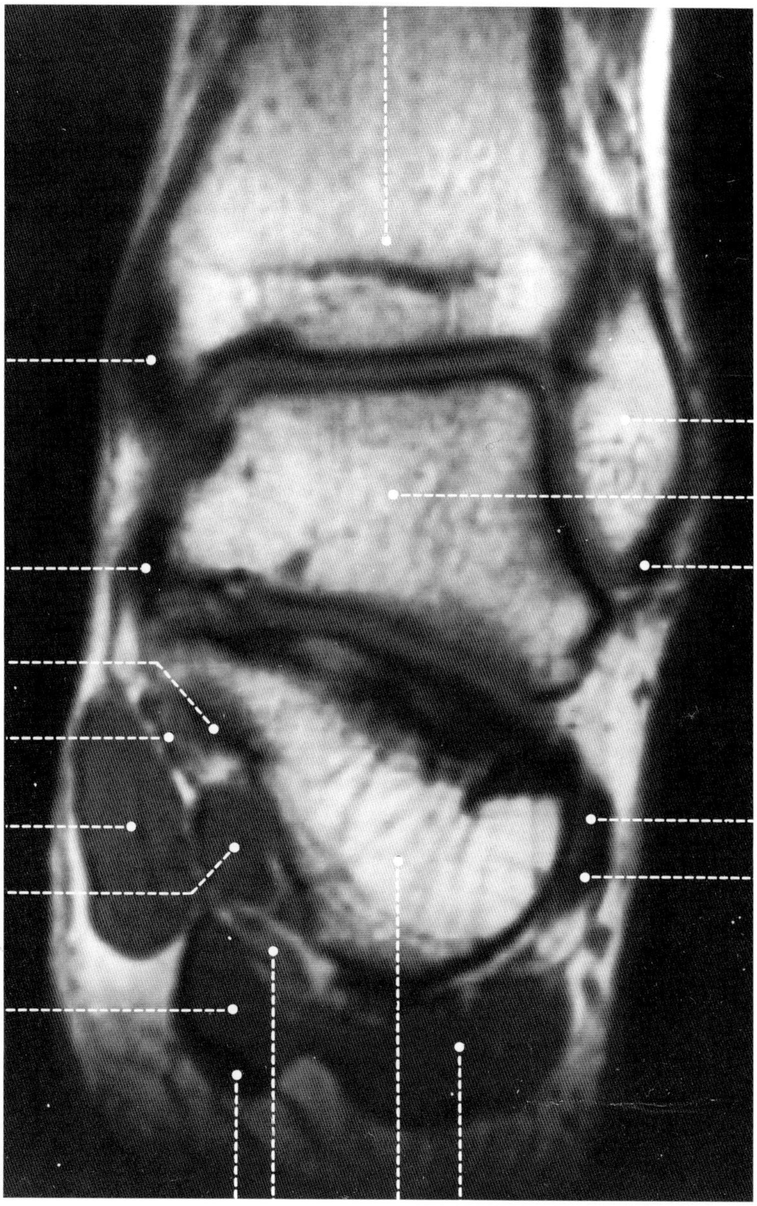

Anatomy and MRI of the Joints   290

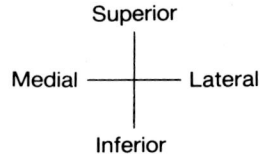

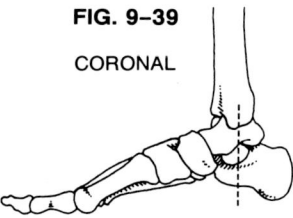

FIG. 9-39

CORONAL

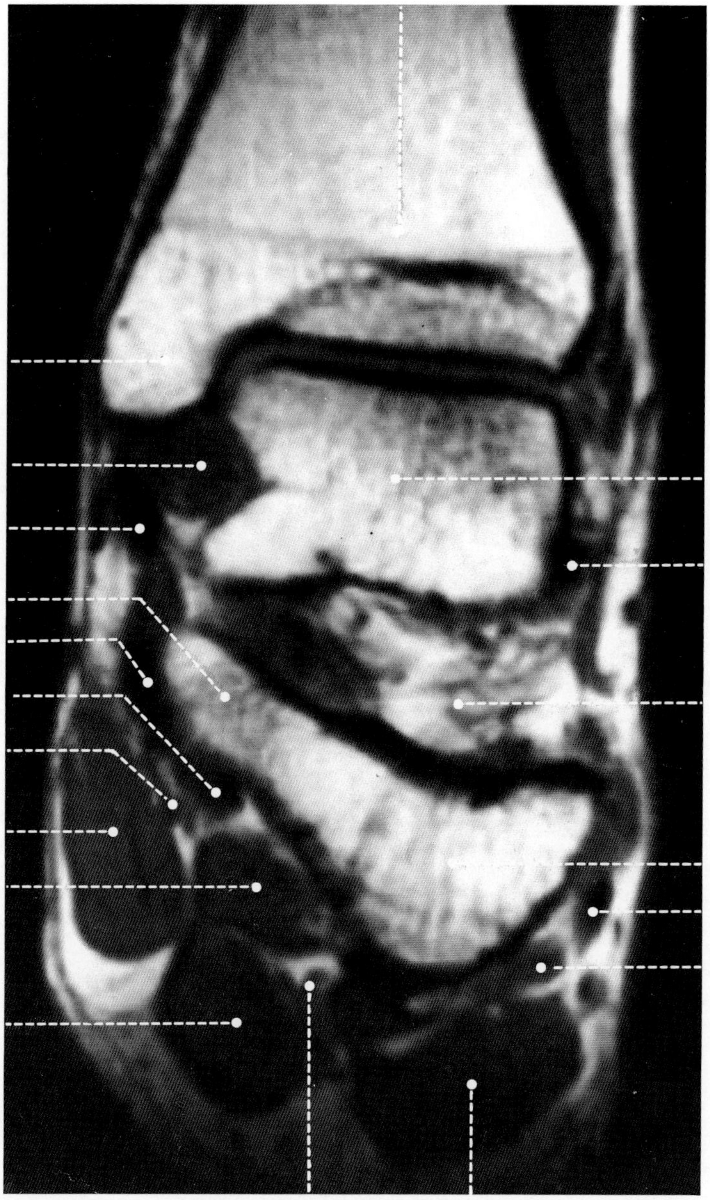

Superior
Medial
Lateral
Inferior

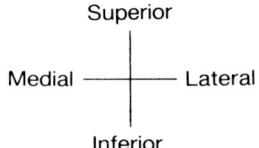

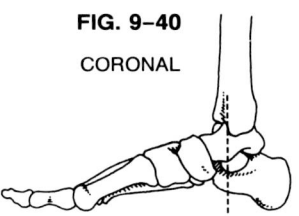

FIG. 9–40

CORONAL

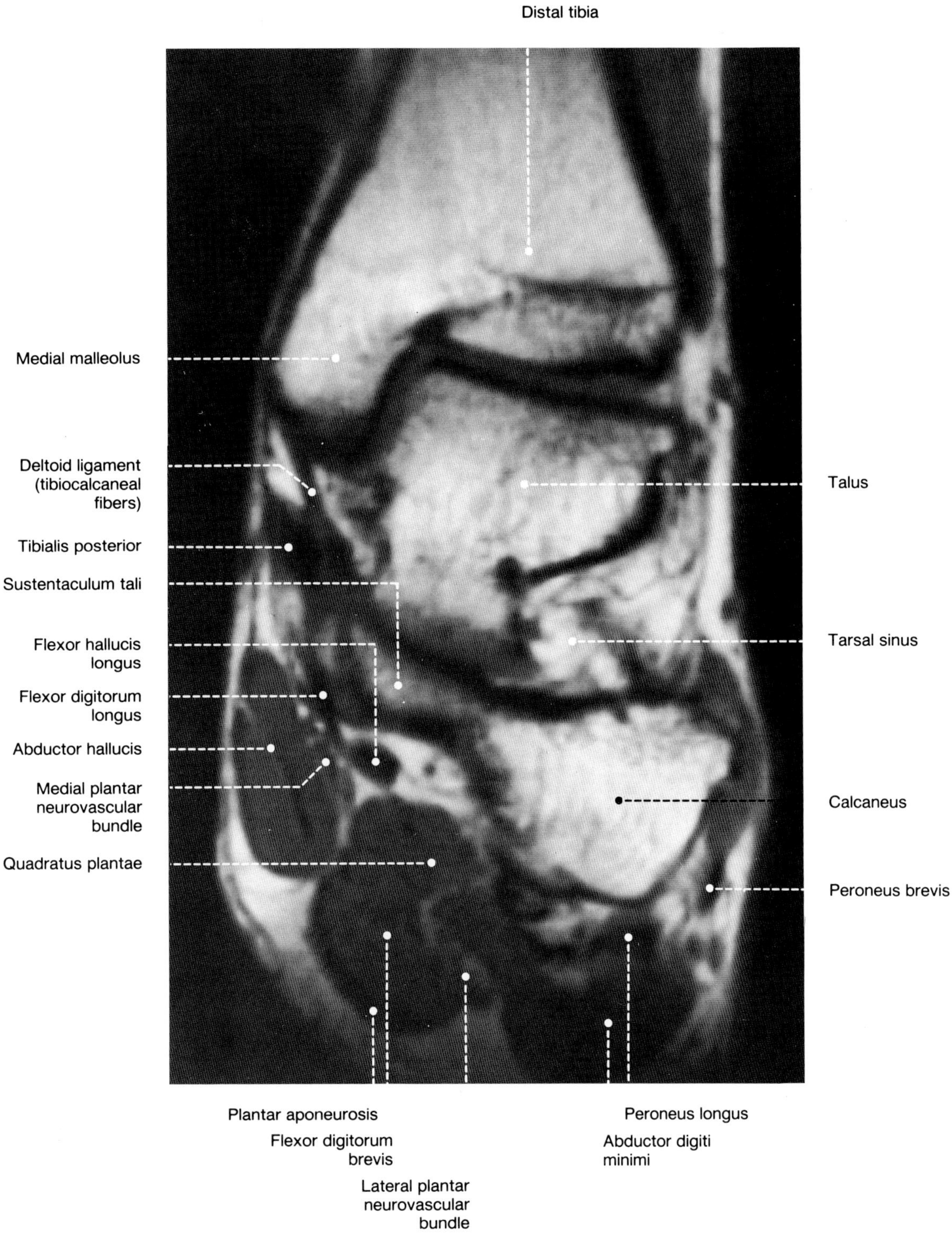

Distal tibia
Medial malleolus
Deltoid ligament (tibiocalcaneal fibers)
Tibialis posterior
Sustentaculum tali
Flexor hallucis longus
Flexor digitorum longus
Abductor hallucis
Medial plantar neurovascular bundle
Quadratus plantae
Talus
Tarsal sinus
Calcaneus
Peroneus brevis
Plantar aponeurosis
Flexor digitorum brevis
Lateral plantar neurovascular bundle
Peroneus longus
Abductor digiti minimi

Anatomy and MRI of the Joints

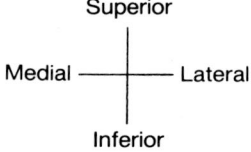

FIG. 9-41
CORONAL
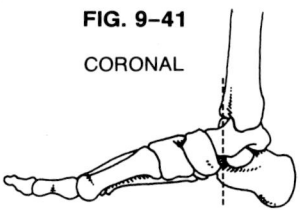

- Medial malleolus
- Tibialis posterior
- Plantar calcaneo-navicular (spring) ligament
- Abductor hallucis
- Flexor digitorum longus
- Flexor hallucis longus
- Medial plantar neurovascular bundle
- Talus
- Peroneus brevis
- Plantar aponeurosis
- Flexor digitorum brevis
- Quadratus plantae

RECOMMENDED READING

General Joint Anatomy

Bharat R, Yeakley JW, Harris JH. *Normal anatomy for multiplanar imaging: the trunk and extremities,* 1st ed. Baltimore: Williams and Wilkins, 1987.

Clemente CD. *Anatomy: a regional atlas of the human body.* Philadelphia: Lea and Febiger, 1975.

Ferner H. *Atlas of topographic and applied human anatomy: volume II. Thorax, abdomen and extremities,* 2nd ed. Baltimore: Urban and Schwarzenberg, 1980.

Hollinshead WH. *Anatomy for surgeons: the back and limbs,* 3rd ed. Philadelphia: Harper and Row, 1982.

Middleton WD, Macrander SJ, Lawson TL, et al. High resolution surface coil MRI of the joints: anatomic correlation. *RadioGraphics* 1987;7:645–683.

Rohen JW, Yokochi C. *Color atlas of anatomy: a photographic study of the human body,* 1st ed. New York: Igaku-Shoin, 1983.

Williams PL, Warwick R. *Gray's anatomy,* 36th ed. Philadelphia: W.B. Saunders, 1980.

The Temporomandibular Joint

Harms SE, Wilk RM. Magnetic resonance imaging of the temporomandibular joint. *RadioGraphics* 1987;7:521–542.

Harms SE, Wilk RM, Wolford LM, Chiles DG, Milam SB. Temporomandibular joint: magnetic resonance imaging using surface coils. *Radiology* 1985;157:133–136.

Kaplan PA, Tu HK, Williams SM, Lydiatt DD. Normal temporomandibular joint: MR and arthrographic correlation. *Radiology* 1987;165:177–178.

Katzberg RW, Bessette RW, Tallents RH, Plewes DB, Manzione JV, Schenck JF, Foster TH, Hart HR. Normal and abnormal temporomandibular joint: MR imaging with surface coil. *Radiology* 1986;158:183–189.

Westesson P-L, Katzberg RW, Tallents RH, et al. CT and MR of the temporomandibular joint: comparison with autopsy specimens. *AJR* 1987;148:1165–1171.

Westesson P-L, Katzberg KW, Tallents RH, Sanchez-Woodworth RE, Svensson SA, Espeland MA. Temporomandibular joint: comparison of MR images with cryosectional anatomy. *Radiology* 1987;164:59–64.

The Shoulder

Huber DJ, Sauter R, Mueller E, Requardt H, Weber H. MR imaging of the normal shoulder. *Radiology* 1986;158:405–408.

Kellman GM, Kneeland JB, Middleton WD, et al. High-resolution magnetic resonance imaging of the supraclavicular region and brachial plexus: normal anatomy. *AJR* 1987;148:77–82.

Kieft GJ, Bloem JL, Obermann WR, Verbout AJ, Rozing PM, Doornbos J. Normal shoulder: MR imaging. *Radiology* 1986;159:741–745.

Middleton WD, Kneeland JB, Carrera GF, et al. High-resolution MR imaging of the normal rotator cuff. *AJR* 1987;148:559–564.

Seeger LL, Ruszkowski JT, Bassett LW, et al. MR imaging of the normal shoulder: anatomic correlation. *AJR* 1987;148:83–91.

Zlatkin MB, Bjorkengren AG, Gylys-Morin V, et al. Pictorial essay: cross-sectional imaging of the capsular mechanism of the glenohumeral joint. *AJR* 1988;150:151–158.

The Elbow

Bunnell DH, Fisher DA, Bassett LW, Gold RH, Ellman H. Elbow joint: normal anatomy on MR images. *Radiology* 1987;165:527–531.

Middleton WD, Macrander S, Kneeland JB, et al. MR imaging of the normal elbow: anatomic correlation. *AJR* 1987;149:543–547.

The Wrist

Baker LL, Hajek PC, Bjorkengren A, et al. High-resolution magnetic resonance imaging of the wrist: normal anatomy. *Skeletal Radiol* 1987;16:128.

Koenig H, Lucas D, Meissner R. Wrist: preliminary report on high-resolution MR imaging. *Radiology* 1986;160:463–467.

Middleton WD, Kneeland JB, Kellman GM, et al. MR imaging of the carpal tunnel: normal anatomy and preliminary findings in the carpal tunnel syndrome. *AJR* 1987;148:307–316.

Weiss KL, Beltran J, Shamam OM, Stilla RF, Levey M. High-field MR surface-coil imaging of the hand and wrist. Part I. Normal anatomy. *Radiology* 1986;160:143–146.

The Finger

Weiss KL, Beltran J, Shamam OM, Stilla RF, Levey M. High-field MR surface-coil imaging of the hand and wrist. Part I. Normal anatomy. *Radiology* 1986;160:143–146.

The Vertebral Column

Berger PE, Atkinson D, Wilson WJ, Wiltse L. High resolution surface coil magnetic resonance imaging of the spine: normal and pathologic anatomy. *RadioGraphics* 1986;6:573.

Clarke LP, Schnitzlein HN, Murtagh FR, et al. High resolution MRI: imaging anatomy of the lumbosacral spine. *Magn Reson Imaging* 1986;4:515.

Daniels DL, Haughton VM, Naidich TP. *Cranial and spinal magnetic resonance imaging: an atlas and guide,* 1st ed. New York: Raven Press, 1987.

Reicher MA, Gold RH, Halbach VV, et al. MR imaging of the lumbar spine: anatomic correlations and the effects of technical variations. *AJR* 1986;147:891–898.

Yu S, Sether L, Haughton VM. Facet joint menisci of the cervical spine: correlative MR imaging and cryomicrotomy study. *Radiology* 1987;164:79–82.

The Hip

Littrup PJ, Aisen AM, Bruanstein EM, Martel W. Magnetic resonance imaging of femoral head development in roentgenographically normal patients. *Skeletal Radiol* 1985;14:159–163.

Totty WG, Murphy WA, Ganz WI, Kumar B, Daum WJ, Siegel BA. Magnetic resonance imaging of the normal and ischemic femoral head. *AJR* 1984;143:1273–1281.

The Knee

Beltran J, Noto AM, Mosure JC, Weiss KL, Zuelzer WA, Christoforidis AJ. Knee: surface-coil MR imaging at 1.5 T. *Radiology* 1986;159:747–751.

Burk DL Jr., Kanal E, Brunberg JA, et al. 1.5 T surface-coil MRI of the knee. *AJR* 1986;147:293–300.

Li DKB, Adams ME, McConkey JP. Magnetic resonance imaging of the ligaments and menisci of the knee. *Radiol Clin North AM* 1986;24:209.

Li KC, Henkelman M, Poon PY, Robenstein J. MR imaging of the normal knee. *J. Comput Assist Tomogr* 1984;8:1147–1154.

Mink JH, Reicher MA, Crues JV. *Magnetic resonance imaging of the knee,* 1st ed. New York: Raven Press, 1987.

Reicher MA, Rauschning W, Gold RH, et al. High-resolution magnetic resonance imaging of the knee joint: normal anatomy. *AJR* 1985;145:895–902.

The Ankle

Betran J. Noto AM, Mosure JC, Shamam OM, Weiss KL, Zuelzer WA. Ankle: surface coil MRI at 1.5 T. *Radiology* 1986;161:203–209.

Hajek PC, Baker LL, Bjorkengren A, et al. High-resolution magnetic resonance imaging of the ankle: normal anatomy. *Skeletal Radiol* 1986;15:536.

Kneeland JB, Macrandar S, Middleton WD, et al. Pictorial essay. MR imaging of the normal ankle: correlation with anatomic sections. *AJR* 1988;151:117–123.

SUBJECT INDEX

Abductor digiti minimi (Ankle), 271, 277–279, 284–286, 288–291
Abductor digiti minimi (Wrist), 84, 111–114, 116–118
Abductor hallucis, 260, 266–268, 273, 283–284, 286–292
Abductor pollicis brevis, 84, 95
Abductor pollicis longus, 85–86, 89–90, 94, 96–98
Acetabulum
   acetabular fossa, 153, 163, 168–170, 190, 200–201
   labrum (cotyloid ligament), 161–163, 169–171, 175–177, 182–183, 189–195, 200–201
   rim, 168–170, 175–176, 182–183, 189, 191, 192, 199–201
   roof, 166, 175–176, 191
Achilles tendon, 251–253, 256–258, 261–264, 269, 273–278
Acromioclavicular ligament, 14
Acromion, 31–33, 37, 39–42, 44–47
Adductor brevis muscle, 165, 174–176, 189–190, 192–195
Adductor muscle, 156
Adductor muscle group, 190, 200
   adductor longus muscle, 156, 164–165, 174
   adductor magnus muscle, 189, 192–194
Adductor pollicis, 84, 93, 99–100, 107, 112–114, 117–118
Anconeus muscle, 52, 57–60, 62–65, 68
Annular ligament, 51, 58
Anterior band, 1, 6–9
Anulus fibrosus, 139–140, 144–151
Articular disc, 4–5, 10–11
Articular eminence, 1, 4–9
Atlas, posterior arch, 146, 149
Auditory meatus, external, 4–9
Axillary artery, 28–29, 35, 42, 46–47
Axillary vein, 29, 35, 42, 46–47
Axis, body, 146, 149

Basiliac vein, 52, 56–57, 61–62
Basivertebral vein, 148
Biceps aponeurosis, 52, 57, 62
Biceps femoris, 206, 208, 210–215, 217–222, 229, 237–238, 244–246
Biceps femoris tendon, 207, 237–238, 245
Biceps tendon (Elbow), 50, 52, 56–58, 60–64, 66–67, 72–73, 76–77, 80
   insertion (Elbow), 52, 60–61, 65, 67, 71, 75, 79
   long head (Shoulder), 14, 22, 26–28, 31–33, 37, 41–43, 47–48
   short head (Shoulder), 14, 26–28, 31, 36

Bilaminar zone, 1
Brachial artery, 52, 56–58, 61–63, 71, 77, 81
Brachial plexus, 29–30, 35, 42, 46
Brachialis, 52, 56–59, 61–64, 66–71, 73, 76–77, 80–81
   insertion, 50, 60, 65–66, 70
Brachioradialis, 50–53, 56–69, 72–74, 76–77, 80–81

Calcaneocuboid ligament, 270
Calcaneofibular ligament, 251–252, 259, 265, 282, 288
Calcaneus, 259–260, 265–266, 268–271, 273–291
Capitate, 83, 90–92, 96–98, 102–103, 108–109, 113–115, 118–120
Capitellum, 49–51, 57, 62, 68–69, 72–73, 75–76, 79
Capsular ligament, 161–165, 168–171, 175–179, 183–184, 187, 189–195, 199, 201–202
Cauda equina, 141, 148
Cephalic vein, 49, 52, 56–57, 61–62
Cerebellum, 149
Cerebrospinal fluid, 150–151
Clavicle, 18–23, 29–30, 35–36, 40–43, 45–48
Collateral ligament (Finger), 121, 124, 126, 128, 130, 136–137
   lateral (Elbow), 205–206, 213–215, 219–222, 239, 246
   lateral (Knee), 206–207, 212, 214–215, 219–221, 239, 246
   medial (Elbow), 50, 79
   medial (Knee), 205–207, 213–215, 219–222, 242, 247–248
Common flexor tendon (Elbow), 50, 56
Coracoacromial ligament, 13–14, 18, 30–32, 37, 42
Coracobrachialis, 14, 26–28, 30–31, 36
Coracoclavicular ligament, 13–14, 23, 29, 35
   conoid portion, 13–14, 41, 46
   trapezoid portion, 13–14, 41, 46
Coracohumeral ligament, 13–14, 30–33, 43, 48
Coracoid process, 21–22, 24–25, 29–30, 35, 42, 47–48
Coronoid fossa, 49, 56, 61
Coronoid process, 66–67, 70–71, 75, 79
Coronoid tubercle, 49, 51
Cruciate ligament, 205–206
   anterior, 205–206, 212–213, 218–219, 227, 234, 240–241, 247–248
   posterior, 205–206, 213, 215, 218–221, 226–227, 233–234, 239–241, 246–248
Cuboid, 270–271, 278–280
Cuneiform
   intermediate, 270, 278

Cuneiform (contd.)
    lateral, 270–271, 278–279
    medial, 267–269, 273–276

Deltoid muscle, 14, 41, 45–46
    anterior, 18–25, 27–38, 43, 48
    lateral, 18–28, 34, 38–40, 42–44, 47–48
    posterior, 19–20, 29–34, 36–38
Deltoid ligament, 251–252, 259, 263–265
    tibiocalcaneal fibers, 252, 258–259, 264, 285, 291
    tibiotalar fibers, 252, 258, 263, 284, 290
Dens, 146, 149
Digital artery, dorsal, 122
Digital nerve, dorsal, 122
Digital vein, dorsal, 122, 124, 128
Disc
    intervertebral, 139, 146–150
    of temporomandibular joint, 1
    intervertebral, fibrous, 151
Dura mater, 146–147

Epicondyle
    lateral, 49–52, 56–57, 61–62, 68, 72, 74–75, 78–79
    medial, 49–53, 56–57, 61–62, 75, 78–79
Extensor carpi radialis brevis (Elbow), 50–52, 58–60, 63–65, 68–69, 73, 75, 78–79
Extensor carpi radialis brevis (Knee), 85–86, 88–100, 107
Extensor carpi radialis brevis (Wrist), 86, 88–90, 92–100, 107
Extensor carpi radialis longus (Elbow), 49–52, 56–65, 68–69, 73, 75, 78–79
Extensor carpi radialis longus (Wrist), 85–86, 88–100, 106–107
Extensor carpi ulnaris (Elbow), 52–53, 58–60, 63–65
Extensor carpi ulnaris (Wrist), 86, 88–92, 94–98, 105
Extensor digiti minimi (Ankle), 285
Extensor digiti minimi (Elbow), 52–53, 60, 65
Extensor digiti minimi (Wrist), 81, 86, 89–98, 104–105, 110
Extensor digitorum (Elbow), 52, 58–59, 63–65, 68, 72, 74, 78, 81
Extensor digitorum brevis (Ankle), 260, 266, 271–272, 280, 286
Extensor digitorum communis (Wrist), 86, 88–99, 102, 108–110
Extensor digitorum longus (Ankle), 253–254, 256–259, 261–265, 271, 286
Extensor digitorum tendon (Finger), 121, 132–133
Extensor expansion (Finger), 121, 125–127, 129–131, 133, 135
Extensor hallucis brevis, 254
Extensor hallucis longus, 253–254, 256–265, 269–271, 278–279, 285–286
Extensor indicis (Wrist), 86, 88–98, 108–109
Extensor pollicis brevis, 85–86, 89–90, 92–98
Extensor pollicis longus, 86, 88–98, 100, 106–107
Extensor retinaculum, 84
Extensor tendon
    common (Elbow), 50–51, 56–57
External obturator muscle, 154–155, 164–165, 172–173, 175–176, 180–183, 189–191, 192, 195, 198–203
    tendon, 163, 177, 185–186

Facet joint, 144–145
Fascia latae, 162, 164–165, 171
Fat pad
    anterior, 66–67, 70–72
    posterior, 66–67, 70–72
Femoral artery, 157, 172, 181
    common, 156–157, 160–164, 166–169, 171–173, 181
    deep, 156–157, 165, 175–176, 190, 195
    superficial, 156–157, 165, 192–195
Femoral condyle, 205
    lateral, 212–213, 218–219, 228, 235–236, 238–239, 244–246, 248
    medial, 212, 218–219, 223–225, 230–232, 239, 245–246, 248
Femoral head, 154, 161
Femoral nerve, 156–157, 160–162, 193, 194
    common, 155, 160–164, 166–169, 171, 173, 195
    deep, 155, 165, 175–176, 190
    superficial, 155, 165, 192–194
Femoral vein, 156–157
    common, 160, 161–164, 166–169, 171–173, 180, 195
    deep, 156–157, 165, 175–176, 190
    superficial, 156–157, 165, 192–194
Femur, 189, 210–211
    distal, 217, 226, 227, 229
    greater trochanter, 153–154, 163–164, 169–173, 178–179, 186–187, 189–191, 197–200
    head, 153–154, 163, 167–171, 175–177, 181–185, 189, 193, 194–195, 199, 201–202
    lesser trochanter, 153–154, 173, 184–185, 190, 198
    neck, 163–164, 171–173, 177–179, 186–187, 199–200
    shaft, 165, 179, 187
Flexor carpi radialis (Elbow), 51–52, 58–60, 63–65, 76–77, 81
Flexor carpi radialis (Wrist), 88–92, 94–98, 100–101, 107, 111–112, 116–117
Flexor carpi ulnaris (Elbow), 52, 57–60, 63–65, 74–75, 78–79
Flexor carpi ulnaris (Wrist), 88–89, 94–95, 105
Flexor digiti minimi brevis, 84
Flexor digitorum brevis (Ankle), 268–270, 274–277, 284–285, 287–292
Flexor digitorum longus (Ankle), 251–253, 256–268, 274–276, 281–288, 290–292
Flexor digitorum profundus (Elbow), 52, 58–60, 63–67, 70
Flexor digitorum profundus (Finger), 112, 121, 125, 127, 129–135
Flexor digitorum profundus (Wrist), 84–85, 88–99, 102–104, 108–110, 116–117
    fourth digit, 124, 128
    second digit, 124
    third digit, 124, 128
Flexor digitorum superficialis (Elbow), 51–52, 57–59, 70, 74
Flexor digitorum superficialis (Finger), 111, 121, 125–127, 129–135
Flexor digitorum superficialis (Wrist), 85, 88–99, 102–104, 108–110, 116
Flexor hallucis longus, 251–253, 256–266, 268–270, 275–278, 281–292
Flexor pollicis brevis, 84
Flexor pollicis longus, 84–85, 88–99, 101, 106–107, 111, 116
Flexor retinaculum, 83, 92, 98, 102–103, 108–109

Gastrocnemius
    lateral head, 206–208, 212, 215–216, 218–222, 226, 228, 236–237, 244–247
    medial head, 206, 208, 212, 214–222, 224–225, 231–234, 237–239, 244–247
Gemelli muscle complex, 188, 196–197
    tendon insertion, 199
Gemellus muscle
    inferior, 155, 163, 175–176, 183, 188, 190, 198
    superior, 155, 162, 168–170, 175–176, 183, 188, 198
Genicular vessels, 207, 233, 235, 237, 244, 248–250
Glenohumeral ligament, 13
Glenoid, 22, 24–28, 30, 36, 39–41, 44–45
Glenoid labrum
    anterior, 22, 25–28
    posterior, 22, 25–28
    superior, 21
Gluteal vessels, inferior, 160–161, 167
Gluteus maximus muscle, 155–156, 160–163, 165–188, 196–199
Gluteus medius muscle, 155–156, 160–162, 166, 168–170, 177–179, 181–183, 185–187, 189–190, 196–203
    tendon, 162, 169, 177–179
    tendon insertion, 188, 197
Gluteus minimus muscle, 154–156, 160–163, 166–169, 177–179, 182–186, 189–193, 194–195, 198–202
    tendon, 161, 178
Gracilis (Hip), 189–190
Gracilis (Knee), 207–208, 210–212, 214–223, 237–246

Hamate, 83, 90–92, 97–98, 103–105, 110, 113–115, 117–120
    hook of, 92, 98, 104, 110–112, 116
Hamstring muscle, 208
    tendon, 182, 188
    tendon insertion, 164–165, 172, 174
Humeral head, 13–14, 19–22, 24–28, 31–34, 37–38, 40–44, 45–48
Hypothenar muscle group, 92–93, 97–99

Iliac artery
    common, 190
    external, 174, 193, 194, 202–203
    internal, branches, 174
Iliac crest, superior, 191
Iliac spine
    anterior inferior, 154, 157, 185
    anterior superior, 154, 157, 186
Iliacus muscle, 175–177, 181, 189, 191, 192, 200–203
Iliac vein
    common, 190
    external, 191–193, 194, 202–203
    internal, branches, 174
Iliac wing, 192–193, 195, 202–203
Iliofemoral ligament, 154–155, 161–164, 168–173, 177, 182, 185–187, 191–195, 200, 202
    insertion, 167
Iliopectineal eminence, 174, 180, 203
Iliopsoas muscle, 155–156, 160–177, 180–184, 189, 191–195, 201–203
    tendon, 160–161, 164–167, 175–176, 193, 194–195

Iliopsoas tendon, 160, 164
Iliopubic eminence, 174, 180, 203
Iliosacral ligament, 188
Iliotibial tract, 206–208, 210–215, 217–222, 240–243, 249–250
Ilium, 153, 155, 157, 160, 174–176, 178–182, 184, 188–190, 193–194, 196–199, 201
Infraspinatus muscle and tendon, 14–15, 18–22, 24–48
Intercondylar eminence, 205, 208
Intermediate zone, 1, 6–9
Internal obturator and gemelli muscle complex, 174, 177–182, 184–186
    ligamentous insertion, 187
Internal obturator muscle, 155, 160–174, 188–203
    tendon, 162, 170, 175–176, 183, 198
Interosseous ligament, 83, 252, 259, 271, 279
Interosseous membrane, 78
Interosseous muscle, 115, 119–121, 124, 132, 134
Interosseous tendon, 124, 128
Interspinous ligament, 139, 141, 147
Intertrochanteric line, 165
Intervertebral disc, 139–140, 146–151
Intervertebral foramen, 139
Ischial spine, 162, 168–170, 174
Ischial tuberosity, 154–156, 163, 171–174, 180–181, 188
Ischium, 153, 155, 165, 175–176, 196–198

Lamina, 139–140, 147–148, 150
Lateral plantar neurovascular bundle, 268, 275–276, 287–291
Latissimus dorsi, 14
Levator ani muscle, 188
Ligamentum capitis femoris, 155
Ligamentum flavum, 139, 146–148, 150
Ligamentum teres, 154–155, 162, 169, 190–194, 201
Longitudinal ligament
    anterior, 139–140, 146–150
    posterior, 139–140, 146–150
Lumbrical muscle (Finger), 121, 132, 134
Lumbrical muscle (Wrist), 84, 112, 117
Lunate, 83, 89, 95, 102–103, 108–109, 112–115, 119

Malleolus
    lateral, 252, 257–258, 262–263, 282–283, 288–289
    medial, 252, 257, 262, 284–285, 290–292
Mandibular condyle, 1, 4–11
Mandibular ramus, 10–11
Masseter muscle, 10–11
Mastoid process, 4–9
Maxillary artery, 1, 8–9
Medial plantar neurovascular bundle, 267–268, 287–292
Median nerve, 52–53, 56–64, 77, 81, 84–86, 88–99
Medulla, 149
Meniscus
    lateral, 205–206, 214, 220, 239–242, 246–249
        anterior horn, 223–226, 230
        posterior horn, 228–229, 235–236
    medial, 205–206, 215, 221, 240–243, 246–250
        anterior horn, 224–225, 230
        posterior horn, 223–225, 230–232
Mid-subtalar joint, 277

Nail bed, 133, 135
Navicular, 260, 266-270, 273-278
Nucleus pulposus, 139-140, 144-151

Oblique cord, 51, 58
Oblique part, 51, 78
Obturator artery, 164
Obturator foramen, 154, 164, 173
Obturator vein, 164
Olecranon, 49, 51, 62, 66-67, 70-71, 74, 78-79, 81
Olecranon fossa, 49-50, 56, 61, 75, 79
Opponens digiti minimi, 111-113, 117
Opponens pollicis, 84

Palmar arch, deep, 120
Palmar digital artery, 122, 124-125, 127-131
Palmar digital nerve, 122, 124-125, 127-131
Palmaris longus, 52, 60, 88-99
Parotid gland, 11
Patella, 205, 211-212, 217-218, 227-229, 233-235
Patellar tendon, 213-216, 220-222, 228-229, 233-235
Pectineus muscle, 155-156, 162-165, 171-176, 180-182, 189-190, 193, 194-195, 201-203
Pectoralis major, 22, 28-30, 35-36
Pectoralis minor muscle, 14, 26-28, 35
Pectoralis minor tendon, 29
Pedicle, 139
Peroneal artery, 254, 261-263
Peroneal nerve, 207, 210-221
  deep, 254, 256-257, 261
Peroneus brevis muscle and tendon, 252-253, 256-266, 271-272, 279-292
Peroneus longus muscle and tendon, 252-253, 256-266, 270-272, 279-291
Peroneus tertius muscle and tendon, 253-254, 256-259, 261-265, 285-286
Piriformis muscle, 155-156, 166-167, 174-176, 180-182, 188, 196-197
  tendon, 160-162, 167-169, 177-179, 184-187, 198-199
Pisiform, 90-91, 96-97, 104-105, 111-112
Pisohamate ligament, 110
Plantar aponeurosis, 269, 283-289, 291-292
Plantar artery
  lateral, 260, 266, 269-270, 274, 283-286
  medial, 260, 266, 273-274, 283-285
Plantar calcaneocuboid ligament, 278
Plantar calcaneonavicular ligament, 251, 260, 265, 266, 286, 292
Plantar ligament
  long, 285
  short, 270
Plantaris, 219-222
Plantar nerve
  lateral, 258-260, 263-266, 269, 274, 281-286
  medial, 258-260, 263-266, 268, 274, 281-285
Popliteal artery, 208, 210-222, 227, 234, 237-239, 244
Popliteus muscle, 206, 216, 228, 238-239
Popliteus tendon, 206-207, 214-215, 219-221, 229, 236, 239-240, 246-247
Posterior band, 1, 6-9

Pronator quadratus, 84, 100-103, 106-107
Pronator teres, 49, 52, 56-67, 70, 75-77, 79-81
Psoas muscle, 175-176
Pterygoid muscle
  lateral, 4-6, 8-11
  medial, 10-11
Pubic ramus, superior, 195, 203
Pubic symphysis, 193, 194
Pubis, 162-163, 165, 170-173, 189-192

Quadratus femoris muscle, 155, 160, 163-165, 171-173, 175-179, 183-185, 188, 196-197
Quadratus plantae, 259-260, 265-266, 269-270, 273-276, 283-292
Quadriceps muscle, 206-208
Quadriceps tendon, 210-211, 217, 227-229, 233-234

Radial artery, 52, 58-60, 64-66, 71, 80, 88-92, 94-98
  superficial palmar branch, 90, 96-97
Radial fossa, 49, 52, 56, 61, 76
Radial head, 49-51, 57-58, 68-69, 72-76, 78-80
Radial neck, 49-50, 62, 68, 73, 76-77
Radial nerve, 52-53, 56, 61, 63, 69, 77
  deep branch, 50-52, 56-60, 62, 64-65
  superficial branch, 50-52, 56-60, 62, 64-65, 68
Radial notch, 49, 51, 57-58, 63, 68, 76
Radial recurrent artery, 51, 57-59, 64
Radial styloid, 89, 95
Radial tuberosity, 49-50, 62, 68, 73, 76-77
Radius, 51, 59, 64, 70, 76, 80, 88, 94, 100-103, 106-109, 113-120
Rectus femoris muscle, 155-156, 161-165, 168-173, 175-179, 182-187, 193, 194-195, 201-203
  tendon, 162, 166-169, 185
Rotator cuff muscle, 14-15

Sacral nerve plexus, 188
Sacroiliac joint, 174-176, 188, 196-197, 199
Sacrospinous ligament, 162, 168-169
Sacrotuberous ligament, 155, 163-165
Sacrum, 174, 188, 196, 198
Sartorius, 155-156, 160-170, 172-174, 177-178, 182-186, 207, 210-222, 237-246
Sartorius tendon, 239
Scaphoid, 83, 89-91, 95-98, 100-101, 106-107, 113-119
  distal, 111-112
Scapula, spine, 18-25, 29-30, 35-36
Scapula, body of, 29
Sciatic nerve, 155-156, 160-176, 180-182, 196, 208
Sciatic plexus, 174
Semimembranosus, 207-208, 210-222, 224-225, 230-234, 237-238, 244-245
Semimembranosus muscle, tendon insertion, 164
Semimembranosus tendon, 223, 230, 237, 244-245
Semitendinosus, 207-208, 210-222, 237-246
Semitendinosus muscle, tendon insertion, 164
Semitendinosus tendon, 223-225, 230-231
Soleus, 237-239
Spinal cord, 141, 144-150

Spine of scapula, *see* Scapula, spine
Spinous process, 139, 146-149, 151
Spring ligament, 251, 259-260, 265-266, 286, 292
Subacromial bursa, 41
Subclavian vein, 43
Subclavius muscle, 21-24, 42-43, 46-48
Subscapularis, 14, 26-30, 35, 39-41, 44-48
Subscapularis tendon, 26-27, 30-31, 36-37, 42-43
Subtalar joint, 251, 277
　anterior, 270, 278
　middle, 259, 265, 269
　posterior, 259, 265, 269-271, 277-278
Superficial temporal artery, 1
Supinator fossa, 49, 76
Supinator muscle, 51
Supracondylar ridge, 49-50, 76-77
Suprascapular artery, 15, 25-28, 35
Suprascapular nerve, 15, 25-28
Supraspinatus, 15, 18-24, 29-32, 35-37, 39-42, 44-48
Supraspinatus tendon, 18-21, 23-24, 30-33, 36-38, 42-43, 47
Supraspinous ligament, 139, 147
Sural nerve, 256-258, 261-264
Sustentaculum tali, 259, 265, 267-268, 270, 275-276, 284, 290-291

Talar dome, 251, 262
Talofibular ligament, 251
　anterior, 252, 283, 289-290
　posterior, 252, 269-272, 278, 282, 287-288
Talus, 251, 257-259, 263-265, 269-271, 276-279, 282-286, 288-292
　head, 251
Tarsal sinus, 285, 290-291
Temporal bone, 10-11
Temporalis muscle, 7, 10-11, 19
Temporal lobe, 6-11
Tensor fascia latae muscle, 155-156, 160-167, 170-173, 178-179, 203
Teres major, 14-15
Teres minor, 15, 29-34, 37, 39-40, 44-46
Teres minor tendon, 38, 41-42
Thenar muscle group, 92-93, 97-101, 106-107
Tibial artery, 257
　anterior, 254, 256-258, 261, 262-264
　posterior, 252, 254, 256-259, 261-265, 267-268, 273, 281-282
Tibialis anterior, 253-254, 256-265, 267-270, 273-278, 285-286

Tibialis posterior, 251-253, 256-268, 273-276, 282-286, 288-292
Tibial nerve (Ankle), 252, 254, 256-257, 261-262, 274
Tibial nerve (Knee), 210-222
　anterior, 258
Tibial plateau, 205, 223-225, 228, 230-235
Tibial vein, posterior, 273
Tibiofibular ligament
　posterior inferior, 252, 270, 271, 278, 281, 287
Transverse acetabular ligament, 154-155, 182-183, 190-194, 199, 201
Trapezius, 18, 29-30, 35, 40-41, 44, 83, 91-92, 97-98, 100, 106, 111-114, 116-118
Trapezoid, 83, 92, 100-101, 106-107, 113-115, 117-120
Triangular fibrocartilage, 104, 110, 113-119
Triangular fibrocartilage complex, 114
Triceps (Elbow), 52, 60-63, 66-73, 81
Triceps (Shoulder), 15
Triceps tendon, 52, 56, 61-62, 66, 68, 70
Triquetrum, 83, 89-91, 96-97, 104-105, 110, 113-115, 117-119
Trochlea, 49, 57, 62, 66-67, 70, 75, 79
Trochlear notch, 49-50, 60, 66, 70, 76
Tubercle talus, medial, 268, 275
Tuberosity, brachialis, 49, 76

Ulnar artery, 52, 58-61, 64-67, 71, 80, 88-99, 110
Ulnar nerve, 52-53, 56-59, 61-65, 69, 74-75, 78-79, 84, 88-91, 94-97
　branches, 84
　deep branch, 92-93, 98-99
　superficial branches, 93, 98-99
Ulnar recurrent artery, 63
　posterior, 81

Vastus intermedius muscle, 164-165, 179, 187, 193-195
Vastus lateralis muscle, 163-165, 171-173, 179, 201-202, 207, 210, 217, 239-242, 248-250
Vastus medialis muscle, 175-176, 187, 190, 207-208, 210, 217, 224-225, 230, 240-243, 248-250
Vertebral arch, 140
Vertebral body, 139, 147, 150
Volar plate, 126, 130, 132-135

Zygomatic arch, 10, 11